Donald School
Textbook of Interventional Ultrasound

Donald School Textbook of Interventional Ultrasound

Editors

Aris J Antsaklis
Professor of Obstetrics and Gynecology
Chairman, 1st Department of Obstetrics and Gynecology
University of Athens, "Alexandra" Hospital, Athens, Greece

Juan M Troyano
Head, Division of US and Fetal Medicine
Department of Obstetrics and Gynecology
University Hospital of Canary Islands
Canary Islands, Spain

JAYPEE BROTHERS MEDICAL PUBLISHERS (P) LTD

New Delhi • Ahmedabad • Bengaluru • Chennai • Hyderabad • Kochi • Kolkata • Lucknow • Mumbai • Nagpur

Published by

Jitendar P Vij
Jaypee Brothers Medical Publishers (P) Ltd

Corporate Office
4838/24 Ansari Road, Daryaganj, **New Delhi** 110002, India, Phone +91-11-43574357

Registered Office
EMCA House, 23/23B Ansari Road, Daryaganj, **New Delhi** 110 002, India
Phones: +91-11-23272143, +91-11-23272703, +91-11-23282021, +91-11-23245672
Fax: +91-11-23276490, +91-11-23245683 Rel: +91-1132558559
e-mail: jaypee@jaypeebrothers.com Visit our website: www.jaypeebrothers.com

Branches

- 2/B, Akruti Society, Jodhpur Gam Road Satellite, **Ahmedabad** 380015
  Phones: +91-79-26926233, Rel: +91-79-32988717 Fax: +91-79-26927094
  e-mail:ahmedabad@jaypeebrothers.com
- 202 Batavia Chambers, 8 Kumara Krupa Road, Kumara Park East,
  Bengaluru 560 001, Phones: +91-80-22285971, +91-80-22382956, +91-80-22372664
  Rel: +91-80-32714073 Fax: +91-80-22281761 e-mail: bangalore@jaypeebrothers.com
- 282 IIIrd Floor, Khaleel Shirazi Estate, Fountain Plaza, Pantheon Road,
  Chennai 600 008, Phones: +91-44-28193265, +91-44-28194897,
  Rel: +91-44-32972089, Fax: +91-44-28193231, e-mail: chennai@jaypeebrothers.com
- 4-2-1067/1-3, Ist Floor, Balaji Building, Ramkote Cross Road, **Hyderabad** 500 095, Phones: +91-40-66610020,
  +91-40-24758498 Rel:+91-40-32940929 Fax: +91-40-24758499, e-mail: hyderabad@jaypeebrothers.com
- No. 41/3098, B & B1, KURUVI Building, St. Vincent Road, **Kochi** 682 018 (Kerala)
  Phones: +91-484-4036109, +91-484-2395739, +91-484-2395740 e-mail: kochi@jaypeebrothers.com
- 1-A Indian Mirror Street, Wellington Square, **Kolkata** 700 013
  Phones: +91-33-22651926, +91-33-22276404, +91-33-22276415 Rel: +91-33-32901926
  Fax: +91-33-22656075, e-mail: jpbcal@dataone.in, kolkata@jaypeebrothers.com
- Lekhraj Market III, B-2, Sector–4, Faizabad Road, Indira Nagar, **Lucknow** 226 016
  Phones: +91-522-3040553, +91-522-3040554 e-mail: lucknow@jaypeebrothers.com
- 06 Amit Industrial Estate, 61 Dr SS Rao Road, Near MGM Hospital, Parel, **Mumbai** 400 012
  Phones: +91-22-24124863, +91-22-24104532, Rel: +91-22-32926896 Fax: +91-22-24160828
  e-mail: mumbai@jaypeebrothers.com
- "Kamalpushpa" 38, Reshimbag Opp Mohota Science College, Umred Road,
  Nagpur 440 009 (MS), Phone: Rel: +91-712-3245220 Fax: +91-712-2704275
  e-mail: nagpur@jaypeebrothers.com

Donald School Textbook of Interventional Ultrasound

First Edition: **2008**

ISBN 978-81-8448-298-0

Typeset at JPBMP typesetting unit
Printed at Ajanta Offset & Packagings Ltd., New Delhi.

CONTRIBUTORS

Aris J Antsaklis
Professor of Obstetrics and Gynecology
Chairman, 1st Department of Obstetrics and Gynecology, University of Athens, "Alexandra" Hospital, Athens, Greece

A Galindo
Ultrasound and Fetal Physiopathology Unit. Department of Obstetrics and Gynaecology. Hospital Universitario "12 de Octubre", Madrid Spain

Bajo-Arenas JM
Head, Department of Obstetrics and Gynecology. University Hospital of Sta Cristina, Madrid Spain

Castagno Romina
Fetal Medicine Unit, Hospital Materno Infantil Vall d´ Hebron, Barcelona, Spain

Carreras Moratonas Elena
Fetal Medicine Unit, Hospital Materno Infantil Vall d´ Hebron, Barcelona, Spain

Eduard Gratacós
Head, Department of Obstetrics, Ultrasound and Fetal Medicine, University Hospital Clinic i Provinial Barcelona, Spain

F Gutiérrez-Larraya
Pediatric Heart Institute. Department of Pediatrics. Hospital Universitario "12 de Octubre", Madrid, Spain

George Makrydimas
Assistant Professor of Obstetrics and Gynecology
Department of Obstetrics and Gynecology
University of Ioanina, Greece

George Daskalakis
Assistant Professor of Obstetrics and Gynecology
1st Department of Obstetrics and Gynecology
University of Athens, "Alexandra" Hospital
Athens, Greece

George A Partsinevelos
Research Fellow
1st Department of Obstetrics and Gynecology
University of Athens, "Alexandra" Hospital
Athens, Greece

Higueras M Teresa
Ultrasonography Department, Hospital Materno Infantil Vall d´ Herbron, Barcelona, Spain

I Martinez-Wallin
Assistant, Division of US and Fetal Medicine
Department of Obstetrics and Gynecology
University Hospital of Canary Islands, Canary Islands, Spain

Juan M Troyano
Head, Division of US and Fetal Medicine
Department of Obstetrics and Gynecology
University Hospital of Canary Islands, Canary Islands, Spain

Juan De León-Luis
Department of Obstrtrics and Gynecology
Gregorio Marañón General Hospital, Madrid Spain

Joaquin Santolaya-Forgas
Center for Fetal Medicine and Prenatal Genetics
Department of Obstetrics and Gynecology Brigham and Women's Hospital, Harvard Medical School
Boston, MA, USA

JM Velasco
Pediatric Heart Institute, Department of Pediatrics
Hospital Universitario "12 de Octubre", Madrid
Spain

M Alvarez de la Rosa
Assistant, Division of US and Fetal Medicine
Department of Obstetrics and Gynecology
University Hospital of Canary Islands, Canary Islands, Spain

Marianna Theodora
Research Fellow
1st Department of Obstetrics and Gynecology
University of Athens, "Alexandra" Hospital
Athens, Greece

Mesogitis Spiros
Associate Professor of Obstetrics and Gynecology
1st Department of Obstetrics and Gynecology
University of Athens, "Alexandra" Hospital
Athens, Greece

Papantoniou Nikolas
Associate Professor of Obstetrics and Gynecology
1st Department of Obstetrics and Gynecology
University of Athens, "Alexandra" Hospital
Athens, Greece

P de la Fuente
Ultrasound and Fetal Physiopathology Unit
Department of Obstetrics and Gynaecology
Hospital Universitario "12 de Octubre", Madrid
Spain

Sánchez Durán M Angeles
Ultrasonography Department, Hospital Materno Infantil Vall d´ Herbron, Barcelona, Spain

S Iniesta
Assistant Doctor. Ultrasound Unit and Fetal Medicine, University Hospital of Sta Cristina
Madrid, Spain

Salazar FJ
Ultrasound Unit and Fetal Medicine
University Hospital of Sta Cristina, Madrid, Spain

Themistoklis Grigoriadis
Research Fellow
1st Department of Obstetrics and Gynecology
University of Athens, "Alexandra" Hospital
Athens, Greece

Toran Nuria
Prenatal Diagnosis Units, Hospital Materno Infantil Vall d´ Hebron, Barcelona, Spain

PREFACE

It is widely accepted that the use of ultrasonography has dramatically changed the obstetrical practice worldwide. As the technology of ultrasound equipment has become more sophisticated, the capability of both diagnostic and therapeutic procedures increased enormously. Moreover, the growing experience and the understanding of pathophysiologic changes both during normal fetal life and in cases of structural abnormal fetuses have given us the possibility of planning and performing different interventions for early diagnosis and therapy.

Interventional procedures for diagnosis have been used since the 1950s although availability and safety were extremely low at the beginning. Since realtime ultrasound became available, visualizations of the placenta, the umbilical cord, the fetus and its vessels were more accurate and the indications for these interventional procedures were broadened. Amniocentesis is the oldest invasive procedure for prenatal diagnosis and remains, even to date, the technique most commonly being used. Chorionic Villus Sampling (CVS) was first introduced in the 1960s and subsequently developed over the last 25 years. The distinct characteristic of CVS is the provision of genetic diagnosis in the first trimester of pregnancy with a comparable safety profile and reliability with the second trimester amniocentesis or fetal cordocentesis, rendering CVS the only established method for prenatal diagnosis in the first trimester. Celocentesis offers the possibility for prenatal diagnosis as early as seven weeks' gestation. Although there are limitations for the use of celocentesis for the diagnosis of aneuploidy, it might be a realistic alternative for the diagnosis of the conditions where the risk for an affected fetus is high, such as β thalassemia. The potential of such an early diagnosis might give the possibility of a timely therapeutic intervention such as *in utero* stem cell therapy.

Fetal medicine today focuses not only on the prenatal diagnosis, but also on the therapy of an affected fetus. Until recently, termination of pregnancy or selective termination of an affected fetus was the option offered to the parents, when a congenital anomaly was diagnosed. Because of our better understanding of fetal physiology and pathology, and the technological improvements implemented during the last decade, many experts in fetal medicine tried to correct the process of a developmental abnormality, early enough in order to prevent a permanent damage to the fetus. Due to the rarity of many conditions in which it is used, the application of fetal therapy is limited at present; however, promising results have been reported in many different trials.

It was not long ago when multiple gestations remained undiagnosed until delivery. Nowadays not only the diagnosis of the presence of more than one fetus *in utero* is possible, but also early detection and management of complex fetal pathological conditions found in twin or even higher-order pregnancies is feasible.

The purpose of this textbook is to provide the obstetricians who are involved in the field of fetomaternal medicine all the uptodate knowledge of indications, complications and results of standard and experimental interventional procedures under ultrasound guidance. It is true that we still have a long way ahead of us until we can be ready to say that diagnosis and fetal therapy are totally clear. Nevertheless, big steps in *in utero* management of the fetus/patient have been accomplished.

Aris J Antsaklis
Juan M Troyano

CONTENTS

CHAPTER

1

Multifetal Pregnancy Reduction and Selective Termination

Aris J Antsaklis

INTRODUCTION

The dramatic increase in the frequency of multiple gestations in the last decade throughout the world, due mainly to the wide spread use of ovulation induction agents and assisted reproductive techniques, is causing medical, ethical, social and economical problems.

In the United States from 1972 to 1974 and from 1985 to 1989 the rate of multifetal births defined as three or more live births increased by 152% among infants of white mothers aged 30 to 34.

The rate of triplets live births increased by 156%, quadruplets by 356% and quintuplets and higher order by 182%.

This increase in multiple gestations is related to the development of assisted reproductive techniques and probably reflects the limitations in the possibilities of controlling the rate of multiple pregnancies.[1, 2]

Depending upon the medications, the incidence of multiples ranges from a low of 7 to 9% with clomiphene citrate, to a high of 39% with human menopausal gonadotropins. Presently, there is consensus that the pregnancy rate improves as the number of embryos or oocytes transferred increases but so does the rate of multiple pregnancies.[3]

More recently, in vitro fertilization centers have specifically aimed at decreasing the multiple pregnancy rate by close monitoring of ovulation induction, limitations in the number of transferred embryos and development in the techniques of blastocyst transfer.

Although assisted reproduction units have recently shown a trend towards reducing the number of embryos replaced, triplets and higher order multiple cannot be completely prevented.

Maternal mortality, perinatal mortality and severe neonatal morbidity rate increased in multiple pregnancies (ESHRE 2000).

The costs of caring for mothers and neonates of multiple births including the costs of treating children with major handicap for life, add a major financial burden for the insurance companies and/or the state.[4] The parents of multiples experience, higher rates of depression and anxiety after the birth of the babies in comparison to parents of singletons are more likely to divorce.[5]

NATURAL HISTORY OF MULTIFETAL GESTATIONS

Most of the perinatal mortality and morbidity associated with a multifetal pregnancy is related to prematurity and birth weight.

In multiple gestations, the length of gestation and infant birth weight are inversely proportional to the number of fetuses.

The published studies contain small numbers of patients and do not include information on the long-term outcome of survivors. Many studies only report on the outcome after 20 to 24 weeks and do not include information on spontaneous losses before this gestational age.

The median gestational age at delivery of twins, triplets and quadruplets is 35, 33 and 30 weeks respectively and the median birth weight is 2,473, 1,666, 1,414 gm respectively.[6]

Despite modern prenatal management, the rate of prematurity rate in multifetal pregnancies has not changed since the 1960s, but perinatal mortality rates have declined due to improved neonatal care.[7]

In most published series of triplets, the average gestational age of delivery in consistently around 33 weeks and approximately 80 to 90% of patients deliver before 37 weeks, 20 to 30% before 32 weeks and 5 to 10% before 28 weeks and perinatal mortality rate has been reported to be 77 per 1000 live births. Very little information is available for the morbidity and the long-term follow-up survivors.

It has been suggested that in multiples the major risk factors for cerebral palsy are preterm birth, intrauterine growth restriction and intrapartum complications, all of which are more common in multiples than in singletons.

Therefore, a patient carrying triplets or high order gestation and who delivers significantly preterm has the potential of having three or even more infants that have major permanent disabilities, including cerebral palsy, mental retardation, chronic seizure disorders, short gut syndrome or blindness.

A number of studies show that risk of cerebral palsy in twins is approximately five times that in singletons and two studies showed that the incidence of cerebral palsy in triplets was 17-fold and 20-fold increased respectively compared with singletons.[8-11]

The relationship of cerebral palsy to preterm delivery and intrauterine growth restriction is of particular relevance. It has been shown that there is an association between perinatal infection and cerebral palsy. In case control studies of infants born before 32 weeks of gestation or with birth weight of 1,500 gm or less, show an increased risk of cerebral palsy related to chorioamnionitis and markers of maternal genital tract infections. Maternal infection has also been associated with preterm birth and periventricular leukomalacia.[12-14]

Several studies have reported that antenatal death of co-multiple *in utero* is the most powerful predictor factor of cerebral palsy of the alive co-multiple.

Greinin and colleagues in 1991[15] reported 13 triplet pregnancies with no perinatal deaths but with a neonatal morbidity in 80% of the infants. Complications included hypebilirubinemia in 51%, hypoglycemia in 30%, respiratory distress syndrome in 28% and intrauterine hemorrhage in 10%. In quadruplets the prematurity rate was quite high and there is very little information about perinatal mortality ,perinatal morbidity and long-term follow-up.

Multiple pregnancies increase the maternal risks. In mothers with triplets there is an incidence of 20% of pregnancy including hypertention, 11 to 35% incidence of anemia, 35% incidence of postpartum hemorrhage, 24% preterm premature rupture of membranes (PPROM), 9% hemolysis, elevated liver enzymes and low platelets (HELLP), 4% acute fatty liver of pregnancy and 1% eclampsia.[16,17]

Multifetal pregnancies are expected to have an increased risk of complications from cardiovascular and pulmonary system because of increased weight gain, increased cardiac output and greater demand of the cardiovascular system.

In triplets there is an increased risk for developing pregnancy-induced hypertention, compares with singletons and twin gestations. The incidence has been reported to be 7% for singletons, 14% for twins and 21% for triplets.[18] Several reasons underlie these differences: First, many mothers with triplets are older than those with singletons; second, many of these are primiparent women who have undergone in assisted reproductions technique; and third, multiple pregnancy is an independent factor for developing pregnancy-induced hypertention.

The number of fetuses and the large placental mass require much larger iron requirements. Bleeding before delivery is increased in multiple pregnancies, since placenta previa and abruptio placenta are increased in multiple gestations. Postpartum hemorrhage is increased and 90 to 100% of triplets are delivered by cesarean section.[19, 20]

There is no agreement about whether there is an increased incidence of gestational diabetes in multifetal pregnancies. Most studies indicate a higher incidence with a greater number of fetuses. A recent study comparing triplets and twin pregnancies after reduction showed 4-fold increased in gestational diabetes in triplets.[21]

Advanced maternal age, infertility due to polycystic ovaries, increased insulin resistance, increased human placental lactogen with larger placentas, all contribute to increase glucose intolerance in triplet pregnancies. The normal adaptation for a singleton pregnancy may be not sufficient for the successful completion of triplets. For the women with an underlying cardiovascular disorder that is borderline, a triplet pregnancy may end in severe maternal sequel. The majority of women with triplets do well despite the increased risk of pregnancy-induced hypertention the postpartum hemorrhage, and the high incidence of cesarean delivery. Careful preconceptional counseling, with good obstetric management can result in healthy mothers and triplets babies.

MULTRIFETAL PREGNANCY REDUCTION

Multifetal pregnancies are at increased risk of preterm delivery and this risk directly correlated with the number of fetuses.

Patients with multifetal pregnancies and their husbands, have three difficult options to choose from. Termination of the entire pregnancy and start a new one which is an unlike choice for a couple who have suffered years of infertility and have probably going through great emotional and financial expenses. A second choice is to continue the high order multiple pregnancy, accepting the high possibility of having a miscarriage or a very preterm delivery, and the increased risk for perinatal mortality and morbidity. The third option is the multifetal pregnancy reduction, where the number of fetuses is reduced in order to lower the likehood of preterm delivery and optimize the chance of a successful outcome.[22, 23]

Multifetal pregnancy reduction has become an alternative in infertility therapy, since its application has allowed physicians to become more aggressive in treating patients resistant to more conservative therapies.[24]

The irony is that many of these women with long standing infertility, now have more fetuses that can be safely carried to viability.

First trimester multifetal pregnancy reduction (MFPR) began in the end 1980s in an attempt to decrease the final number of fetuses in order to decrease the incidence of prematurity.

The main reason for a second trimester selective termination was the case where one fetus in a multiple pregnancy was affected or had serious abnormalities and is reduced to improve the outcome of the remaining fetuses. There are fundamental differences between the two procedures. The procedure of reducing the number of fetuses in an otherwise normal multifetal gestation is called MFPR.

The technique of selectively termination of the affected fetus in a multiple pregnancy during the first or second trimester was introduced with different names such as selective reduction, selective termination, selective feticide, selective embryocide, selective abortion, selective birth, etc.

Bercowitz and Lynch[25] covered the term "reduction" since the term illustrates the nature of the procedure and disassociates it from the "selective termination" of targeted fetuses. Selective termination is the case of terminating a malformed or compromised fetus. The ethical considerations surrounding the "selective termination" of a structurally affected fetus differ from those raised in the multifetal pregnancy reduction.

The first report of first trimester multifetal pregnancy reduction published in 1986 by Dumez and Oury.[26] They presented the first series of selective abortion in multifetal pregnancies, reduced to 4 singletons, 10 set of twins and 1 set of triplets. The procedures were performed by dilating the cervix, and aspirating one or more sacs transvaginally, under ultrasound guidance. Of the 11 completed pregnancies, 4 patients delivered at term, three delivered between 33 and 36 weeks, one delivered at 30 weeks and two lost their pregnancies in the second trimester. This technique was quickly abandoned because of high complication rate.

The same year Kanhai and colleagues (1986) reported the reduction of a quintuplet pregnancy to twins, by thoracic puncture under ultrasound guidance.[27]

Boulot and colleagues (1993) published a series of 61 women who had undergone MFPR, 35 by transabdominal approach and 26 by transcervical sac perforation and crushing of the embryo if size permitted. Fetal loss rate was 13.1% and preterm labor rate was 56.6%. Since that time the majority of the centers, which perform the technique, utilize transabdominal approach with intrathoracic injection of potassium chloride under ultrasound guidance.[28]

TECHNICAL ASPECTS

Each patient before the procedure undergoes an extensive consultation and the risks and benefits of MFPR are discusses in detail. It should be explained to the patients, and the patient should be reassured that this solution is not carried any risks for the other fetuses, and that is essentially harmless to the remaining fetuses. The procedure is performed in the ultrasound unit. A very details ultrasound examination is recommended before the procedure in order to determine the number and location of all the fetuses, their interrelationship and location in relation to the internal cervic os, ascertain fetal viability, measure the crown-rump length of each fetus, localize the placentas and rule out major structural anomalies.

The evaluation of chorionicity is a very important part of this detailed ultrasound examination. Separate placentas are obviously dichorionic. If the placentas are fused, chorionicity can be determined by ultrasonographic appearance of the thickness of the dividing membranes (thick dichorionic, thin monochorionic) during the first trimester of pregnancy and the presence of chorionic villi between layers of a dichorionic membrane (twin peak sign, lamda sign).[29]

Transabdominal approach is usually performed using the free hand technique without using a needle guide.

The fetus in the lower sac is not reduced, unless it has detectable anomalies or is one twin of a monochorionic set of twins. A 22-gauge, 9 cm long, spinal needle is introduced transabdominally under ultrasound guidance into the fetal thorax in the longitudinal plane and 2 to 3 mEq potassium chloride (2 mEq/ml concentration) is injected slowly so as not to dislodge the needle tip.[30] A pleural effusion should be seen as well as an asystole. The cardiac activity is carefully observed for at least 2 minutes and if cardiac activity persists, more potassium chloride is injected. About 0.5 ml of potassium chloride solution is usually sufficient to stop the heartbeat. The selection of the fetuses to be reduced is based on the technical ease with which the procedure can be performed. In transabdominal approach, the fetus in the sac over the internal cervical os is left alone unless abnormalities are noted in that fetus. In trandabdominal approach, it is most common to reduce fetuses located in the middle or upper part of the uterine cavity.

A new needle injection is required to terminate each fetus. We avoid transversing the sac of a fetus in order to terminate the fetus directly beneath. It has been suggested to avoid termination of more than three fetuses at one session; therefore, women with six fetuses have their procedures performed during two or more sessions generally one week apart.

In case of monochorionic-diamniotic, or monoamniotic twins in a dichorionic-diamniotic, or dichorionic-triamniotic triplet pregnancy, the monochorionic twins will need to be considered for reduction, due to the fact that these may develop future signs of twin to twin transfusion syndrome (TTTS). After the procedure, the patient is observed for one hour to monitor for evidence of progressive uterine contraction vaginal bleeding or leakage of amniotic fluid.

The ultrasound examination is repeated in order to confirm normal cardiac activity in the non-reduced fetuses, and the asystol in the reduce fetuses.

MFPR in most centers is performed between 10 and 14 weeks gestation. Before 10 weeks, it is technically more difficult because of the small size of the fetuses and greater distance from the maternal abdominal wall to the fetuses. Waiting until 10 weeks, spontaneous loss of a fetus could occur, which would obviate the need to perform MFPR, especially in triplets. If MFRP performed too late the risk of premature delivery may be greater.

There is no advantage in delaying the procedure beyond the 12th week of gestation, because if all fetuses are alive and are of appropriate size at that time, spontaneous losses are not likely in the next few weeks. Moreover, the later in pregnancy the termination is performed, the more probable it is that fetal resorption will be incomplete, and maybe the rare chance, that maternal disseminated intravascular coagulation will develop.[31] Delay beyond 12 weeks is unnecessary and the risk of miscarriage or preterm rupture of membranes is increased.

In 1993 Timor-Trisch and colleagues reported their experience with 134 patients undergoing MFPR by transvaginal puncture and potassium chloride injection. They used a spring-loaded device with a 21-gauge needle attached to the transvaginal ultrasound probe. The placement of the needle was very accurate and the procedure was painless because of the high velocity entry of the needle. The uncorrected loss rate was 12.6% and there was no difference in the loss rate in those patients whose fetuses in the sac over the internal os were targeted for reduction, as opposed to the others.[32]

Other authors have also reported transvaginal needle embryo aspiration. Itskovits and colleagues (1992) reported two quadruplet pregnancies successfully reduced to twins by transvaginal ultrasound guided aspiration of the gestational sacs. This procedure was similar to transvaginal oocytes retrieval and is performed at an earlier gestational age.[33]

Mansour and colleagues (1999) recently reported a modification of the technique of transvaginal MFPR. This modification involved eliminating the use of KCl. After introducing the needle into fetal echoes between 6 and 9 weeks of gestation, suction was applied with a 20 ml syringe until all or most of the embryonic parts were aspirated. The loss rate in this group was 8.8%.[34]

The first series of ultrasound-guided transabdominal MFPR with intrauterine potassium chloride injection was reported by Berkowitz and colleagues in 1988.[23] In that series the first three patients had transcervical procedure while in the rest nine cases the procedure was performed transabdominally with a total loss rate of 33%. In 1990 Wapner et al reported selective reduction in 46 multiple pregnancies with loss rate 3% and the 81% of the cases delivered after 36 weeks.[34]

The experience with the first 200 cases of tranabdominal MFPR from a single center was reported in 1993. At the time of the procedure, 88 women had triplets, 89 had quadruplets, 16 had quintuplets and seven had six to nine fetuses. Reduction to triplets was done at the patient´s request and reduction to singleton was only done for medical indications. The pregnancy loss rates were 7.9% for those who presented with three or four fetuses, 12.5% for those with five and 42.9 for those with six or more.[30]

The first collaborative data published in 1993 by Evans and colleagues[35] covered the years from 1988 through early 1991, included all cases performed transabdominally with introthoracic potassium chloride injection.

The total pregnancy loss rates were 4% at two or less post-procedure, 5% at four weeks or less and 16.4% through 24 completed weeks´ gestation.[35] The loss rates were 7%, 15% and 30% for patients presenting with triplets, quadruplets and quintuplets respectively and who where reduced to twins. The total loss rate was 14% in patients reduced to twins compared with singletons (25%) and triplets (27%). From these first series could be concluded that:

1. The total pregnancy loss is correlated with the initial and final number of fetuses.
2. Gestational age at delivery is inversely correlated with the initial and final number of fetuses.
3. Gestational age at the time of procedure within 10 to 12 weeks has no effect on pregnancy loss. Procedures performed after 12 weeks´ gestation

may be associated with higher rates of prematurity.
4. Maternal complications have not been reported.
5. Risk of congenital anomalies in survivors is not increased.

The second collaborative study in 1994 compared the transabdominal to transcervical approach for MFPR. The experience on 1,000 patients showed a significant decrease in the overall pregnancy loss rate in cases preformed transabdominally from16 to 8% and in the transvaginal/transcervical cases a loss rate of approximately 13%. The prematurity rate between 25 and 28 weeks´s gestation was 5,5%, 10% of the patients delivered at 29 to 32 weeks´ and 50% of all patients reached 37 weeks´ gestation. It has been also suggested that there is an inverse relationship of starting and finishing number of fetuses to the loss rate.[36]

The latest collaborative study published in 1996 described 1,789 completed pregnancies after MFPR. The results obtained from nine centers in five countries. The overall pregnancy loss rate in this study was 11.7% and varied from 7.6% in cases of reduction of triplets to twins and increased to 22.9% for sextuplets to twins.[37]

In the most recent international collaborative series, Evans et al (2003) reported on 3,513 MFPR. All procedures were performed by transabdominal potassium chloride injection, except 331 that were done transvaginally by one group. The overall loss rate was 9.6%, with loss rate varying depending on the starting and finishing number of fetuses. Data by the finishing number of fetuses demonstrated that twins had the best outcomes. Although difference between twins and singletons was small, both groups had significantly lower loss rates than did the group ending with triplets.

CONTROVERSIES IN MFPR

There are several issues reporting multifetal pregnancy reduction:
1. Are there medical indications to reduce triplets?
2. Multifetal pregnancy reduction to a singleton.
3. Does genetic amniocentesis or chorionic villus sampling presenting an excess risk for patients before or after MFPR?
4. The value of nuchal translucency in screening.
5. The effect of MFPR on the maternal clotting factors.

Fetal Reduction in Triplets

Although MFPR has proved to be effective in reducing preterm delivery and perinatal loss in quadruplets and high order multiples, there is an on going debate about the benefits of embryo reduction in triplet pregnancies.[38-40]

This is due to the fact that the progress in the management of multiple pregnancies and in neonatal care has improved the perianatal outcome in triplets.[41, 42]

Most authors in cases of reduced triplets to twins report improvement in maternal complications, length of gestation, severe prematurity and low birth weight, although a significant improvement in perinatal mortality has not been noted.[43-46] The question remains: is there medical indication to reduce triplets and since some studies find a better obstetric outcome in reduced pregnancies,[28, 47] whereas other studies do not.[48,49]

Macones and his group (1993) published their experience in comparing the perinatal outcome of triple pregnancies reduced to twins with the outcome of continuing triplet pregnancies and twin pregnancies. The mean gestational age at delivery for the reduced triplets was 35.6 weeks compared with 31.2 weeks in the nonreduced triplets. The perinatal mortality rate was 30/1000 in the reduction group and 210/1000 in the nonreduced triplets. The mean birth weight of the nonreduced triplets compared to the triplets reduced to twins and to nonreduced twins were 1,593, 2,279 and 2,293 respectively.[50]

Antsaklis and colleagues (1998) compared the outcome of 158 sets of twins obtained by MFPR compared with 135 control twin pregnancies. The spontaneous loss rate in reduction group was 10.6% vs 9.5% in the control pregnancies. The mean gestational ages at delivery were 35.1 weeks and 35.7 weeks respectively.[51]

Yaron and colleagues (1999) compared the outcomes of triplet pregnancies undergoing reduction to twins with outcomes of nonreduced twin gestation and expectantly managed triplet gestation. They found that reduction of triplets to twins significantly reduces the risk for prematurity and low birth weight and may also be associated with a reduction in overall pregnancy loss. This suggests that MFPR of triplets to twin is a medically justifiable procedure not only from medical viewpoint but also from the ethical perspective of supporting patients´ autonomy and in respect of patients individual circumstances.[52]

Antsaklis and colleagues (2004) examined retrospectively 225 trichorionic triplet pregnancy, of which 185 had embryo reduction to twins and 70 were managed expectantly. The rates of pretern delivery were significantly lower in the reduced group (11.17% vs 36.76% for delivery at ≤ 32 weeks and 40.58% vs 83.82% for delivery at ≤ 35 weeks reduced vs non-reduced group).

Total fetal loss was significantly higher in the reduced group than in the nonreduced group (15.41% and 4.76% respectively) and the difference was mainly due to the higher miscarriage rate in the reduced group (8.11% vs 2.86% in the nonreduced group). With the expected rates of handicap in preterm infants we would anticipate 0.63% of severely handicapped children due to extreme prematurity in the reduced group and 1.64% in the nonreduced group. They concluded that MFPR significantly reduces the risk of severe preterm delivery and very low birth weight by about 1/3, increase the total fetal loss by about one-quarter and reduce the risk of having a severely handicapped child due to extreme prematurity.[53]

In 1996, Lipitz and colleagues compared the outcome of 43 triplet pregnancies reduced to twin which had reached at least 24 weeks' gestation to 34 dichorionic twin pregnancies. In general, the outcome between the two groups did not differ significantly from those of the naturally occurring twin pregnancy. There was a higher incidence of premature rupture of the membranes in the reduced cases compared to the natural twins (18.6% vs 8.2%). The mean gestational age was similar in the two groups. They concluded that the outcome of triplet pregnancies reduced to twins did not differ substantially from that of nonreduced twin pregnancy.[54]

Leondires and colleagues in 2000 retrospectively reviewed 127 triplet pregnancies. Thirty-six percent of patients chose MFPR. In the expectant management group, 13.6% were reduced spontaneously after 9 weeks of gestation. The mean gestational ages at delivery for MFPR group and expectant management group were 33.25 ± 1.03 weeks and 32.04 ± 0.58 weeks and the mean birth weights of infants delivered at >24 weeks of gestation were 2,226 ± 79 gm and 1,796 ± 44 gm respectively (p<0001). There were no significant differences in perinatal mortality gestational age at delivery or "take home" infant per delivery rates between these groups and they concluded that MFPR does not have a significant impact on the probability of live birth or on gestational age at delivery for women with triplets.[55]

Kadhel and colleagues (1998) in a retrospective study compared the outcome of a group of on-going triplet pregnancies, and a group of triplets reduced to twins. Prematurity rate was lower in the reduced pregnancies group (62.5% vs 95.6% P <0.05). Severe prematurity was not different in the two groups. No significant difference was observed for perinatal mortality. The authors concluded that the difference observed does not seem to represent a dicisive benefit for reducing triplet pregnancies. Due to the progress in the management of multiple pregnancies and neonatal intensive care they think that MFPR should no longer be justified by obstetric benefit but rather as a possibility offered to couples who could be confronted with the potential severe psychological, social and economic problems of triple births.[56]

Alexander and colleagues in 1995 compared the obstetric outcomes of twin pregnancies obtained as a result of MFPR to those in which this procedure had not been used. They concluded that fetal growth of the reduced group seems to be improved independently of gestational age at which delivery occurred and this article introduced a degree of uncertainty for the benefits of MFPR in triplet pregnancies.[57]

The preterm delivery and growth restriction in 127 multiple pregnancies reduced to twins was examined. In 16 (12.6%) of the 127 multifetal pregnancies reduced to twins, there was a miscarriage of both fetuses before 24 weeks. Both fetal loss before 24 weeks and the interval between embryo reduction and delivery were significantly associated with the gestation at reduction. In the pregnancies reduced to twins compared to the nonreduced twins, the percentage of miscarriages was higher than mean gestation at delivery was lower.[58]

The most likely cause of pregnancy loss and severe preterm delivery in MFPR is the development of an inflammatory response to the resorbing dead feto-placental tissue with subsequent release of cytokines and stimulation of prostaglandins.[59]

In conclusion, it seems that there is a good evidence that reduction from triplets to twins or to singletons improves the outcome of the pregnancy by reducing the risk of severe prematurity at the expense of a higher fetal loss rate and is likely to reduce the risk of serious handicap in surviving children.

Patients with triplets should receive all the information available and the option of multifetal pregnancy reduction should be offered. The decreased rate of maternal complication in reduced triplets should also be discussed.

Multifetal Pregnancy Reduction to a Singleton

There is an agreement between the number of fetuses to be left (two fetuses left has the best outcome) and the choice of which fetuses to terminate is governed by a number of variables. The majority of patients undergoing MFPR reduce to a twin fetus, but there is increasing number of patients with a multiple pregnancy who are interested in carrying a singleton pregnancy. No data suggest that this produces significantly improved perinatal outcome, unless specific medical factors, such as important maternal cardiac disease, a prior history of incompetent cervix, uterine abnormalities or prior early preterm delivery. When information regarding the risk of the procedure became available, reduction to singleton is performed for purely elective reason. Stone and colleagues[60] in 1998 reported the outcome of 64 patients undergoing MFRP to a singleton. Twenty-eight patients undergoing MFPR for medical indication and 36 for elective reasons. The overall loss rate was 4.7% and all occurred in the medically indicated group. The results suggested a low loss rate in patients reducing to singleton, particularly when the indication was elective. However, the small number of patients suggests that there is not enough data to recommend deduction to singleton. However, reduction to a singleton will be undertaken if after counseling the couple still wish to do so. In case of patients with triplets in which there is a monochorionic twin gestation, because of the increased risk of monochorionicity, the patients are advised to consider reducing the monochorionic twins and continuing with singleton gestation.[61]

Prenatal Diagnosis and MFPR

Very frequently the MFPR performed in women who at the time of delivery will be 35 years or older making these candidates for prenatal diagnosis. Patients with multifetal pregnancies who are at risk for chromosomal abnormalities or genetic disease, have two options available for prenatal diagnosis. One option is to undergo MFPR and then 4 weeks later to undergo amniocentesis on the remaining fetuses. The second option is to have chorionic villus sampling (CVS) performed before the MFPR, there by having the ability to leave karyotypically normal fetuses concerning the first option.

Tabsh and Theroux in 1995 reported their experience in 53 women who reduced their higher order multifetal pregnancies to twins and subsequently underwent genetic amniocentesis. Five of these patients (9.4%) lost their entire pregnancy 2 to 14 days following amniocentesis. The authors hypothesized that it is possible that the MFPR causes some alteration in the intrauterine environments that they predispose the patients to a higher risk of spontaneous rupture of the membranes and for infections following genetic amniocentesis.[62]

Women carrying multifetal pregnancies are also at higher risk of having a chromosomally abnormal fetuses than are women carrying singletons, and this risk is even higher in infertility patients because of advanced maternal age. Therefore, it is not unusual with twin pregnancies who have undergone MFPR, to also seek prenatal diagnosis. In such cases amniocentesis is the method of choice in most centers.

Antsaklis and colleagues in 2000[63] compared the results of 73 genetic amniocentesis in twin pregnancies followed by multifetal pregnancy reduction, to 434 genetic amniocenteses in twins without reduction. The median maternal age of the MFPR group was 36.3 years and of the controls was 36.1 years. The rate of pregnancy loss did not differ significantly between the reduced group (4.1%) and controls (3.32%). The compared rate of pregnancy loss in the entire study population was 3.4%. Only 35.7% of patients in MFPR group delivered at term compared with 56.5% of the controls. This difference was mainly attributed to deliveries occurring between 25 and 28 week's gestation (17.1% and 1.3%).

It has been reported that amniocentesis in multrifetal pregnancies reduced to twins significantly increases the risk of preterm delivery especially before 29 weeks´ gestation. A crucial question is whether this increase in prematurity rate is attributable to amniocentesis or to MFPR. The current literature suggests that it is mainly related to the MFPR process. The likehood of fetal loss secondary to genetic amniocentesis in twin pregnancies after MFPR seems to be at the same order of magnitude, as that in non reduced twin gestation and amniocentesis in appropriate candidates who have undergone MFPR and have a genetic indication was strongly suggested.

The major drawback to amniocentesis after MFPR is that if one of the remaining fetuses after MFPR is found to be chromosomally abnormal, the patient is forced to undergo yet another procedure to selectively terminate the abnormal fetus.

Concerning the second option, it seems important to offer pre-procedure noninvasive genetic screening and detailed ultrasound scanning using nuchal translucency (NT) measurements especially for those patients (advanced maternal age) with significantly increased risk of chromosomal abnormalities. Screening by NT measurements, as a part of pre-procedure noninvasive testing, before embryo reduction, lowering the probability of leaving an affected fetus after the procedure and the current policy includes a routine ultrasound examination for detection of fetal structure abnormalities and NT measurements. The identification of a visible anomaly or a smaller than expected CRL or abnormal NT, influences the decision about which fetus to remove. However, it has been suggested that in high risk group for chromosomal aneuploidy, CVS should be affected before embryo reduction is employed.

CVS procedure was associated with 1.2% sampling error which is similar to the background risk for aneuoploidy in this group.[64,65]

CVS pre-reduction has also some disadvantages such as: the increased risk of miscarriage, the difficulties and complication of sampling a triplet pregnancy, the difficulty of identifying the affected fetuses to be reduced within few days of taking the sample and the higher stress level in patients caused by two invasive procedures within few days.[66, 67]

Brambati and colleagues in 1995, in queries of 69 women who underwent CVS before MFPR, showed no additional loss rate after CVS and MFPR when compared with patients undergoing MFPR without CVS.[64]

Eddleman et al (2000) reported their results on 86 patients undergoing CVS before MFPR. CVS was successfully completed in 85 patients. Three out of 164 fetuses (1.8%) had abnormal chromosomes. They suggested that CVS before MFPR is technically feasible and accurate, with an acceptably low sampling error rate, and pregnancy loss rate, and is the method of choice in patients undergoing prenatal diagnosis and MFPR.[65]

Selective Termination

The diagnosis of a severe abnormality in a twin or triplet pregnancy often leads to a management dilemma. Patients with this problem have three options: (i) continue the pregnancy with both the normal and the abnormal fetuses, (ii) terminate the entire pregnancy and terminate a healthy fetus and (iii) selectively terminate the abnormal fetuses. When termination is an option, selective termination should be considered. Selective reduction or selective termination or selective feticide of an abnormal multiple is a unique problem with its own issues and controversies. In selective reduction we face the problem of terminating a handicapped fetus but at the same time attempting to protect a healthy one.[68, 69]

The technique of selective termination is similar to that at the first trimester multifetal pregnancy reduction but the potassium chloride injection must be performed directly into the fetal heart. The dose of potassium chloride increases with gestational age, but rarely exceeds 3 ml.[70]

Before undergoing ST, all patients need ultrasound confirmation of dichorionicity. This procedure should not be done in monochorionic twins because of intrafetal vascular anastomoses and the risk of injury to the remaining fetuses. Potential options for ST in monochorionic twins include cord ligation, cord coagulation or laser cord occlusion.[71, 72]

Selective termination is a serious problem with additional medical and ethical issues such as the correct identification of the affected fetus following the initial diagnostic procedure. Selective termination might occur several weeks after an amniocentesis or CVS, so documentation including *in utero* mapping of all fetuses and placentas is critical at the time of CVS or amniocentesis. If identification is difficult or uncertain by using the fetal and the placental location, the fetal sex or the presence of detectable structural malformations, in one twin, further diagnostic testing by cordocentesis, or amniocentesis should be performed prior to the reduction for rapid determination of karyotype by direct preparation or fluorescence *in situ* hybridization on amniocytes is appropriate.

The first report of selective termination in a twin pregnancy with Hurler´s syndrome was made in 1979.[73] The authors utilized cardiac puncture at 24 weeks gestation. The normal twin was delivered prematurely at 33 weeks. A second report of selective termination resulting in a term delivery of a normal child, published by Beck and colleagues. In this case hysterotomy was performed to remove the affected fetus at 22 weeks of gestation.[74]

In 1981, Kerenyi and Chithara reported on a selective reduction of one twin with Down syndrome when the mother threatened to abort the normal and the affected twin. This case has been discussed widely as an alternative to aborting the healthy fetus together with the affected one.

Chitkara and colleagues (1989) reported on 17 patients undergoing second trimester selective termination. In the first seven cases termination was achieved by cardiac puncture with either exsanguination (one patient) or embolism (five patients) or cardiac tamponade (one patient). Four of those pregnancies were lost completely. The remaining 10 procedures were performed by injecting intracardiac potassium chloride and all pregnancies resulted in the birth of healthy singletons.[75]

In 1994, Evans and colleagues compiled data on 183 completed cases of selective termination using a variety of techniques. These cases included 169 twins, 11 triplets and three quadruplets. Twenty-three of the 183 pregnancies (12.6%) were lost completely before 24 weeks' gestation. If the procedure was performed at ≤ 16 weeks the loss rate was 5.4% and increased to 14.4% if the procedures were performed at ≥ 17 weeks, 83.8% of the pregnancies were delivered after 33 weeks.

Antsaklis and colleagues (2001) were investigated the pregnancy outcome of selective termination when it is performed in the second trimester and compared the results with those when it is performed in the first. In pregnancies in which selective termination was performed before 12 weeks' gestation the miscarriage rate was 5.6% while in those in which it was performed in second trimester the rate was 8.3% ($p > 0.05$ NS). The mean gestational age at delivery was 36.7 weeks for the first trimester group and 35.1 weeks for the second trimester group. The rate of cesarean section was not statistically different and there was no perinatal mortality in either group.[76]

The authors concluded that selective feticide of an affected fetus is as safe in the second trimester as it is in the first trimester.

Selective termination of a fetus with lethal malformation is only indicated if the continuation of the pregnancy with such a lethal defect, presents greater hazard to the co-twin than does the risk of termination. Selective termination in these situations would potentially improve the outcome by eliminating the possibility of polyhydramnios and premature delivery.[77]

Another very important ethical issue is the fact that in some countries late termination is a legal procedure under certain circumstances. Lipitz and colleagues in 1996 reported the results and the follow-up of 37 dichorionic twin gestations in which ST was performed late between 24 and 33 weeks showed favorable outcomes with rates of prematurity less than 31 weeks, less than 34 weeks and less than 37 weeks of 5.7%, 14.3% and 22.9% respectively.[78]

In 1996, Lynch et al examined the rate of preterm delivery after selective termination in 69 consecutive twin pregnancies and the fetal loss rate was 3%.

Effect of MFPR and ST on the Maternal Clotting Factors

Another very important issue concerning the MFPR and the selective termination is the effect of these procedures on the maternal clotting factors. The demise of one fetus in a multiple gestation has been known to be a theoretical, real risk to the mother for developing disseminated intravascular coagulopathy due to release of thromboplastic material from the dead fetus into maternal circulation. This risk is felt to be different for the first versus second trimester reduction procedures.

In a study by Skrablin and colleagues (1994) with 26 multifetal pregnancies with single fetal demise after 12 weeks of gestation where fibrinogen levels in maternal blood were estimated weekly. In three of 13 cases, heparin in doses of 15000 IU daily was administrated prophylactically while in others no therapy was given. One untreated women developed severe fibrinogenemia.[79]

Lynch and Berkowitz (1993)[31] investigated coagulation profiles in 17 of their first trimester reduction patients. The studies included platelet count, partial thromboplastic time, prothrombin time, fibrinogen and fibrin split products and were drawn between 2 and 5 weeks after reduction. Over 200 reduction patients, no clinical disseminated intravascular coagulopathy has been encountered. Recent studies concluded that there is no threat to the health of patients undergoing multifetal pregnancy reduction from the changing levels of clotting factors.[79]

CONCLUSION

Over the last 25 years MFRP and ST have become a well accepted procedures to reduce the perinatal mortality and morbidity associated with higher order multiple gestation (MFPR) and to selectively terminate on affected twin or triplet in multiple pregnancy (ST).

The gained experience suggests that the trans-abdominal approach undertaken between 10 and 12 weeks gestation is preferred. Both procedures have been shown to be technically safe and result in acceptable pregnancy loss rate.

With increasing experience the risks associated with MFRP are small and similar to risks of carrying multiple gestations without MFPR.

Prenatal diagnosis after MFPR performing by amniocentesis 4 weeks later or before prenatal diagnosis MFPR by performing CVS, is feasible and safe. The excellent pregnancy outcome associated with MFPR, CVS before MFPR and amniocentesis after MFPR are obtained in centers with vast experience with these procedures, with a relatively limited number of operators adhering to a strict common protocol. These procedures should not be generalized to all centers and patients should be extensively counseled for the advantages and disadvantages of MFPR the risk and the complications and the option of ST should be offered even in the setting of a lethal anomaly.

Although MFPR would appear to be of benefit for triplets and higher order gestation, the more logical approach would be prevention of their occurrence through the more judicious use in the future of newer assisted reproductive techniques.

REFERENCES

1. Kiely JL, Kleinman JC, Kiely M. Triplets and higher order multiple births time trends and infant mortality. Am J Disorders in Childs 1990; 46: 862-8.
2. Lynch L. Multifetal pregnancy reduction in fetal therapy: invasive and transplacental. Fisk N, Moise K Cambridge University Press 1997; pp 60-71.

3. Shenker J G, Yarkoni S, Granat M: Multiple pregnancies following induction of ovulation. Fertil Steril 1981; 35: 105.
4. Elster N and the Institute of Science Low and technology Working Group on reproductive technology: Less in more: the risks of multiple births. Fertil Steril 2000; 74:617-23.
5. Craigo SD. Triplet pregnancy and multifetal reduction: a rational view of the data. Contemp Ob Gyn 1998 April; 78.
6. Itzkowic D. A survey of 59 triplet pregnancies. Br J Obstet Gynecol 1976; 83:967-73.
7. Kiely J, Kleinman J, Kiely M. Triplets and higher order multiple births: time trends and infant mortality. Am J Diseas Child 1992; 146: 862-8.
8. Pharaoh PO, Cooke T. Cerebral palsy and multiple births. Arch Dis Child Fetal Neonat Ed 1996; 75: F174-7.
9. Yokohama Y, Shimizu T, Hayakawa K. Prevalence of cerebral palsy in twins, triplets and quadruplets. Int J Epidemial 1995; 24: 943-8.
10. Nelson KB, Ellenberg JH. Chilhood neurological disorders in twins. Pediatr Perinat Epidemiol 1995; 9:135-45.
11. Petterson B, Nelson KB, Watson L, Stanley F. Twins, triplets and cerebral palsy in birth in Western Australia in the 1980´s. Br Med J 1993; 307:1239-43.
12. Stanley F, Blair E, Alberman E. Pathways to cerebral palsy involving very preterm birth. In cerebral palsy. Epidemiology and causal pathways. London: Mackeith Press 2000; 60-82.
13. Murphy DS, Sellers S, Mackenzie IZ, Yudkin PL, Johnson AM. Case control study of antenatal and intrapartum risk factors cerebral palsy in very preterm singleton babies. Lancet 1995; 346:1449-54.
14. O´Shea TM, Klinepeter KL, Meis PJ, Pillard RG. Intrauterine infection and the risk of cerebral palsy in very low birth weight infants. Pediatric Perinat Epidemiol 1998; 12:72-83.
15. Greinin H, Katz M, Laros R. Triplet pregnancy: changes in morbidity and mortality. Journal of Perinatal 1991; 111:207-12.
16. Lynch L, Bercowitz R. Multifetal pregnancy reduction. Ultrasonography in reproductive medicine 1991; 2:771-81.
17. Klein VR. Maternal complications associated with triplet pregnancies in triplet pregnancies and their consequences. Ed. L. Êeith I. Blickstein, The Parthenon Publ Group 2002; 215-24.
18. Lynch A, McDuffier R, Murphy J, Fabar K, Orleans M. Preeclampsia in multiple gestation: the role of assisted reproductive technologies. Obstet Gynecol 2002; 99:445-51.
19. Newman RB, Luke B. Multiple pregnancy: A Hand Book for Care of the Pregnant Patient. Philadelphia: Lippincott Williams and Wilkins 2000; 173-91.
20. Devine PC, Malone FD, Athanassin A, Harvey-Wilkes K, D´ Alton ME. Maternal and neonatal outcome of 100 consecutive triplet pregnancies. Am J Perinatal 2001; 18:225-35.
21. Sivan E, Maman E, Hamko CJ, Lipitz S, Cohen S, Schiff E. Impact of the fetal reduction on the incidence of gestational diabetes. Obstet Gynecol 2002; 99:91-4.
22. Evans MI, Dommergnes M, Wapner R, et al. Selective reduction of multifetal pregnancy in the first trimester.
23. Berkowitz RL, Lynch L, Chitkara V, et al. Selective reduction of multifetal pregnancy in the first trimester. N Eng J Med 1988; 318: 1043-7.
24. Evans MI, Hume RF, Yaron Y, Kromer RL, Johnson MP. Multifetal pregnancy reduction. Bailliere´s Clin Obstet Gynecol 1998; 12:147-59.
25. Lerner JP, Timor-Tritsch IE, Monteagndo A. First and second trimester multifetal pregnancy reduction. In Monteagndo A, Timor-Tritsch IE (Eds): Ultrasound and Multifetal Pregnancy. Parthenon Publishing: New York, London 1998; pp 179-200.
26. Dumez Y, Oury J: Method for first trimester selective abortion in multiple pregnancy. Contribution to Gynecology and Obstetrics 1986; 15:50-3.
27. Kanhai HH, van Rijssel EJ, Meerman RJ, Bennebroaek-Gravenhorst J. Selective termination in quintuplet pregnancy during first trimester. Lancet I 1986: 1447.
28. Boulot P, Hedon B, Pelliccia G, et al. Effects of selective reduction in triplet gestation: a cooperative study of cases with or without this procedure. Fertil Steril 1993; 60:497-503.
29. Sepulveda W, Sebire NJ, Odibo D, et al. Prenatal determination of chorionicity in triplets pregnancy by ultrasound graphic examination of the epsilon zone. Obstet Gynecol 1996; 88: 855-8.
30. Berkowitz RL, Lynch L, Lapiski R, Bergh P. First trimester transabdominal multifetal pregnancy reduction: a report of two hundred completed cases. Am J Obstet Gynecol 1993; 169:17-21.
31. Lynch L, Berkowitz R. Maternal serum alpha – fetoprotein and coagulation profiles after multifetal pregnancy reduction. Am J Obstet Gynecol 1993; 169:987-90.
32. Timor-Tritsch IE, Peisner DB, Monteagndo A, Lerner JP, Sharma S. Multifetal pregnancy reduction by transvaginal puncture: evaluation of the technique use in 134 cases. Am J Obstet Gynecol 1993; 168:799-804.
33. Itskovits-Eldor J, Drugan A, Levron J, Thaler I, Bromdes J. Transvaginal embryo aspiration a safe method for selective reduction in multiple pregnancies. Fertil Steril 1992; 58: 351-5.
34. Mansour RT, Aboulghar M, Serour G, et al. Multifetal pregnancies reduction modification of the technique and analysis of the outcome. Fertil Steril 1999; 71:380-4.
35. Evans M, Dommergues M, Wapner RL, Lynch L, Dumez Y, Goldberg J, Zador MS, Nicolaides K, Jonhson MP, Colbus MS, Boulot R, Bercowitz R. Efficacy of transabdominal multifetal pregnancy reduction: collaborative experience among the World´s largest centers. Obstet Gynecol 1993; 82:61-6.
36. Evans M, Dommergues M, Timor-Tritsch I, Zador IE, Wapner RL, Lynch L, Dumez Y, Goldberg J, Zador MS, Nicolaides K, Jonhson MP, Colbus MS. Boulot R, Akin AJ,

Monteagudo A, Bercowitz R. Transabdominal versus trascervical and transvaginal multifetal pregnancy reduction: international collaborative experience of more than one thousand cases. Am J Obstet Gynecol 1994; 170:902-9.

37. Evans M, Dommergues M, Wapner RL, Goldberg, Lynch L, Zador MS, Carpenter R, Timor-Tritsch I, Brambati B, Nicolaides K, Dumez Y, Monteagudo A, Jonhson M, Colbus M, Tuhci L, Polak S, Bercowitz R. International collaborative experience of 1789 patients having multrifetal pregnancy reduction: a plateauing of risk and outcome. J Soc Gynecol Invest 1996; 3:23-6.
38. Evans J, Krivchenie EL, Gelber SE, Wapner RJ. Selective reduction. Clin Perinatal 2003; 30:103-11.
39. Stone J, Eddleman K, Lynch L, Bercowitz R. A single center experience with 1000 consecutive cases of multifetal pregnancy reduction. Am J Obstet Gynecol 2002; 187:1163-7.
40. Boulot P, Virgal J, Verges C, et al. Multifetal reduction of triplets to twins a prospective comparison of pregnancy outcome. Hum Reprod 2000; 15:1619-23.
41. Lipitz S, Reichman B, Parel G, et al. The improving outcome of triple pregnancy. Am J Obstet Gynecol 1989; 161:1279-84.
42. Albrecht JL, Tomich RG. The maternal and neonatal outcome of triplet gestation. Am J Obstet Gynecol 1996; 174:1551-6.
43. Lipitz S, Reichman B, Uval J. A prospective comparison of the outcome of triplet pregnancies managed expectantly by multifetal reduction to twins. Am J Obstet Gynecol 1994; 170:874-9.
44. Macones GA, Schemmer G, Pritts E, et al. Multifetal reduction of triples to twins improves perinatal outcome. Am J Obstet Gynecol 1993; 196:982-6.
45. Berkowitz RL, Lynch L, Stone J, Alvarez M. The current status of multiple reduction. Am J Obstet Gynecol 1996; 174: 1265-72.
46. Evans M, Dommergues M, Wapner R, et al. Efficacy of transabdominal multifetal pregnancy reduction: collaborative experience among world´s largest centers. Obst Gynecol 1993; 82:61-6.
47. Lipitz S, Reichman B, Uval J, et al. A prospective comparison of the outcome of triples pregnancy managed expectantly or by multifetal reduction to twin. Am J Obstet Gynecol 1994; 170:874-9.
48. Dommergues M, Nisand I, Mondelbrot L. Embryo reduction in multifetal pregnancies after infertility therapy: obstetrical risks and perinatal benefits are related to operative strategy. Fertility Sterility 1991; 55:805-11.
49. Porreco RP, Burke MS, Hendrix ML. Multifetal reduction of triplets and pregnancy outcome. Obstet Gynecol 1991; 78:335-8.
50. Macones GA, Schemmer G, Pritts E, et al. Multifetal pregnancy reduction of triples to twins improves perinatal outcome. Am J Obstet Gynecol 1994; 169:982-6.
51. Antsaklis A, Drakakis R, Vlazakis G, Michalas S. Reduction of multifetal pregnancies to twins does not increase obstetric or perinatal risks. Hum Reprod 1998; 4:1338-40.
52. Yaron Y, Bryont-Greenwood P, Dave N, Moldenhauer J, Krimer R, Johnson M, Evans M. Multifetal pregnancy reduction of triplets to twins: comparison with non-reduced triplets and twins. Am J Obstet Gynecol 1999; 180:1268-71.
53. Antsaklis A Souka A, Daskalakis G, Papantoniou N, Koutra P, Kavalakis J, Mesogitis S. Embryo reduction versus expectant management in triplet pregnancies. J Mater Fet and Neonat Medic 2004; 16:219-22.
54. Lipitz S, Uval J, Achiron R, Schiff E, Lushy A, Reichman B. Outcome of twin pregnancies reduced from triple compared with non-reduced twin gestations. Obstet Gynecol 1996; 87:511-4.
55. Leondires M, Erust S, Miller B, Scott R. Triplets: outcome of expectant management versus multifetal pregnancy reduction for 127 pregnancies. MA J Obstet Gynecol 2000; 183:454-9.
56. Kadhel PH, Olivennes F, Fernandez H, Nal M, Frydman R. Are there still obstetric and perinatal benefits for selective embryo reduction of triplet pregnancies. Hum Reprod 1998; 13:3555-9.
57. Alexander JM, Hammand KR, Steinkompf MP. Multifetal reduction of high order multifetal pregnancy: comparison of obstetrical outcome with non reduced twin gestation. Fertil Steril 1995; 64:1201-3.
58. Evans M, Hume RF, Yaron Y, Kromer RL, Johnson MD. Multifetal pregnancy reduction. Bailliere´s Clin Obstet Gynecol 1998; 12:147-59.
59. Sebire N, Sherod C, Abbas A, Snijders R, Nikolaides K. Preterm delivery and growth restriction in multifetal pregnancies reduced to twins. Hum Reproduct 1997; 12:173-5.
60. Stone J, Eddlemom K, Gallouses F, Berkowitz R. Pregnancy outcome after first trimester MPR to a single fetus [abstract]. Am J Obstet Gynecol 1998;178:521.
61. Bush M and Eddleman K. Multifetal pregnancy reduction and selective termination. Clin Periantal 2003; 30: 623-41.
62. Tabsh KMA, Theronx NL. Genetic amniocentesis following multifetal pregnancy reduction to twins: assessing the risk. Prenat Diagn 1995; 15:221-3.
63. Antsaklis A, Daskalakis G, Papantoniou N. Genetic amniocentesis in multifetal pregnancy reduced to twins compared with non-reduced twin gestations. Fertil Steril 2000; 74:1051-2.
64. Brambati B, Tului L, Baldi M, et al. Genetic analysis prior to selective fetal reduction in multiple pregnancy. Technical aspects and clinical outcome. Hum Report 1995; 10:818-25.
65. Eddleman KA, Stone JL, Lynch L, Berkowitz R. Chorionic villus sampling before multifetal pregnancy reduction. Am J Obstet Gynecol 2000; 183:1078-81.
66. Monni G, Zoppi MA, Can G, et al. Importance of nuchal translucency measurements in multifetal pregnancy reduction [letter] Ultrasound Obst Gynec 1999; 13:377-8.
67. Wapner R, Davis G, Johnson A, et al. Selective reduction of multifetal reduction of multifetal pregnancies. Lancet 1990; 335:90-3.
68. Antsaklis A, Politis J, Karagiannopoulos C, Kaskarelis D. Selective survival of only the healthy fetus following perinatal diagnosis of thalassemia major in binocular twin gestation. Prenat Diagn 1984; 4:489-96.

69. Boulot P, Hedon B, Pelliccia G, et al. Obstetrical results after embryonic reductions performed on 34 multiple pregnancies. Hum Reprod 1990; 5:1009-13.
70. Evans M, Littmann L, King M, Fletcher JC. Multifetal gestation: the role of multiple pregnancy reduction and selective termination. Am Perinatal 1992; 19:345-56.
71. De Catte L, Camus M, Foulon W: Monochorionic high order multiple pregnancy and multifetal pregnancy reduction. Obstet Gynecol 2002; 100 (3):561-6.
72. Quintero R, Romero R, Reich H, Groucalves L, Johnson M, Carreno C, et al. *In utero* percutaneous umbilical cord ligation in the management of complicated monochorionic multiples gestations. J Ultras Obstet Gynecol 1996; 8:16-22.
73. Aberg A, Mitelman F, Cantz M, Gehler J. A cardiac puncture of fetus with Hurler´s disease avoiding abortion of unaffected co-twin [letter]. Lancet 1978; 2:990-1.
74. Beck L, Terinde R, Daff M. Zwillingsschwangerschaft mit freier Trisomie 21 eines kindes: sectio parra mit Enteferung des kranker und Sparete gebert des gesunden kindes. Geburtsh Fraunheilkd 1980; 40:397.
75. Chitkara U, Berkowitz R, Ivilking IA. Selective second trimester termination of the anomalous fetus in twin pregnancies. Obstet Gyneocol 1989; 73:690-4.
76. Antsaklis A, Drakakis P, Vlazakis G, Michalas S. Selective feticide of an affected fetus in the second trimester has comparable risks to those in the first trimester. Prenat Diagn 2001; 21:135-7.
77. Romero R, Duffy DP, Berkowitz RL, Chang E, Hobbins J. Prolongation of a preterm pregnancy complicated death of a singleton in utero and disseminated intravascular coagulation. N Engl J Med 1984; 310:772-4.
78. Lipitz S, Shalev E, Meizuer I, Yagel S, Weinranb Z, Jaffe A, et al. Late selective termination of fetal abnormalities in twin pregnancies, a multicenter report. Br Obst Gynecol 1996; 103(12):1212-6.
79. Skrablin S, Kuracic I, Fuduric I, Hodzi C. Antenatal fetal demise in multiple gestation: the outcome of surviving fetus at one to four years of age. Eur J Obstet Gynecol 1994; 56:15-9.

CHAPTER

2

Interventional Fetal Cardiology

A Galindo, F Gutiérrez-Larraya
JM Velasco, P de la Fuente

INTRODUCTION

The cardiovascular system begins to develop during the third week and it is not fully developed until the second year of life. During fetal development, two periods—early and late—can be distinguished in the formation of the heart. In the early stage, between weeks 5 and 8, the primitive heart undergoes a process of folding, remodeling, and septation. By the end of the eighth week partitioning is completed, the semilunar valves of both great arteries are differentiated and the fetal heart is formed. After this early period of cardiac organogenesis, another important and more prolonged stage of flow-dependent cardiac morphogenesis begins during which the human heart acquires its final shape, size and function: as a normal forward flow over the course of gestation is required for a normal growth of the cardiac chambers and great arteries, altered pressure and flow relationships may result in significant damage to the developing heart[1]. Although the critical period of heart development is from about day 30 to day 50, in which defects in signaling left their usually irreversibly mark, there are numerous critical events during cardiac development, and deviation from the normal pattern at any one time may produce one or more congenital heart defects (CHDs).

Over the past two decades, fetal echocardiography has emerged as an accurate tool to diagnose and study the evolution of congenital heart disease during fetal life and we are now seeing an attempt to ascertain the impact that prenatal diagnosis has had on the outcomes of fetuses with CHDs. Three are the main benefits offered by prenatal diagnosis: first, by the timely detection of a fetus with CHD, obstetric health care providers often have sufficient time to categorize the disorder fully including the recognition of associated anomalies. Second, prenatal diagnosis can be beneficial to parents and other family members by providing them with time to prepare for the medical, emotional, and socioeconomic consequences of a child with CHD. Third (and most important), the antenatal diagnosis of CHDs has more value since it can have a substantial impact on the management and outcome of an affected pregnancy, including both termination of pregnancy and perinatal management of the affected child. Although, the main impact of diagnosing CHDs prenatally is a decrease in the incidence of live born affected infants due to the high rate of terminations following the diagnosis, fetal echocardiography has impacted on the management strategy for many of these lesions with intrauterine therapy being a real option for some cardiac diseases[2].

It has become clear that some CHDs tend to undergo progression *in utero* and these key observations concerning the natural history of cardiac defects are among the most important points concerning the prenatal diagnosis of CHDs. Several reports have documented how naive is to think that the anatomical and hemodynamical abnormalities are fully established from the beginning.[3-5] Although we are unable to image the heart diagnostically until about 12 to 14 weeks of gestation using modern ultrasound techniques, we can already appreciate the effect that abnormal flow patterns have begun to play in further remodeling valves, their supporting ventricles and great arteries.[6] The more aggressive progression of disease is seen in CHDs with severe semilunar valvar obstructions that may inflict progressive secondary damage to the affected ventricle and associated cardiovascular structures often resulting in hypoplasia of the supporting ventricle, thus precluding biventricular circulation after delivery and significantly increasing postnatal mortality and morbidity.

Currently, standard management of prenatally diagnosed CHDs involves vigilant monitoring of the progression of the cardiac defect. Babies with hypoplastic left heart syndrome (HLHS) or right ventricle hypoplasia have a single ventricle physiology and associated hypoplasia of the great arteries continue to be a challenge in terms of management and survival. Although significant improvements in survival rates have been reported by some centers in recent years, others still have discouraging low results in terms of survival with significant ongoing life long morbidity among survivors.[7] The frustration arising from watching the prenatal progression of severe obstruction of the semilunar valves well before fetal maturity has prompted the interest in exploring the feasibility of fetal cardiac intervention. The prenatal modification of the natural course of these heart diseases might reduce the severity of secondary cardiovascular injury and, if this goal is achieved, postnatally reconstructive (rather than palliative) surgical procedures would be possible. Fetal cardiac interventions have been anticipated for many years but only recently have been developed for palliation of CHDs *in utero*. From the pioneering interventions in early 1990s,[8,9] several groups have attempted fetal cardiac interventions worldwide with limited technical success.[10] These catheter interventions in the human fetus have not consistently led to modification of prenatally detected CHDs or improved outcomes. However, balloon valvuloplasties of severe stenosis of semilunar valves have been affirmed to be conceptually valid and therefore deserving of further investigation. Accordingly, several large centers most of them in western countries are currently offering *in utero* these procedures although the accumulated experience until date is not enough to provide a conclusive efficacy figure. These fetal cardiac interventions must be included within the spectrum of fetal interventions and should not be considered as an extension of invasive pediatric cardiology nor even a viable alternative to conventional neonatal repair. However, as with all fetal interventions, there is a need for teamwork with involvement of a pediatric cardiologist as a key figure in this process.[11,12]

There are a variety of cardiac defects that can be considered to be candidates for fetal intervention. To date, the predominant defects include severe aortic stenosis with evolving HLHS, critical stenosis or atresia of the pulmonary valve with intact ventricular septum (PS-PA/IVS) with evolving hypoplastic right ventricle or heart failure and HLHS with intact or restrictive atrial septum and thus impaired pulmonary venous return. In all these cases, early diagnosis and referral of patients who are to be considered for a fetal intervention procedure is imperative. Fetal cardiac intervention includes the process of identifying fetuses who are candidates for such a procedure and taking the steps to make treatment available to them. However, in many cases the procedures offered are later refused by the parents. Therefore, records of clinical experience in fetal cardiac intervention should include all those cases in which there was an intention to treat and not only those fetuses that are finally intervened. Paramount importance in the selection process as well as in peri-interventional fetal monitoring and during the procedure itself have the ultrasound techniques as they are the primary diagnostic and monitoring modalities in fetal cardiology.

Several issues will be discussed in this chapter: the rationale for fetal cardiac intervention, the criteria for patient selection and the technical aspects of intervention including current limitations and shortcomings, the defects that are suitable for these procedures, the available evidence about their results and finally, the future perspectives in the technology of intervention of the fetal heart.

RATIONALE FOR FETAL CARDIAC INTERVENTION

Most CHDs can now be repaired successfully in the postnatal period with excellent results in terms both of mortality and long-term outcome. Therefore, for these defects there would be no need for fetal intervention. Moreover, minimally invasive procedures have been strongly developed in recent years with postnatal balloon aortic valvuloplasty becoming the procedure of choice for children of all ages with congenital valvar aortic stenosis in many centers.[13,14] However, for other CHDs, often representing the more severe form of the defect, only palliative repair could be offered in the postnatal period and these surgical strategies are associated with high mortality with many of these patients also showing life-long morbidity.[7] It is also important to emphasize that most fetuses with CHDs considered suitable for *in utero* intervention will survive until term gestation and therefore these techniques must not be interpreted as life-saving procedures. Moreover, it must also be kept in mind that cardiac interventions in the prenatal period might be not only technically unsuccessful but also followed by fetal intrauterine death or other obstetric complications leading to a very preterm delivery with its associated complications for the patient. The ultimate aim of fetal cardiac intervention is to improve postnatal surgical options and overall prognosis. Although more procedures will most likely be required postnatally, fetal cardiac intervention may ameliorate the natural history of the cardiac defect to such an extent that catheter interventions of reconstructive biventricular instead of palliative univentricular surgical procedures become possible. However, even with technically successful fetal cardiac interventions, the ultimate success will be determined by the long-term outcome after biventricular surgical repair in comparison with currently available postnatal procedures.[15]

As for many other *in utero* invasive procedures, the risks of fetal cardiac intervention must be weighed against the potential benefits offered by the technique. Moreover, the healthy mother is involved in the procedure, as in all fetal interventions, and is in an extremely vulnerable position. The following items must be taken into account systematically before any fetal cardiac intervention:

- The cardiac defect should have an unsatisfactory postnatal outcome with high mortality and significant morbidity
- The proposed procedure should be intended to significantly modify the defect and thereby improve the outcome
- The cardiac defect should be identified and intervention undertaken at a fetal age sufficiently early to alter the course of hemodynamic changes, and before the development of irreversible ventricular damage. When the fetal myocardium is severely damaged by the time of initial diagnosis the results will be poor even if fetal intervention is attempted
- There must be a technically feasible *in utero* therapeutic option available with little or no collateral tissue damage
- The mother would not be put at undue risk by the procedure.

In terms of modifying disease there are several CHDs that in theory could benefit from *in utero* therapy because current postnatal options are suboptimal. The evolving nature of these CHDs continues to have significant morbidity and mortality in the early postnatal period and therefore there seems to be good clinical reasons to further attempt prenatal cardiac interventions to improve these conditions.[3,4,7,16-18] Significant progression may be defined as secondary damage to the heart and lungs, resulting from abnormalities of growth and flow, to an extent that biventricular circulation is no longer possible after delivery. In this setting, the primary aim of prenatal intervention would be to reverse the pathological process to preserve cardiac and lung structure and function, thereby improving postnatal course. A secondary objective might be to modify the severity of the disease to enhance postnatal surgical outcomes.

As a normal forward flow over the course of gestation is required for a normal growth of the cardiac chambers and great arteries, altered pressure and flow relationships that accompany severe semilunar valvar stenosis may result in significant secondary damage to the developing heart, including hypoplasia of the supporting ventricle and thus precluding its use in the postnatal period. These types of defects include aortic or mitral valve stenosis and critical PS-PA/IVS. Subnormal growth of the left ventricle with advancing gestation can be seen in fetuses with severe mitral or aortic valve stenosis, so that, by term, the left ventricle and aorta may be severily hypoplastic.[4,17] In such cases, the left heart structures may be incapable of supporting the systemic circulation and management will be akin to other forms of HLHS.[16,19,20] This evolution implies a significant change in prognosis as defects that rely on univentricular repair have the worst outcomes. Similarly, abnormal anterograde flow during pregnancy through the pulmonary valve is responsible for the progressive obstruction at the level of infundibulum and pulmonary valve and the progressive arrest of the pulmonary artery growth and its branches, leading even to pulmonary atresia.[3,21] Severe pulmonary valve stenosis or atresia as a primary lesion has also the potential to retard the growth of the right ventricle leading to hypoplastic right heart syndrome during gestation or other flow abnormalities, such as tricuspid regurgitation and large ventriculo-coronary connections, therefore complicating postnatal management and worsening outcome.[22] It has also been proven that a restrictive foramen ovale in the setting of HLHS, with secondary left atrial hypertension is one of the most critical factors that has an impact on the outcome of HLHS for both staged reconstruction and heart transplantation. These neonates develop profound cyanosis and pulmonary edema immediately after delivery with standard resuscitative measures often being unsuccessful.[18] This may be due in part to associated intrapulmonary anatomic abnormalities, with "arterialization" of the pulmonary veins and lymphatic dilation, which have been attributed to left atrial hypertension *in utero*.[23] Therefore, decompression of the fetal left atrium by creating an atrial septal defect seems to be the best way to improve the outcome of these patients.[24]

The main arguments to support the performance of fetal cardiac interventions are based upon the following concepts: first, the restoration of normal flow promotes growth, and reduction in ventricular pressure enables more normal development and function, minimizing secondary damage. Second, biventricular circulation provides a better quality of life than univentricular circulation.

Concerning the first concept, the measurement of valve and ventricular dimensions in fetuses with valvular obstruction demonstrates that cardiac growth falls below normal charts.[20] Moreover, there is evidence that postnatal restoration of forward flow in the neonate by valvuloplasty restores the original growth potential. Although postnatal studies documenting ventricular growth after aortic and pulmonary valvuloplasty differ in their conclusions, in the majority normalization both of the dimensions of the affected structures and hemodynamics has been observed. A large retrospective study of 113 patients with critical aortic stenosis who underwent balloon aortic valvuloplasty in the first two months of life with 91 early survivors with two-ventricle circulation showed that in almost all patients with a baseline aortic annulus Z score less than 1, the annulus diameter increased to within the normal range within 1 to 2 years. Similarly, left ventricular end-diastolic dimension Z scores, which ranged from 5 to 7.5 before valvuloplasty, normalized within 1 to 2 years in nearly all patients with a predilation Z score less than 1.[14] This is also in agreement with another series where seven of nine surviving patients with PS-PA/IVS showed right ventricular length within the normal range 5 years after a surgical procedure to establish a right ventricular to pulmonary artery communication in the neonatal period.[25] These studies are partially in contrast to one that documented no significant change of the tricuspid valve Z score or right ventricular length Z score with time (mean follow-up time 28 ± 24 months) following neonatal balloon valvuloplasty for PS-PA/IVS; however, despite apparently inadequate right ventricle size, a biventricular circulation was achievable in many patients, suggesting that a "normal"-sized right heart is not required to maintain, at least at rest, a normal pulmonary blood flow after the normalization of intracardiac pressures post-valvuloplasty.[26] Selection bias (measurements of cardiac growth performed in patients with biventricular circulation and excluding those cases with a worst anatomy) may also contribute to explain these partially conflicting results. Unfortunately, there is still little evidence that valvuloplasty in the fetus restores the original growth potential as seen after postnatal procedures. However, in the largest series published to date of balloon dilation of severe aortic stenosis in the fetus, ongoing left-heart growth was documented by multidimensional measurements of the left ventricle in fetuses with technically successful procedures while in cases technically unsuccessful and in those who declined development of HLHS was noted in follow-up.[27]

It is well known that severe semilunar valvar stenosis may provoke significant secondary damage in the fetal heart. One important mechanism of ventricular damage results from the impairment of coronary perfusion to the myocardium. The endocardial fibroelastosis commonly seen in fetuses with critical aortic stenosis is multifactorial and may be attributed to the reduced coronary perfusion secondary to elevation of ventricular end-diastolic pressure, the myocardial perfusion with desaturated blood coming from the arterial duct and the high intraventricular pressure itself.[12] Doppler echocardiography has recently been used in the assessment of coronary flow dynamics before and after balloon valvuloplasty in neonates with critical aortic stenosis and an increase in coronary flow volume/left ventricular mass ratio after the procedure, suggesting the improvement of myocardial blood perfusion.[28] As it has been mentioned before, pulmonary vascular development is also affected by increased left atrial pressure associated with progressive aortic valve stenosis and closure of the foramen ovale in HLHS and transposition of great arteries (TGA). This results in an increase in vascular smooth muscle and vessel number, and hence elevated pulmonary vascular resistance. In a series of 33 neonates with HLHS and intact or restrictive atrial septum who underwent transcatheter atrial septostomy in the first two days of life, the pulmonary vascular resistance and pulmonary arterial pressure were normal in the group of patients who survived the neonatal period and underwent subsequent bidirectional Glenn and Fontan operations. These patients had degrees of left atrial hypertension similar to that of patients who died in the neonatal period. From a clinical point of view this suggests that the damage to the pulmonary vasculature in the setting of pulmonary venous hypertension *in utero* may be reversible over time, although the reversibility of the histopathological pulmonary vascular changes observed in patients with HLHS and left atrial hypertension have not been still fully documented.[18] Ultrasound-guided fetal atrial septoplasty to create an interatrial communication is feasible with a high rate of technical success. Unfortunately, no positive clinical impact has been still demonstrated to date with this procedure.[24] Moreover, fetal PS-PA/IVS with restrictive foramen ovale can lead to hydrops fetalis. In this setting, fetal pulmonary valvuloplasty could be life saving.[29] The reversibility of prehydropic features in these fetuses such as cardiomegaly, pericardial effusion, holosystolic tricuspid regurgitation and/or abnormal venous Doppler has been reported in several case reports.[30,31]

The second important concept is that biventricular circulation provides a better quality of life than a univentricular circulation. Assessment of quality of life includes more than the superior functional ability and cognitive development associated with a biventricular circulation. Over the past two decades, advances in congenital heart surgery, pediatric cardiology, and intensive care medicine have dramatically increased the survival of infants with single-ventricle physiology. Despite these improvements, significant morbidity remains after the Fontan completion, including myocardial systolic and diastolic dysfunction, systemic arterial and venous hemodynamic abnormalities, diminished exercise capacity, arrhythmias, protein-losing enteropathy, somatic growth retardation, neo-aortic valve root dilation and insufficiency, thromboembolic complications, and below-average cognitive development. However, emerging data indicate that these neurocognitive difficulties are not only attributable to the consecutive operations performed in these patients and that may be influenced by other factors such as associated structural abnormalities of the brain, the intrinsic hemodynamic abnormality of the cardiac defect itself or even a genetic predisposition of the patient to neurological injury.[7,32] Fetal intervention has been shown to restore forward flow through the aortic arch in cases of critical aortic stenosis, and thus may improve the delivery of blood flow to the cerebral circulation. This may theoretically reduce the risk of neurological damage associated with major cardiac defects.

The early experience of cardiac interventions was poor with few survivors. More recent experience has thus far been more encouraging and advances have clearly been made, particularly in the field of interdisciplinary cooperation for an adequate planning and performance of the intervention. Although the hypotheses mentioned above to justify fetal cardiac interventions are physiologically sound, there is currently little practical evidence that relieving semilunar valve stenosis or performing an atrial septostomy in the fetus will halt or reverse the evolution of the heart disease. Although *in utero* aortic and pulmonary valvuloplasties have been attempted for more than a decade, these attempts have been frequently affected by limited technical success, variable patient selection and timing of procedure. Indeed, the results of attempted intrauterine transcatheter techniques have been poor so far with no increase in ejection fraction post-procedure and only a little change in left ventricular end-diastolic volume. To date, few successful therapeutic cardiac interventions have been performed world wide. Many of the procedures reported in the literature were performed in the third trimester, which was possibly too late in gestation to modify the natural course of the disease. Therefore, it has been noticed that fetal cardiac interventions will likely have to be performed earlier in gestation to have its desired effect. Performing such a challenging procedure in the smaller fetus might not only be more difficult, but it might spur the development of the equipment specifically designed for this purpose. The significance of early detection of CHDs suitable for fetal interventions applies particularly to aortic or pulmonary valve stenosis, in which there is likely a window of opportunity (probably around 20 weeks) when the ventricular growth can be normalized.[29]

PATIENT SELECTION, LIMITATIONS AND INACCURACIES

Current prenatal detection of CHDs is based upon mostly in two-dimensional ultrasound for anatomical features and complemented with Doppler and M-mode capabilities for functional evaluation. In spite of technological improvements, fetal echocardiography is a diagnostic tool with its own limitations to be added to those other clinical factors affecting the sonologists ability to achieve a successful imaging. These affect not only the examination of the fetal heart but the whole fetal anatomy. If the high rate of associated extracardiac anomalies that accompany CHDs in fetal life and the difficulties for their detection are taken into account, the difficulties to give prognostic information to the parents that might not only depend on the CHDs will be clearly understand. Despite recent advances, prenatal detection and accuracy of diagnosis still remain problematic. Paramount in the approach to the fetus with CHD is the multidisciplinary team with involvement of a pediatric cardiologist to improve diagnostic accuracy and allow the parents to obtain the most accurate counseling about the defect, including the likely course and treatment. As mentioned above, some cardiac lesions may evolve during pregnancy and therefore clarification of the fetal cardiac findings and outcome may not be possible until late gestation or even the postnatal period. Although the team approach broadens the competence in parental counseling, these diagnostic inaccuracies notably affect the prognostic information given to the parents that in some cardiac conditions will be accompanied, in some degree, by uncertainty. The uncertain prognosis for these prenatally diagnosed lesions should be explained to the parents as early as possible to ensure that they are in a position to make a fully informed decision about management of the defect. Their options will depend on the gestational age at diagnosis and the presence or absence of other fetal anomalies with most of the parents opting for termination of pregnancy or supportive postnatal care when a cardiac lesion which may progress in severity and might require a postnatal surgical univentricular palliation is detected antenatally.[2]

In general, the prenatal diagnostic accuracy improves with the severity of the CHD.[33] However, it must be emphasized that although the prenatal diagnosis of the specific defect may be partially incorrect, neither the prognosis nor the patient care are significantly affected as the prenatal precise detection of the main defect allows an accurate estimation of the severity in most cases. Agreement rate between prenatal and postnatal findings ranges widely, showing those in which a pediatric cardiologist is involved in the prenatal diagnosis of CHDs better diagnostic accuracies.[33,34]

These difficulties are remarked when the sonographers or pediatric cardiologists are asked to assess the adequacy of ventricular size and function with a view to future suitability for bi- or univentricular repair in some forms of CHDs. Reliable antenatal predictive criteria for critically progressive CHD to further justify fetal cardiac intervention are an essential part of the decision to proceed with *in utero* valve dilation and still have to be defined. A possible definition of critically progressive disease is that necessitating univentricular surgical palliation or causing death in the first months of life. However, these features may not be obvious in the first half of pregnancy, mainly because the process of arrest of growth of the cardiac chambers and/or great vessels is not significant enough to be detected, and becomes discernible only in late gestation and, therefore, making prognostication early in pregnancy extremely difficult. So, to give an accurate prognosis, sequential studies every 4 to 6 weeks until delivery are required whenever a CHD is detected to monitor for ventricular dysfunction, valvular regurgitation, and the growth rate of the structures affected by abnormal forward flow. This monitoring may be made most easily using a combination of morphological and physiological parameters. There are a few studies that document the natural history of cardiac growth for some fetal malformations providing helpful information on growth of valves and ventricles throughout gestation.[3,4,16,17,19] CHDs in the fetus are associated with abnormalities of flow through the atrioventricular and semilunar valves, reversal of flow in the arterial duct and aortic isthmus, and abnormalities of flow both in the ductus venosus and in the pulmonary veins. Reversal of flow with atrial contraction in venous duct waveforms may be seen as a result of increased right atrial pressure when atrioventricular regurgitation is severe or the foramen ovale is restrictive.[29] Serial studies of pulmonary venous Doppler are useful to assess left atrial pressure where there is a restrictive interatrial septum. Abnormal waveform patterns, characterized by reversal of flow in late diastole, may be seen in association with HLHS or critical aortic stenosis due to raised left atrial pressure.[35] This complication may also arise in fetuses with simple TGA and therefore serial Doppler evaluation of the pulmonary venous and foramen ovale flows is mandatory for early detection of those patients at risk to develop pulmonary venous congestion and hemorrhage.[24] Chronic elevation of ventricular pressure in the setting of severe semilunar valvar stenosis may damage the fetal myocardium with biventricular repair being an unsuitable option due to poor ventricular performance.[36] Fetuses with both mitral and aortic atresia usually have severe disease at presentation and they are not candidates for fetal intervention. In some cases, the size of the ventricular chamber may be within normal limits but with well-established endocardial fibroelastosis, impairing contractile and relaxation properties of the fetal heart. In this setting it is unlikely to obtain a major benefit from prenatal intervention. Antenatal intervention has been performed for aortic valve stenosis/atresia, pulmonary valve stenosis/atresia and defects associated with restriction or closure of the interatrial septum. Therefore, the number of fetuses suitable for intervention is not too large. Critical pulmonary and aortic stenosis or atresia will each affect 4 to 5% of fetuses with CHDs[37] and the incidence of intact atrial septum in the setting of HLHS has been estimated at 6%.[23,24]

In order to describe the severity of the cardiovascular compromise following a systemic way, Huhta et al[38] have proposed the use of the cardiovascular profile score to describe the state of fetal wellness. This assessment tool includes the Doppler evaluation of the umbilical vein, ductus venosus and umbilical artery, the measurement of the heart size and the cardiac function evaluating both systolic and diastolic properties. These authors firmly believe that following this evaluation the fetus can be treated before the onset of hydrops fetalis and permanent organ injury.

The underlying anatomy, and not only the progression of the disease itself, may also play a key role in the poor outcome showed by some fetuses. Critical PS-PA/IVS can also lead to a progressive underdevelopment of the right ventricle. The severity of this condition and the degree of right ventricle hypoplasia are mainly dependent on the time of onset of the anatomical defect. Moreover, the anomalies of the coronary arteries frequently associated to this lesion complicate treatment even further as decompression of the ventricle via the fistula in fetal life probably contributes to the reduced growth of the tricuspid valve. In cases of severe semilunar valvar stenosis, the valves are often poorly developed, and unicommisural valves are reported in about one-third of neonates requiring balloon valvuloplasty for critical aortic stenosis.[12]

Concerning extracardiac abnormalities, counseling may be difficult, particularly in early gestation or when the imaging is suboptimal. Some major malformations or genetic syndromes may only become apparent later in gestation or even in the postnatal period, and these conditions may have a significant impact on postnatal outcome. Moreover, the information given to the parents regarding the current results in the management of the specific cardiac defects may not be based solely in postnatal series, where the majority of the patients included have not been diagnosed in fetal life. It is well known that the more complex and severe defects, with the more dramatic anomalies of the intracardiac structure, predominate in fetal life. Therefore, it is more appropriate to counsel parents based on the series that document the outcome of all, including those detected prenatally, many of whom do not reach the surgeon. The results reported in these series are often much less optimistic.[2,39]

TECHNIQUES FOR FETAL CARDIAC INTERVENTION

With the application of the balloon catheter dilatation procedures to the fetus, the unique circumstances of approaching one patient through another individual must be considered. The complexity of the procedure makes necessary the multidisciplinary approach, including obstetrician, perinatologist, fetal cardiologist, and surgeon. The techniques for fetal cardiac intervention vary slightly from group to group and most have been performed by percutaneous direct approaches under ultrasound guidance. Mini-laparotomy is rarely needed although in cases with poor imaging quality due to maternal habitus the direct application of the transducer on the uterine wall may optimize the intervention. Obviously, the procedures should be performed by an experienced team both in fetal cardiology and intrauterine interventions, and therefore capable of dealing with any emergency situation that might threaten the life of the mother or fetus.[40]

All the procedures to date have been performed in the second half of pregnancy, ranging from 20 to 34 weeks.[10,15,24,27,30,31,41] To perform these procedures, direct insertion of a needle through the maternal abdomen into the uterus and from there through the fetal chest wall into the cardiac region of interest is monitored by two-dimensional ultrasound imaging (Figure 2.1). Following the appropriate intracardiac positioning of the needle, interventional devices (floppy-tipped guide wire, balloon coronary catheter) are introduced and advanced through the needle shaft towards the affected structure with the balloon centered over the stenotic lesion. Usually one to three inflations are done to assure that the stenotic lesion is appropriately enlarged. The needle needs to be at least 15 cm long, with or without sharpening at the end and with a flexible sheath that can be left in the fetal heart while the balloon is fed through it over a wire, allowing the repositioning if the needle becomes dislodged. A variety of needle sizes have been used ranging from 16- to 20-gauge depending on the size and profile of the balloons used. The guide wire is usually 0.014-inch. Currently a balloon diameter to valve diameter ratio of 1.2 is used. With the increasing operator experience there is a tendency toward the use of larger balloons in order to avoid restenosis of the fetal valve in spite of promoting valve regurgitation. However, it has been observed that within weeks this valve regurgitation regresses and often disappears.[29] The major technical limitations associated with the direct transthoracic approach may be summarized in two points; first, in approximately 50% of the cases is impossible to achieve correct alignment of the device with the outflow tract once the needle has been inserted directly in the fetal heart. Second, the echocardiographic guidance of the device is difficult due to the diffraction of the ultrasound beam secondary to the presence of the needle.[27] To avoid the risks associated to a poor image control of the devices, it should be important to premeasure and mark the cannula, guide wires, and balloon shafts before the introduction in the fetal heart so that positioning within the heart is known.

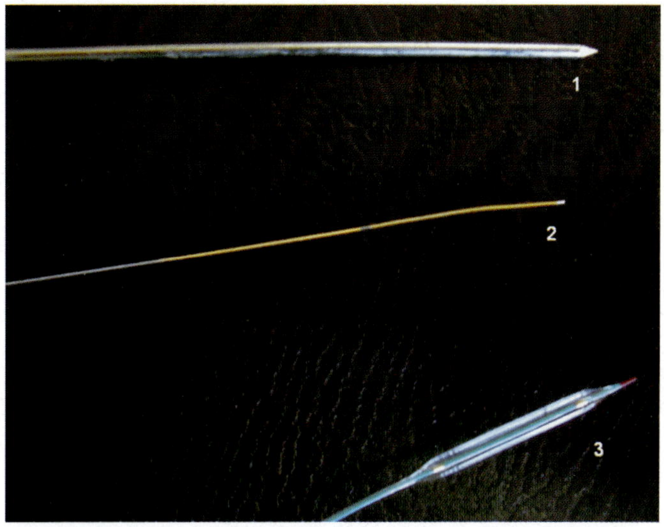

Figure 2.1: Basic material necessary for fetal cardiac intervention. 1. An 18-gauge needle with a stylet, without sharpening end. 2. A 0.014 coronary guide wire. 3. A 15 mm long and 3.5 mm diameter balloon

A brief and self-limited episode of bradycardia is commonly observed during the procedure. However, either epinephrine or atropine should be available for immediate intramuscular or intracardiac injection in the setting of sustained fetal bradycardia. Following the intervention and after verifying the improvement in the antegrade flow through the stenotic valve, both needle and wire are withdrawn and if hemopericardium is observed it may then be aspirated. Even during realtime imaging the differentiation between needle shaft and catheter is extremely difficult and this may result in balloon rupture as the balloon is torn by the edges of the catheter shaft during inflation.[15] This balloon rupture was a complication observed in up to 50% of the earliest procedures.[10] One group has used both ultrasound and fetoscopy to perform aortic valvuloplasty[42] and laser to perform an atrial septostomy.[41]

For the success of these interventions, adequate fetal position and excellent imaging quality are of paramount importance. The fetus should lie in dorso-posterior position and with no limbs between the uterine wall and the chest. For an adequate guidance of the course of the needle toward the fetal chest wall is also of importance to have an adequate amount of amniotic fluid between the uterine wall and the fetus. The fetus receives anesthesia by way of the placenta but, once the fetus lies in the appropriate position, additional intramuscular injection of nondepolarizing muscle relaxants together with analgesics and atropine under ultrasound guidance may help maintain the desired fetal lie, suppress fetal stress responses and reflex movements that may result in bleeding complications or dislodging of interventional devices. These agents have also been given directly into the fetal heart at the time of cardiac puncture. Currently, the majority of the procedures are performed under local anesthetics together with sedation and administration of opioid analgesics (fentanyl). However, some procedures have been performed under general anesthesia, in order to provide more uterine relaxation, thus allowing manipulation of the fetus into a favorable position. This increases the length of the procedures considerably and multiplies the risk to both mother and fetus.[10-12,15,27,43]

Concerning the timing of the intervention, it is desirable the performance soon after the diagnosis and the appropriate selection of the suitable cases have been made in order to avoid significant secondary damage in the fetal myocardium. However, it is important to provide an adequate amount of time to the parents for counseling and decision making. The limited clinical experience with which any of these procedures have been performed, the lack of appropriately tested devices for fetal cardiac intervention, and the selection of the worst cases have been contributing factors to the limited success observed to date with significant fetal morbidity and mortality.[43]

Following valvuloplasty, the fetus will likely require as much time as possible *in utero* for the ventricle to recover, thus any procedure that would substantially increase the likelihood of premature delivery would be counterproductive. The mother must be monitored closely for clinical and ultrasound evidence of placental abruption, intra-abdominal bleeding, or amniotic fluid leakage. Premature rupture of the membranes is likely to occur in up to 7% of the procedures. Fetal wellbeing should also be monitorized as well as the improvement in the antegrade flow through the stenotic valve and the associated hemodynamical status including significant pericardial effusions, valve regurgitation and/or fetal hydrops. Restenosis of the valve is a real option and this must be carefully monitored throughout pregnancy. Once this complication is detected, the management should be based on the same principles that guided the original procedure and will depend in last instance on gestational age at which it occurs.[10-12,15,43]

The development of open and fetoscopic techniques for fetal cardiac surgery has the potential to improve the technical success rate of fetal valvuloplasties and other cardiac procedures not amenable to percutaneous ultrasound-guided approaches. However, the most invasive technique, as used in open fetal surgery, includes a uterine incision and fetal exposure. The fetal heart can then be accessed with traditional techniques (femoral, umbilical cord, carotid artery); but, once a uterine incision is made, maternal morbidity increases significantly and premature delivery is likely. Therefore, this approach has been performed only rarely in humans and it is not currently recommended for fetal cardiac intervention.[15] Adopting techniques from endoscopic surgery, Kohl et al[15,44,45] have developed innovative techniques in animals using fetoscopy and umbilical cord access to perform balloon valvuloplasty in fetal lambs. Fetoscopic fetal cardiac surgery is achieved by percutaneous intra-amniotic placement of endoscopic cannula guided by transesophageal or intra-amniotic fetal echocardiography, which improves the imaging of the balloon catheter inside the heart. During fetal cardiac procedures, conventional maternal transabdominal fetal echocardiography is precluded because it interferes with the operative approach or may not be possible after gaseous insufflation of the amniotic cavity. Ultrasound catheters advanced within the esophagus permit accurate definition of fetal cardiac anatomy. These catheters have a shaft diameter ranging from 6.5 to 19 French and can be inserted in human fetuses from 20 weeks onwards. These transducers lack Doppler capabilities and, therefore, assessment of fetal hemodynamics during intervention is made indirectly by means of changes in cardiac size and foramen ovale patency. The decreased depth penetration and the lack of Doppler information limit the application of these ultrasound systems but these limitations may be overcome in the future by intravascular ultrasound technology.

Critical Aortic Stenosis

Critical aortic stenosis (AS) has a high mortality whether treated by surgery or valvuloplasty in spite of current technical advances.[20,40] With the severe obstruction to blood flow across the aortic valve, the infant is frequently unstable with progressive, and often intractable, congestive heart failure and metabolic acidosis shortly following birth, resulting in death without aggressive early intervention. Even with intervention, the left ventricle often fails to maintain an adequate output, related to the degree of ventricular dysfunction and associated endocardial fibroelastosis.[40] Valvulotomy of any type is a palliative procedure and reintervention remains frequent; in the neonatal group with critical or severe aortic stenosis only 29% of patients survive to 14.4 years without intervention and only 35% surviving without a second procedure.[46] It is due to the progressive underdevelopment of the left ventricle *in utero* secondary to fetal blood flow diversion or the unability of this ventricle to support systemic circulation even after relief of valvular obstruction, ultimately resulting in HLHS. Even with current technology and strategies, mid- and long-term results of HLHS surgery are discouraging;[47] after successful palliative surgeries, the child with HLHS is left with single ventricle circulation. This supports the interest of the concept of intrauterine valvuloplasty to prevent unfavorable left ventricle maturation or development.

Currently neonatal balloon aortic valvuloplasty is the procedure of choice in most cardiological centers. After prenatal diagnosis immediate delivery and postnatal surgical or transcatheter intervention are not a real option because of the low birth weight, immaturity and poor ventricular function; surgical relief of severe aortic stenosis has to be performed on cardiopulmonary bypass and inherits a high risk below 1600 gm bodyweight; transcatheter balloon dilatation below 2000 gm also involves a high risk and the results are questionable.[48]

In some mid-gestation fetuses with severe AS, the size of the left ventricle is normal or even dilated but as gestation progresses the left heart growth is retarded (Figure 2.2). In this group of fetuses primary left outflow tract obstruction results in progressive ventricle compromise throughout gestation with second-trimester ultrasonography revealing the obstructed outflow and dysfunctional contractility of the left ventricle wall. As has been mentioned above, one important mechanism of ventricular damage results from the effect of reduced coronary perfusion to myocardium: fetuses with critical aortic stenosis and HLHS have reduced or no forward flow through the aortic root and the coronary perfusion predominantly depends on the relatively desaturated retrograde flow from the arterial duct. In the fetus, 75% of the resistance to coronary flow is due to intraventricular pressure, with the remaining 25% due to myocardial contraction and tissue pressure. As such, elevation of ventricular end-diastolic pressure associated with aortic stenosis is a potent determinant for fibrosis development.[12] Myocardial response to aortic valve closure includes division and hypertrophy with redistribution of cytoskeletal and stress protein expression; pressure load upregulates the angiotensin-converting enzyme gen and transforming growth factor beta-1, both of which are potent regulators of fibrosis and have close correlation with myocyte degeneration.[49]

It is essential to identify those fetuses who will be candidates to intrauterine palliation: AS must be the dominant lesion, the left ventricle length should not be <2 SD of normal for gestational age, and Doppler blood flow patterns should demonstrate left to right shunt across the atrial septum and retrograde flow in the transverse aortic arch. Doppler-derived gradients across the stenotic valve in the fetus can be misleading, and a low gradient in the face of a stenotic valve can be a sign of poor ventricular function. Moreover, the measured gradient can be affected by the competitive retrograde flow in the

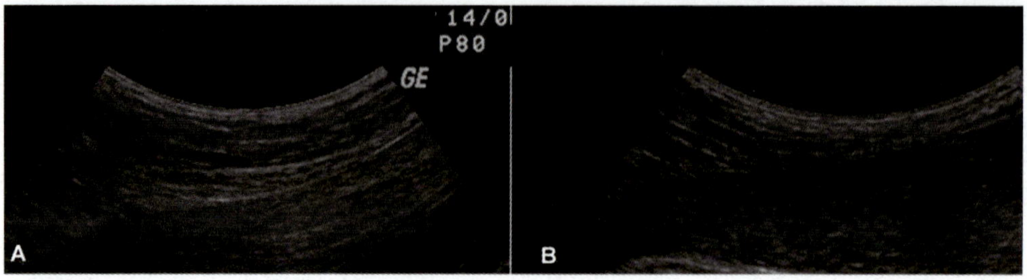

Figures 2.2A and B: A. Four-chamber cardiac image in a fetus with a suitable left ventricle in the setting of aortic stenosis. B. Hypoplastic left ventricle unsuitable for biventricular surgical repair. RV, right ventricle; LV, left ventricle; RA, right atrium; LA, left atrium

aortic arch supplied by the arterial duct. It has been suggested that if a high aortic velocity is observed in the last 10 weeks of gestation there would be enough residual left ventricular function to wait until birth for treatment.[9]

It has been observed that when the transition from a normal-sized left ventricle to HLHS in fetuses with AS can be documented, it almost always occurs in the second or early third trimester. Therefore, interventional tools and techniques should be performed earlier than previously reported, probably before 28 weeks.[27] Most of the fetal aortic valvuloplasties have been performed by maternal transabdominal puncture with an 18 G or 19 G 11.5 cm long needle gaining the left ventricle across the anterior fetal left thoracic wall, then the stilet is removed and a 0.014 steerable guide wire is passed into the left ventricle and advanced across the aortic valve; a convenient first balloon catheter chosen to keep a balloon to aortic annulus diameters ratio around 0.9 is passed over the wire and advanced into the valve ring an the balloon is then inflated. This technique is very similar to the surgical technique described several years ago.[50]

The aim of valvuloplasty in AS is to prevent HLHS but today it still has not been consistently documented that a successful *in utero* technique would restore adequate flow to permit left heart growth *in utero*. First reports of fetal cardiac intervention for severe AS appeared in 1991[8] and a multiinstitutional report of 12 cases was published in 2000,[10] but in 2004 only 2 of these 12 babies were alive and the only one survivor with a two-ventricle circulation had intervention near term (33 weeks) and had a marked enlarged left ventricle at that time, making it unlikely that this fetus would have progressed from severe AS to HLHS; all the procedures were performed in the third trimester. In 2004 Tworetzky et al[27] published the results of their prospective protocol began in 2000: after offering the alternative of fetal cardiac intervention to 24 selected mothers with severe fetal AS and with the left heart potentially salvageable and judged to progress to HLHS if left untreated, they finally performed 20 *in utero* valvuloplasties (10 percutaneously through maternal abdominal wall and 10 via a minilaparotomy) at a mean gestational age of 23.9 +/–2.3 weeks. Technical success (defined by ultrasound visualization of balloon insufflation across the aortic annulus and increase in postdilation aortic valve flow) was achieved in 14 of the 20 fetuses. Three had two-ventricle physiologies at 1 month of age, and two additional infants underwent surgical repair but have maintained two-ventricle circulation; two fetuses were lost postprocedure and the remaining seven fetuses developed HLHS; of the six fetuses with technically unsuccesful interventions, and in those who declined, serial echocardiograms noted arrest of left ventricle growth and development of HLHS.[51] These authors conclude that successful aortic valve dilation prevents left heart growth arrest, and may result in normal ventricular anatomy and function at birth.

Pulmonary Atresia/Critical Pulmonary Stenosis

Critical PS-PA/IVS is an uncommon condition accounting for about 1 to 3% of all CHDs in pediatric series. On the other hand, its incidence in fetal life is higher, with figures close to 5%.[52] Similar to the underdevelopment of the left ventricle with severe aortic valvular stenosis, the natural history of critical pulmonary valvular stenosis can lead to a progressive underdevelopment of the right ventricle, tricuspid valve, right ventricular outflow tract, and pulmonary artery.[53] The severity of this condition, the degree of right ventricle hypoplasia and its hemodynamic disturbances are mainly dependent on the time of onset of the anatomical defect. Tricuspid regurgitation is a common feature in fetuses with this cardiac defect. It is usually severe and constitutes one of the main hemodynamical disturbances making it unique from other right heart obstructive diseases (i.e. tricuspid atresia).

Different treatment strategies are available within a wide anatomic and clinical spectrum, with the ultimate aim being the achievement of biventricular circulation. This can be achieved in milder cases through early intervention with balloon valvuloplasty and surgical palliation at birth. However, the presence of a significantly hypoplastic right ventricle at birth adversely affects the results obtained by valvuloplasty. Moreover, the anomalies of the coronary arteries frequently associated to this lesion resulting from the persistence of embryonic sinusoids complicate treatment even further as right ventricle decompression can lead to fatal coronary artery insufficiency. These severe forms of the defect will require single ventricle palliation. As a consequence, the overall mortality in live born infants with this defect is close to 50% with well-documented prenatal deaths. These may explain the different levels of incidence reported in pre and postnatal series. Moreover, only one-third of survivors had a biventricular circulation.[54]

Current development of diagnostic tools in fetal echocardiography, invasive procedures and interventional cardiac technology make it possible to offer, in selected cases, an intrauterine approach to improve their natural history, aimed at achieving biventricular circulation. The outlet portion of the right ventricle may have thin membranous atresia with an open outflow tract below the valve and with reasonable sized main and branch pulmonary arteries and this is the only cardiac anatomy that is amenable to fetal intervention. However, those fetuses without an open outflow tract in the right ventricle with a long segment muscular atresia or a very hypertrophied, high pressure right ventricle (often with coronary fistulae) are usually not suitable for interventional procedures.[30] Selection criteria for intervention in this condition have been proposed by Huhta et al[38] where selection is based on a cardiovascular score profile. The heart failure score is 10 if there are no abnormal signs and reflects two points for each of five categories: hydrops (none, 2 points; ascites or pleural or pericardial effusion, –1 point; hydrops, –2 points), venous Doppler (normal, 2 points; end-diastolic reversal flow in ductus venosus, –1 point; umbilical vein pulsations, –2 points), heart size by means of the ratio heart area/chest area (< 0.35, 2 points; 0.35 to 0.50, –1 point; > 0.50, –2 points), cardiac function by means of flow through atrioventricular valves and shortening fraction (normal, 2 points; holosystolic tricuspid regurgitation or shortening fraction < 0.28, –1 point; holosystolic mitral or tricuspid regurgitation or monophasic filling, –2 points), and Doppler in the umbilical artery (normal, 2 points; absent end-diastolic velocity, –1 point; reversed end-diastolic velocity, –2 points). In the setting of critical stenosis or atresia of the pulmonary valve with intact ventricular septum, a cardiovascular profile score of 7 or less, reflecting impending or established congestive heart failure, should constitute an indication to perform fetal pulmonary valvuloplasty, in order to prevent development of non-immune hydrops and fetal death (Figure 2.3). In fetuses with pulmonary atresia and intact ventricular septum congestive heart failure may arise when the interatrial shunting is restrictive or due to massive tricuspid regurgitation with septal displacement in the ventricle impairing left ventricular filling and function. By establishing antegrade flow across the pulmonary valve it is likely to observe an improvement in the filling and growth of the right ventricle, a lesser degree of reversal flow through the arterial duct, a decrease in central venous pressure, and, thereby increasing the chances of a biventricular outcome (Figure 2.4). Indeed, fetal pulmonary

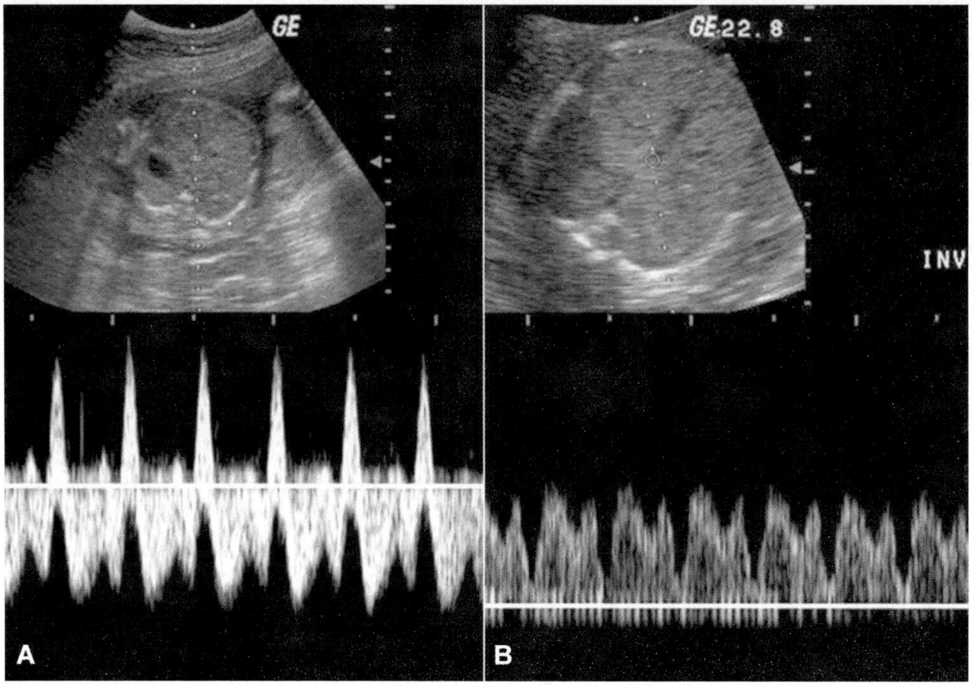

Figures 2.3A and B: A. Transverse view of the fetal abdomen in a fetus with critical pulmonary stenosis and intact ventricular septum with end-diastolic reversed flow in the ductus venosus. B. Transverse view of the fetal abdomen post-valvuloplasty showing a normal flow in the ductus venosus

valvuloplasty has been shown to fulfil all these objectives and may help to prolong pregnancy in better fetal condition. Several procedures have been performed to date with technical success leading to biventricular repair in the majority of the cases.[30,31] In all cases, authors are well aware that the limited experience available to date precludes any general recommendations to be concluded. In this particular disease, as well as in many others in fetal and pediatric cardiology, the low incidence and prevalence limits the possibility of adequate statistical analysis. For example, it is unrealistic to randomize the management of those fetuses with critical PS/PA-IVS. Fortunately, in most of the cases the result of postnatal treatment of children with this congenital heart defect is excellent. However, the deterioration in the venous Doppler, a finding that it is not observed in all fetuses with the same disease, reflecting worsening disease with cardiac compromise and increase central venous pressure should constitute an indication to perform intrauterine pulmonary valvuloplasty.

The other indication to attempt this procedure is to avoid the development of a hypoplastic, non-functional right ventricle, in the setting of an adequate foramen ovale.[53] Given that patients who have the mild or moderate form of the disease can undergo right ventricle decompression postnatally with potential for right ventricle growth, it has been speculated that early in utero valvulotomy may result in better growth of the right ventricle making it more amenable to biventricular repair. However, for an adequate selection of the candidates for valve dilation it will be precise to define a better method of assessing the growth potential of the right ventricle. Huhta et al[30] have proposed the use of an inotropic agent such as terbutaline to increase the cardiac output and analyze the reserve of the right ventricle to select the appropriate candidates for opening the outflow tract of the ventricle.[29] Evidence of significant pressure gradient across the stenotic semilunar valve or in the ventricle on tricuspid valve jet measurements would be indicators of an adequate ventricular reserve. After technically successful fetal pulmonary valvuloplasties, ongoing growth of the pulmonary valve, tricuspid valve and right ventricle have been documented. Therefore, it seems that this procedure might be able

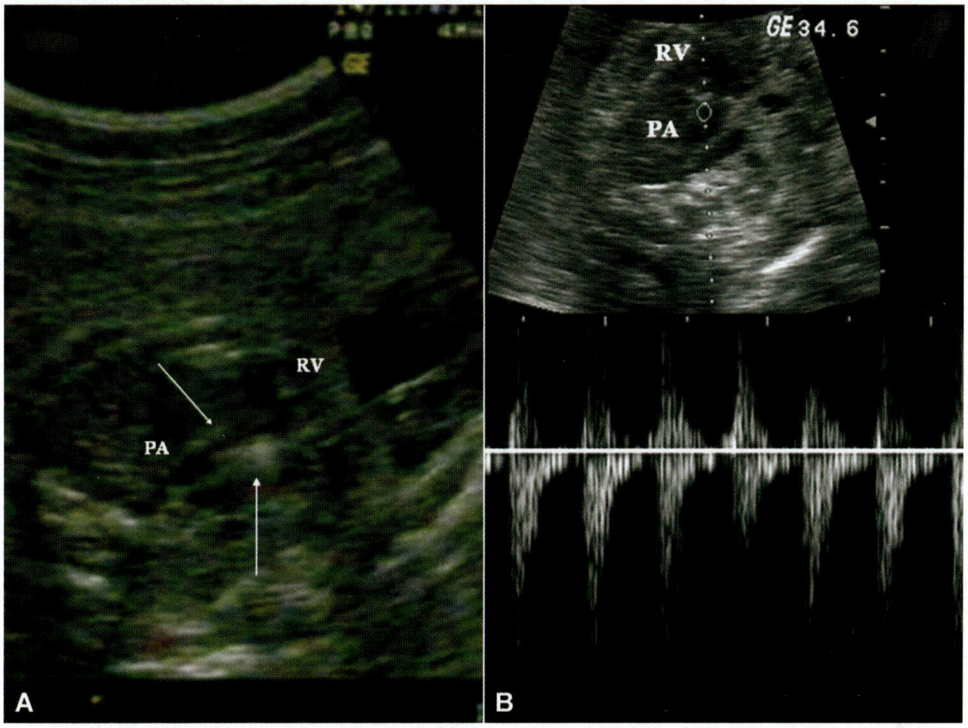

Figures 2.4A and B: A. Coronary balloon (arrow) partially inflated across the pulmonary valve (open arrow). B. Improvement in the antegrade pulmonary flow after balloon valvuloplasty. PA, pulmonary artery; RV, right ventricle

to alter the prenatal natural history, prevent secondary damage to the fetal heart and enable sufficient right ventricle growth to save fetuses with PS-PA/IVS from a life with single ventricle physiology thus improving their quality of life.

Restrictive/intact Atrial Septum

A highly restrictive or intact atrial septum with secondary left atrial hypertension is one of the most critical factors that have an impact on the outcome of HLHS for both staged reconstruction and heart transplantation. Restrictive atrial septum places the neonate at risk of severe pulmonary hypertension and lung congestion, which complicates the perioperative course and may alter single-ventricle palliation results.[23,35] The incidence of intact atrial septum in the setting of HLHS has been estimated at 6%, with some degree of atrial septal restriction occurring in up to 22% of cases.[23,24] These neonates develop profound cyanosis and pulmonary edema shortly after birth. Given the usually ineffectiveness of standard resuscitative measures, some centers have performed emergent Norwood procedures to improve the condition of these newborns. However, only 17% of the patients managed in this fashion survived at 6 months.[23] Even among neonates undergoing early transcatheter procedures to relieve atrial septum obstruction before surgical palliation, the preoperative and early postoperative mortality is 48%.[18] This high mortality may also be due to associated intrapulmonary anatomic abnormalities, including "arterialization" of the pulmonary veins and lymphatic dilation.[23,55] This complication may also be observed in fetuses with simple TGA.

Prenatal recognition of highly restrictive or intact atrial septum in fetuses with HLHS provides not only the opportunity to plan the delivery and immediate postnatal intervention but also raises the possibility of decompressing the left atrium prenatally. If an atrial septal defect could be created *in utero*, the postnatal pulmonary venous flow may improve, reducing the need for additional or urgent procedures and improving the infant's preoperative situation and surgical outcome.[24] Moreover, decompressing the left atrium prenatally the changes in the pulmonary vasculature might be avoided.

Direct evaluation of the atrial septum in fetuses with HLHS may be difficult because of a high and posterior position of the interatrial communication, which is commonly seen in this condition, or difficult fetal position. Even when direct anatomic and Doppler observations of the foramen ovale can be performed, it has been observed that these correlate poorly with the degree of left atrial hypertension after birth.[23] Some evaluation of the state of the pulmonary vascular bed can be obtained by examining the pulmonary arterial and venous Doppler. The pulmonary arterial Doppler in HLHS is known to be normal and increased pulsatility index in central pulmonary arteries suggests elevated resistance.[29] Doppler assessment of venous flow patterns has been shown to indirectly reflect downstream atrial filling pressures (Figures 2.5 and 2.6). Increased reversal flow during atrial contraction in the pulmonary veins correlates closely with increased left atrial pressures in fetuses.[35]

Intrauterine balloon atrial septostomy is performed by direct right atrial wall puncture under continuous ultrasound guidance. An 18- or 19-gauge introducer cannula is percutaneously advanced from the maternal abdomen into the fetal right atrium and then positioned against the atrial septum. The obturator is then removed and is replaced by a 22-

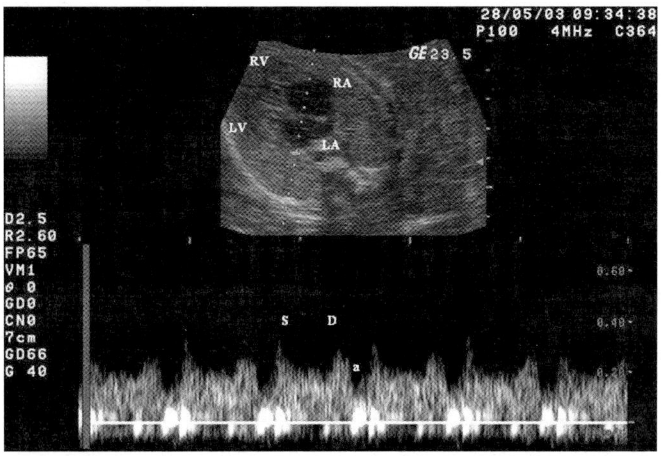

Figure 2.5: Normal triphasic flow in a pulmonary vein in a fetus in the third trimester of pregnancy. Note the presence of antegrade flow during the whole cardiac cycle. RV, right ventricle; LV, left ventricle; RA, right atrium; LA, left atrium; S, systolic flow; D, diastolic flow; a, atrial contraction

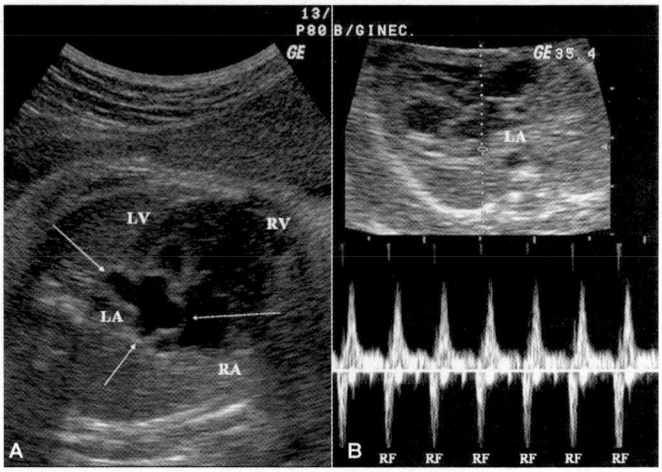

Figures 2.6A and B: A. Four-chamber view in a fetus with hypoplastic left heart syndrome and intact atrial septum showing a marked bulging into the right atrium (open arrow) and enlarged pulmonary veins (arrows). B. Pulmonary venous flow in a fetus with intact atrial septum demonstrating flow reversal. RV, right ventricle; LV, left ventricle; RA, right atrium; LA, left atrium; RF, reversal flow

gauge Chiba needle which punctures the atrial septum and introduced in the left atrium. Finally, through the Chiba needle the wire is entered in the left atrium or a pulmonary vein and over the wire the Chiba needle is exchanged for a balloon angioplasty catheter. Marshall et al[24] have performed 7 procedures with one death between 26 and 34 weeks gestation. Six procedures were successful technically (defined as one in which passage and inflation of a balloon across the atrial septum were documented by ultrasound and flow was subsequently detected across a new atrial septal defect) and of the six that were live born at term, four died as neonates. One of the six fetuses with technically successful procedure is alive after Norwood procedure. The perinatal mortality rate in these cases that were treated *in utero* was similar to that reported for neonates who underwent a similar palliative procedure postnatally.[23] It is possible that the procedures were performed too late when the pulmonary damage has already occurred or the defect created was too small as the pulmonary reversal flow persisted in all cases. This kind of compromises between the devices used to reach the clinical objective without inducing significant traumatic tissue injury often arise in fetal interventions. Difficulties may also arise in fetuses with thicker interatrial septum that may make ineffective the static dilation with septal recoil after balloon deflation. Other complications may arise after the procedure such as severe hemorrhage following puncture of the atrial wall. Nevertheless, although no significant clinical impact has been observed to date, the feasibility of performing an atrial septostomy *in utero* has been demonstrated with a high rate of technical success and no maternal morbidity. Critical issues that deserve further investigation include the patient selection, timing of intervention, the effective size of the interatrial communication, and development of new devices to create larger defects and alternative techniques for thicker interatrial septa.

Indeed, it has been observed that *in utero* laser atrial septostomy is feasible.[41] This approach has the advantage of producing an interatrial defect that is not subject to reduction in size because of tissue recoil. However, the outcome of the case reported was poor and the procedure also showed to be ineffective in alleviating the hemodynamic problems that are commonly observed in these patients.

Counseling

In spite of some successful case reports and small series, invasive cardiac interventions in fetal life remain investigational and should be considered palliative, until the benefits are determined by well-controlled clinical trials. Physicians and their patients who are considering these procedures must be made fully aware of the potential risks to both mother and fetus and the parents should be advised realistically regarding the risk of fetal demise due to the procedure. Maternal morbidity is not insignificant and complications may include wound infection, hemorrhage and thrombosis. Furthermore, manipulation of the fetus may lead to placental abruption with fetal loss. Renowned authors do not share the enthusiasm regarding the ability of fetal echocardiography to adequate select the patients eligible for fetal catheterization at mid-gestation. In addition, some small left ventricles may grow during late gestation or during the postnatal period following the postnatal relief of aortic stenosis, becoming the prenatal invasive procedure even more questionable.[56]

There are many technical difficulties, most of which are currently unavoidable and limit the ultimate patient outcome. They are mainly related to fetal approach as well as catheter, needle, and guide wire sizes. These interventions, however, may change the adverse natural history of some heart diseases and allow for fetal maturity to be reached in better conditions. Although both parents and physicians should be aware that in many of the cases one or more additional postnatal procedures will be required for adequate management of this defect,[57] improvement in fetal conditions must also result in an improvement in morbidity and mortality figures. Obviously, some affirmations cannot be proved, and more studies and longer follow-up are needed to answer all the questions that currently remain unresolved. However, published data support the concept that the natural history of all flow-dependent diseases consistently tends to deteriorate resulting in an unfavorable postnatal scenario.

Extensive informed counseling of the parents about alternative postnatal options for treatment remains critical. Fortunately, medical advances allow offering postnatal surgical strategies to a great many of the infants with CHDs with an average mortality of open cardiac surgery lower than 10% in good centers. Although the length and quality of life are highly dependent on the severity of the CHD, good long-term outcomes are achievable in most cases. The prognostic evaluations and available pre- and postnatal surgical options should be explained, modified and updated accordingly as they constantly change in individual categories. Recent series have demonstrated that mortality and morbidity after staged palliation of HLHS have improved significantly and should have a favorable impact on perinatal counseling.[7,47] Anyway, the parents must be fully supported in their decision whatever their choice.

FUTURE PERSPECTIVES

The field of interventional transcatheter repair or palliation of obstructive cardiac defects appears to have a significant potential for favorably altering the adverse hemodynamics during the development of the fetus through later pregnancy. In theory, this could provide a significant improvement in outcome for the more severe obstructive cardiac defects by preventing the development of the secondary changes considered to result from the decreased or altered flow patterns. The challenges for the future with this technique are to ensure that an accurate diagnosis can be made at an appropriately early stage of development before irreversible changes have occurred and to demonstrate that effective intervention initiated at an appropriate time that can favorably alter the course of the cardiac defect. The creation of an unselected database based on intention to treat is one way to determine whether fetuses with similar morphology and physiology might benefit from a fetal intervention, over and above the natural history of the disease process. In Europe, most fetuses with HLHS or PS-PA/IVS will be terminated.[2,52] It is not known how the offer of a fetal intervention might alter their decision making but the experience shows that these procedures are usually refused by the parents due to uncertainties concerning the efficacy of the intervention. Until the results of such a database are available for scrutiny, selection of cases must be made on the limited experience of specialists in fetal cardiology.

Further developments in the technology of intrauterine intervention both in fetal imaging and interventional devices designed for the very small heart are necessary for this potential to attain a more reasonable degree of reality and also are sure to come. Current improvements in intrauterine ultrasound (catheters placed on the fetal abdomen or into the esophagus) and endoscopy, providing the ability to visualize directly the site of intended intervention in the heart, would be a great advance if it could be done safely. Moreover, the miniaturization of the interventional catheters in order to allow an earlier application of these interventions *in utero* would minimize the changes in the fetal heart secondary to the primary defect. It is reasonable to suggest that the earlier these procedures are performed the better the results and outcome will be. For example, early experience suggests that treatment of PS-PA/IVS may be needed before 20 weeks to prevent the development of ventriculocoronary connections.

REFERENCES

1. Dudek RW. Cardiac embryology. In Hess DB, Hess LW (Eds): Fetal Echocardiography. Appleton & Lange, Stamford: Connecticut, 1999; 1-32.
2. Galindo A, Gutiérrez-Larraya F, de la Fuente P. Congenital heart defects in fetal life: an overview. Ultrasound Rev Obstet Gynecol 2004; 4:194-207.
3. Hornberger LK, Benacerraf BR, Bromley BS, Spevak PJ, Sanders SP. Prenatal detection of severe right ventricular outflow tract obstruction: pulmonary stenosis and pulmonary atresia. J Ultrasound Med 1994; 13:743-50.
4. Hornberger LK, Sanders SP, Rein AJ, Spevak PJ, Parness IA, Colan SD. Left heart obstructive lesions and left ventricular growth in the midtrimester fetus: a longitudinal study. Circulation 1995; 92:1531-8.
5. Simpson JA. Hypoplastic left heart syndrome. Ultrasound Obstet Gynecol 000; 15:271-8.
6. Comas C, Galindo A, Martínez JM, Carrera JM, Gutiérrez-Larraya F, De la Fuente P, Puerto B, Borrell A. Early prenatal diagnosis of major cardiac anomalies in a high-risk population. Prenat Diagn 2002; 22:586-93.
7. Rychik J. Hypoplastic left heart syndrome: from *in-utero* diagnosis to school age. Semin Fetal Neonatal Med 2005; 10:553-66.
8. Maxwell D, Allan LD, Tynan MJ. Balloon dilatation of the aortic valve in the fetus: a report of two cases. Br Heart J 1991; 65:256-58.
9. Allan LD, Maxwell DJ, Carminati M, Tynan MJ. Survival after fetal aortic balloon valvoplasty. Ultrasound Obstet Gynecol 1995; 5:90-1.
10. Kohl T, Sharland G, Allan LD, Gembruch U, Chaoui R, Lopes LM, Zielinsky P, Huhta J, Silverman NH. World experience of percutaneous ultrasound-guided balloon valvuloplasty in human fetuses with severe aortic valve obstruction. Am J Cardiol 2000; 85:1230-3.
11. Tworetzki W, Marshall AC. Balloon valvuloplasty for congenital heart disease in the fetus. Clin Perinatol 2003; 30:541-50.
12. Gardiner HM. Progression of fetal heart disease and rationale for fetal intracardiac interventions. Semin Fetal Neonatal Med 2005; 10:578-85.
13. Hawkins JA, Minich LL, Tani LY, Day RW, Judd VE, Shaddy RE, McGough EC. Late results and reintervention after aortic valvotomy for critical aortic stenosis in neonates and infants. Ann Thorac Surg 1998; 65:1758-62.
14. McElhinney DB, Lock JE, Keane JF, Moran AM, Colan SD. Left heart growth, function, and reintervention after balloon aortic valvuloplasty for neonatal aortic stenosis. Circulation 2005; 111:451-8.
15. Kohl T. Fetal echocardiography: new grounds to explore during fetal cardiac intervention. Pediatr Cardiol 2002; 23:334-46.
16. Allan LD, Sharland G, Tynan MJ. The natural history of the hypoplastic left heart syndrome. Int J Cardiol 1989; 25:341-3.
17. Simpson JM, Sharland GK. Natural history and outcome of aortic stenosis diagnosed prenatally. Heart 1997; 77:205-10.

18. Vlahos AP, Lock JE, McElhinney DB, van der Velde ME. Hypoplastic left heart syndrome with intact or highly restrictive atrial septum. Outcome after neonatal transcatheter atrial septostomy. Circulation 2004; 109:2326-30.
19. Danford DA, Cronican P. Hypoplastic left heart syndrome: progression of left ventricular dilation and dysfunction to left ventricular hypoplasia in utero. Am Heart J 1992; 123:1712-6.
20. Simpson JA. Hypoplastic left heart syndrome. Ultrasound Obstet Gynecol 2000; 15:271-8.
21. Cohen MS. Fetal diagnosis and management of congenital heart disease. Clin Perinatol 2001; 28:11-29.
22. Maeno YV, Boutin C, Hornberger LK, McCrindle BW, Cavalle-Garrido T, Gladman G, Smallhorn JF. Prenatal diagnosis of right ventricular outflow tract obstruction with intact ventricular septum, and detection of ventriculocoronary connections. Heart 1999; 81:661-8.
23. Rychik J, Rome JJ, Collins MH, DeCampli WM, Spray TL. The hypoplastic left heart syndrome with intact atrial septum: atrial morphology, pulmonary vascular histopathology and outcome. J Am Coll Cardiol 1999; 34:554-60.
24. Marshall AC, van der Velde ME, Tworetzky W, Gomez CA, Wilkins-Haug L, Benson CB, Jennings RW, Lock JE. Creation of an atrial septal defect *in utero* for fetuses with hypoplastic left heart syndrome and intact or highly restrictive atrial septum. Circulation 2004; 110:253-8.
25. Hanseus K, Bjorkhem G, Lundstrom NR, Laurin S. Cross-sectional echocardiographic measurements of right ventricular size and growth in patients with pulmonary atresia and intact ventricular septum. Pediatr Cardiol 1991; 12:135-42.
26. Tilman H, Soderberg B, McCrindle B, Nykanen D, Freedom R, Williams W, Benson L. Percutaneous balloon valvotomy in pulmonary atresia with intact ventricular septum: impact on patient care. Circulation 2003; 108:826-32.
27. Tworetzky W, Wilkins-Haug L, Jennings RW, van der Velde ME, Marshall AC, Marx GR, Colan SD, Benson CB, Lock JE, Perry SB. Balloon dilation of severe aortic stenosis in the fetus: potential for prevention of hypoplastic left heart syndrome: candidate selection, technique, and results of successful intervention. Circulation 2004; 110:2125-31.
28. Harada K, Toyono M, Tamura M. Effects of balloon valvuloplasty on left anterior descending coronary artery blood flow in a neonate with critical aortic stenosis with transthoracic doppler echocardiography. J Am Soc Echocardiogr 2003; 16:88-90.
29. Huhta J, Quintero RA, Suh E, Bader R. Advances in fetal cardiac intervention. Curr Opin Pediatr 2004; 16:487-93.
30. Tulzer G, Arzt W, Franklin RC, Loughna PV, Mair R, Gardiner HM. Fetal pulmonary valvuloplasty for critical pulmonary stenosis with intact septum. Lancet 2002; 360:1567-8.
31. Galindo A, Gutiérrez-Larraya F, Velasco JM, de la Fuente P. Pulmonary balloon valvuloplasty in a fetus with critical pulmonary stenosis/atresia with intact ventricular septum and heart failure. Fetal Diagn Ther 2006; 21:100-104.
32. Marino BS. Outcomes after the Fontan procedure. Curr Opin Pediatr 2002; 14:620-6.
33. Berghella V, Pagotto L, Kaufman M, Huhta JC, Wapner RJ. Accuracy of Prenatal Diagnosis of Congenital Heart Defects. Fetal Diagn Ther 2001; 16:407-12.
34. Paladini D, Calabro R, Palmieri S, D'Andrea T. Prenatal diagnosis of congenital heart disease and fetal karyotyping. Obstet Gynecol 1993; 81:679-82.
35. Taketazu M, Barrea C, Smallhorn JF, Wilson GJ, Hornberger LK. Intrauterine pulmonary venous flow and restrictive foramen ovale in fetal hypoplastic left heart syndrome. J Am Coll Cardiol 2004; 43:1902-7.
36. Brackley KJ, Kilby MD, Wright JG, Brawn WJ, Sethia B, Stumper O, Holder R, Wyldes MP, Whittle MJ. Outcome after prenatal diagnosis of hypoplastic left-heart syndrome: a case series. Lancet 2000; 356:1143-7.
37. Allan LD, Sharland GK, Milburn A, Lockhart SM, Groves AM, Anderson RH, Cook AC, Fagg NL. Prospective diagnosis of 1006 consecutive cases of congenital heart disease in the fetus. J Am Coll Cardiol 1994; 23:1452-8.
38. Huhta JC. Guidelines for the evaluation of heart failure in the fetus with or without hydrops. Pediatr Cardiol 2004; 25:274-86.
39. Andrews R, Tulloh R, Sharland GK, Simpson J, Rollings S, Baker E, Qureshi S, Rosenthal E, Austin C, Anderson D. Outcome of staged reconstructive surgery for hypoplastic left heart syndrome following antenatal diagnosis. Arch Dis Child 2001; 85:474-7.
40. Carter GA. Interventional cardiology in the fetus. In Hess DB, Hess LW (Eds): Fetal Echocardiography.Appleton & Lange, Stamford: Connecticut, 1999; 295-8.
41. Quintero RA, Huhta JC. Suh E, Chmait R, Romero R, Angel J. *In utero* cardiac fetal surgery: laser atrial septotomy in the treatment of hypoplastic left heart syndrome with intact atrial septum. Am J Obstet Gynecol 2005; 193:1424-8.
42. Quintero RA, Suh E, Huhta JC, Chmait R, Angel J, Lichtenstein S. Percutaneous fetal aortic valvulotomy with intracardiac endoscopy for the treatment of critical aortic valve stenosis. Ultrasound Obstet Gynecol 2004; 24:279.
43. Meyer-Wittkopf M. Interventional fetal cardiac therapy-possible perspectives and current shortcomings. Ultrasound Obstet Gynecol 2002; 20:527-31.
44. Kohl T, Strumper D, Witteler R, Merschhoff G, Alexiene R, Callenbeck C, Asfour B, Reckers J, Aryee S, Vahlhaus C, Vogt J, van Aken H, Scheld HH. Fetoscopic direct fetal cardiac access in sheep: an important experimental milestone along the route to human fetal cardiac intervention. Circulation 2000; 102:1602-4.
45. Kohl T, Witteler R, Strümper D, Gogarten W, Asfour B, Reckers J, Merschhoff G, Marcus AE, Weyand M, Van Aken H, Vogt J, Scheld HH. Operative techniques and strategies for minimally invasive fetoscopic fetal cardiac interventions in sheep. Surg Endosc 2000; 14:424-30.
46. Thomson JDR. Management of aortic stenosis in children. Heart 2004; 90:5-6.
47. Twedell JS, Hoffman GM, Mussato KA, Fedderly RT, Berger S, Jaquiss RDB, Ghanayem NS, Frisbee SJ, Litwin

SB. Improved survival of patients undergoing palliation of hypoplastic left heart syndrome: lessons learned from 115 consecutive patients. Circulation 2002; 106(suppl 1):I-82-9.

48. Schmider A, Henrich W, Dähnert I, Dudenhausen JW. Prenatal therapy of non immunologic hydrops fetalis caused by severe aortic stenosis. Ultrasound Obstet Gynecol 2000; 16:275-8.
49. Gardiner H. Response of the fetal heart to changes in load: from hyperplasia to heart failure. Heart 2005; 91:871-3.
50. Neish SR, O´Laughlin MP, Nihill MR, Ott DA, Cooley DA. Intraoperative balloon valvuloplasty for critical aortic valvular stenosis in neonates. Am J Cardiol 1991; 68:807-10.
51. Wilkins-Haug LE, Benson CB, Tworetzky W, Marshall AC, Jennings RW, Locks JE. In-utero interventions for hypoplastic left heart syndrome—a perinatologist´s perspective. Ultrasound Obstet Gynecol 2005; 26:482-6.
52. Todros T, Paladini D, Chiappa E, Russo MG, Gaglioti P, Pacileo G, Cau MA, Martinelli P. Pulmonary stenosis and atresia with intact ventricular septum during prenatal life. Ultrasound Obstet Gynecol 2003; 21:228-33.
53. Freedom R: How can something so small cause so much grief? Some thoughts about the underdeveloped right ventricle in pulmonary atresia and intact ventricular septum. J Am Coll Cardiol 1992; 19:1038-40.
54. Daubeney PE, Delany DJ, Anderson RH, Sandor GG, Slavik Z, Keeton BR, Webber SA; United Kingdom and Ireland Collaborative Study of Pulmonary Atresia with Intact Ventricular Septum. Pulmonary atresia with intact ventricular septum: range of morphology in a population-based study. J Am Coll Cardiol 2002; 39:1670-9.
55. Graziano JN, Heidelberger KP, Ensing GJ, Gomez CA, Ludomirsky A. The influence of a restrictive atrial septal defect on pulmonary vascular morphology in patients with hypoplastic left heart syndrome. Pediatr Cardiol 2002; 23:146-51.
56. Jouannic JM, Boudjemline Y, Benifla JL, Bonnet D. Re: In-utero intervention for hypoplastic left heart syndrome: for which fetus and for what? Ultrasound Obstet Gynecol 2006; 27:101-3.
57. Allen HD, Beekman RH, Garson A, Hijazi ZM, Mullins C, O' Laughlin M, Taubert KA. Pediatric therapeutic cardiac catheterization. Circulation 1998; 97:609-25.

CHAPTER 3

Congenital Diaphragmatic Hernia

Eduard Gratacós

DEFINITION AND EPIDEMIOLOGY

Congenital diaphragmatic hernia (CDH) is a defect in the diaphragm, which results from incomplete fusion of the embryonic structures that form the diaphragm. The main consequence of this condition is herniation of the abdominal organs into the chest cavity, which prevents normal pulmonary development and may result in lethal pulmonary hypoplasia at birth.

CDH usually occurs by the ninth to tenth week of gestation.[1] The most common mechanism causing the defect is failure of the pleuroperitoneal membranes to fuse with the septum transversum and the dorsal esophageal mesentery, resulting in persistence of the pleuroperitoneal canal. After the physiological closure of the umbilical hernia by the eleventh week, herniation of the abdominal viscera will and will definitely prevent closure of the pleuroperitoneal canal. Congenital diaphragmatic hernia is unilateral in more than 95% of cases, among which 80% occur on the left side and 20% on the right.[2] The predominance of left defects is thought to be due to later closure of the pleuroperitoneal canal on this side.

CDH occurs in approximately one out of 2400 pregnancies.[2] In about one-third of cases there are associated chromosomal defects, other malformations or genetic syndromes (Table 3.1).[3] In the other two-thirds, CDH is an isolated malformation.

Table 3.1: Genetic syndromes and chromosomal defects most commonly associated with CDH

- Associated malformations (30-35 %): rule out particularly:
  - Cardiac malformations (in 50 %)
  - Genetic syndromes
    - Fryns (craneofacial anomalies, limb hypoplasia, internal malformations)
    - Pallister-Killian (abnormal facies, long bones dysplasia)
- Chromosomal defects (10-15%, normally associated with malformations)
  - Trisomy 18 (more commonly)
  - Trisomy 13
  - Trisomy 21
  - Tetrasomy 12p (Sd. Pallister Killian) (to be diagnosed with FISH)

Isolated CDH is usually a sporadic condition. It has been reported in association with the intake of antiepileptic agents, thalidomide, and other rare medications, but no teratogenic agents or epidemiological associations have been consistently identified.

PATHOPHYSIOLOGY AND NATURAL HISTORY

The main consequence of CDH is pulmonary hypoplasia, by a mechanism of external compression. Since CDH precedes complete formation of the bronchial tree, it interferes with essential steps in pulmonary development, with variable degrees of severity that mainly depend on the size of the defect and, consequently, on the magnitude of visceral herniation. The most prominent changes occur in the lung ipsilateral to the defect, but the contralateral lung is also affected. The main features of the pulmonary histological abnormalities and their clinical correlates are summarized in Table 3.2.[4]

Table 3.2: Pathophysiological features and their clinical correlates in CDH

Histological features	*Clinical features*
• Alteration in pulmonary development: hypoplasia	Severe respiratory insufficiency
• Deficit in the generation of bronchial branches	
• Deficit in alveoli and exchange surface	
• Vascular alteration	Pulmonary hypertension
• Reduced vascular tree	
• Arteriolar muscular hyperplasia	
• Maturational alteration	Reduced surfactant
• Relative deficit in pneumocyte II	

Isolated CDH diagnosed *in utero* is associated with an overall perinatal mortality of about 50%, regardless of intensive neonatal care.[5] Most babies will survive to term and will be born alive. The essential clinical feature is respiratory insufficiency, ranging from mild to extremely severe cases. In addition to respiratory problems, pulmonary hypertension complicates a large number of cases. Despite intensive neonatal care, a considerable number of prenatally diagnosed infants die in the neonatal period as a consequence of severe respiratory insufficiency and/or pulmonary hypertension.[4, 5]

In about 75% the prenatal course is complicated by increased amniotic fluid, generally in the third trimester, possibly due to impaired fetal swallowing induced by displacement of the esophagus and stomach, the presence of frank polyhydramnios is less common.[5] Pleural effusion, and more uncommonly hydrops, may be associated with large diaphragmatic defects.

ULTRASOUND DIAGNOSIS

Gestational Age, Ultrasound View and Main Features for the Diagnosis

Although severe CDH can theoretically be diagnosed earlier, the condition is generally detected at 18- to 23-week anomaly scan. The standard sonographic section is the four-chamber view, in which the integrity of the lung parenchyma is evaluated. In particularly mild cases the diagnosis cannot be established until the third trimester, but these infants generally have a very good prognosis.

In the standard four-chamber view, the most striking features are a loss of the uniform echogenicity of the lungs, together with marked mediastinal shift. The heart is pushed to the side contralateral to the hernia and the angle of the heart axis, usually at 45°, is inverted and approaches 0° with respect to the anteroposterior axis (Figure 3.1). Once the diagnosis is made, other ultrasound views, such as coronal sections of the chest and abdomen, can be helpful for assessing important features of the herniated viscera (Figure 3.2). The diaphragm is easily identified in the coronal section as an anechoic linear structure dividing the thorax and abdomen. However, the diagnosis of CDH on the basis of this image may be misleading; except in patients with agenesis of the diaphragm, anterior coronal sections may show an apparently normal diaphragmatic image, which actually corresponds to the remaining anterior flaps of the diaphragm.

Side Affected and Abdominal Contents

Left CDH

Left CDH is easier to recognize than right-sided defects. The four-chamber view is markedly abnormal, with obvious mediastinal shift and heterogeneous contents replacing the uniformly echogenic lung. The presence of abdominal viscera can be identified.[6]

- *Intestines* (90%): Occasionally with dilated loops due to compression.

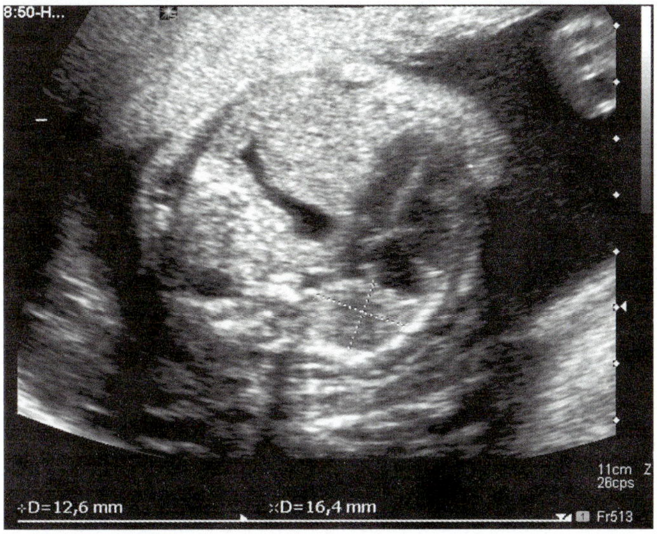

Figure 3.1: Left CDH in a transverse view

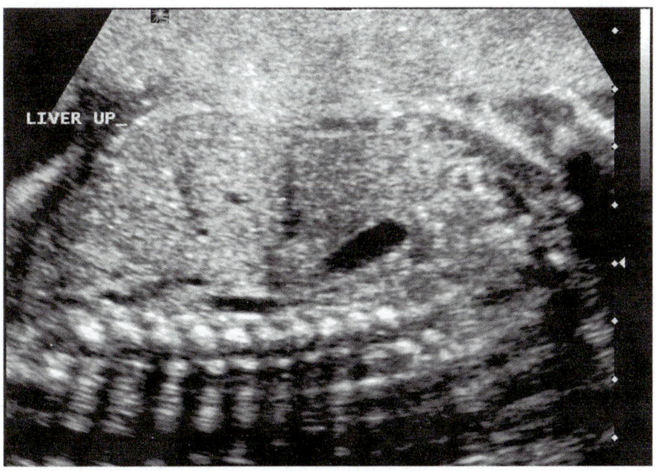

Figure 3.2: Coronal section of a fetus with CDH and clear liver herniation

- *Stomach* (60%-70%): Easily identified as a hypoechogenic chamber, it may present atypical morphology and occasionally be only partially herniated. A posterior location in the thorax normally indicates the existence of liver herniation. In very large diaphragmatic defects, the stomach may be found in the contralateral hemithorax, behind the heart.
- *Liver* (15%-20%): Used as one of the parameters to establish the prognosis. Aside from indirect signs (stomach posterior), the liver can be identified in transverse or coronal sections with ultrasound. Color-Doppler can be used to demonstrate kinking of the intra-abdominal umbilical vein and cephalad displacement of the hepatic vessels (Figure 3.3). In contrast, normal configuration of the intrahepatic umbilical vein in the transverse section, and normal arrangement of the hepatic vasculature in the coronal view, indicate that liver herniation is unlikely.

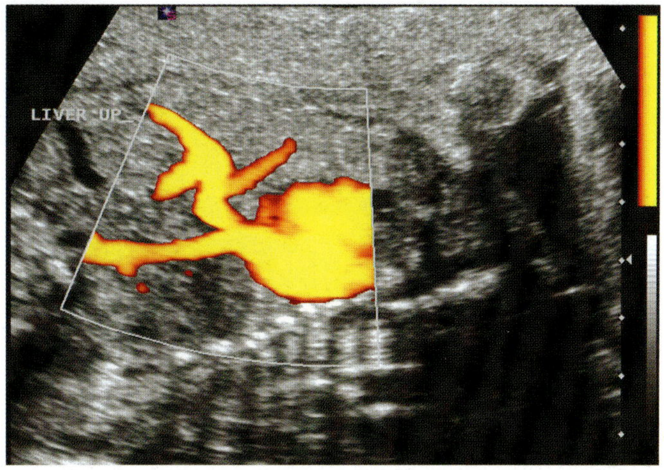

Figure 3.3: Coronal section of the same fetus as in Figure 3.2, with power Doppler showing displacement of hepatic vasculature into the thorax

- *Other viscera:* The adrenal gland can be identified in severe cases, and, less commonly, the kidney can be partially or totally herniated. The spleen may also be herniated in severe cases, but the ultrasound appearance is confusing, making the spleen difficult to distinguish from other viscera.

Right CDH

The diagnosis may be more difficult in these cases because of the similar echogenicity of the liver and lung. Once again, the presumptive diagnosis can be established on the four-chamber view if attention is paid to the position of the heart, since significant mediastinal shift is almost invariably present (Figure 3.4).

The *liver* is the herniated organ by definition; in severe defects a large portion of the liver is herniated into the chest cavity. Herniation can be identified in coronal sections according to the same views and concepts defined above for left-sided defects, using gray-scale ultrasound and Doppler. Apart from the liver, other viscera can also be identified. The *gallbladder* with its typical hypoechogenic appearance is present, but often adopts a different disposition. *Intestines* can be identified in large defects, occupying much less space than they do in left lesions. *Adrenal* and *right kidney* are more rarely identified. Very

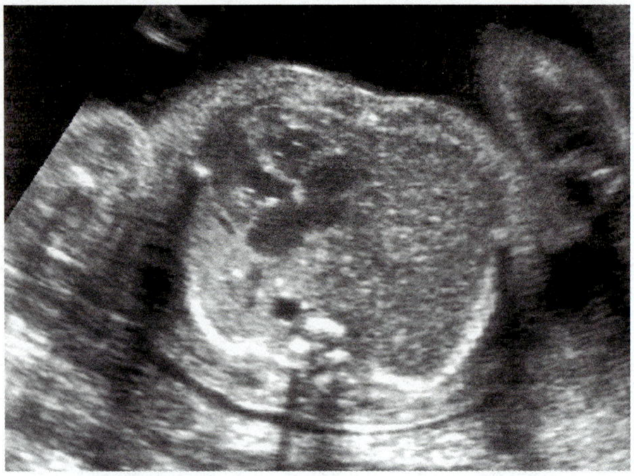

Figure 3.4: Right CDH. The heart is shifted toward the left, which may hamper recognition of this condition. The right hemithorax is occupied by a solid mass (liver) and the left lung is markedly reduced

uncommonly, in large defects or diaphragmatic agenesis, the *stomach* may also herniate into the thorax.

Bilateral CDH

Bilateral CDH is very rare, and has usually been reported in association with other defects. Prenatal diagnosis of a bilateral condition is difficult; most reported cases were initially oriented as left-sided defects, the diagnosis of bilateral hernia being established postnatally.[7]

Lung Identification and Size

The lung *contralateral* to the hernia can be visualized in all cases of CDH, invariably in a position behind the heart in the four-chamber view (see Figures 3.1 and 3.4). The lung is compressed and its form is more or less preserved depending on the severity of the hernia. The contralateral lung size is used to calculate the lung-to-head ratio (LHR),[8] an essential parameter for estimating the degree of hypoplasia and the prognosis for postnatal survival. LHR must be calculated in a four-chamber view, measuring the anterior and transverse diameter of the lung (Figure 3.5). The measurement is more difficult when the shape of the lung in a transverse section is not rounded, since this may raise doubts as to how to perform the measurement. Another shortcoming is that it does not takes into account the ipsilateral lung, which is occasionally visible on ultrasound. Despite these limitations, the interobserver correlation is acceptable and is particularly good for small lungs, a fact that has clinical relevance.

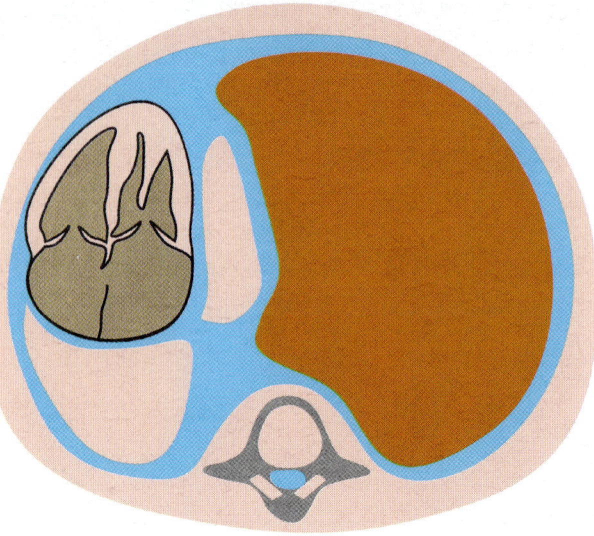

Figure 3.5: Schematic view of the section obtained for measuring the contralateral lung, behing the heart, in order to calculate the LHR

The *ipsilateral* lung can be identified in less severe cases, usually in high transverse or coronal sections, and is generally located in an anterior position due to rotation of the entire cardiopulmonary block induced by visceral herniation.

Doppler can be used to follow the course of the pulmonary main vessels and branches and identify the contralateral lung, but it is not absolutely necessary and requires specific training.

DIFFERENTIAL DIAGNOSIS

The differential diagnosis has to be established essentially with other causes of pulmonary masses, mainly CCAM and bronchopulmonary sequestration.

PROTOCOL FOR PRENATAL ASSESSMENT AND FOLLOW-UP

The prenatal protocol should focus on ruling out other malformations or syndromes, and in the case of isolated hernia, on establishing the prognosis for survival.

1. *Karyotyping:* Aside from full karyotyping studies, specific defects potentially associated with CDH can be searched (i.e. 12p tetrasomy (Pallister-Killian syndrome) with FISH analysis where available.

2. *Sonography:* Detailed examinations (exclude signs consistent with most commonly associated syndromes or chromosomal disorders), calculation of the LHR and assessment of hepatic herniation.
3. *Magnetic resonance imaging (MRI):* Confirmation of the diagnosis and the herniated viscera. Potentially useful in the confirmation/identification of viscerae which may be difficult to distinguish with ultrasound (i.e. spleen). Currently the most important contribution of this imaging technique is calculation of lung volume, which correlates significantly with the LHR.[9] The calculation most commonly used is the percentage relative to the theoretical volume corrected by GA. Up to now, this parameter has not been integrated in the calculation of risk, but in the future it may allow a more precise estimation. Additionally, the technique may offer valuable information in the monitoring of lung growth response following *in utero* therapy.
4. *Assessment of prognosis:* Essentially carried out by ultrasound evaluation, although MRI may help to confirm hepatic herniation. Currently, prognosis is established on two main parameters:
   - Lung-to-head ratio
   - Presence or absence of hepatic herniation

With these data a relatively accurate prognosis for the likelihood of survival with conventional management can be established (Table 3.3),[5] and counseling can be adapted accordingly. It must be stressed that these figures apply to centres with optimal postnatal care.

Table 3.3: Survival prognosis on the basis of LHR and presence/absence of liver herniation in a consecutive multicenter series of prenatally diagnosed left CDH[5]

LHR	*Liver*	*survival*	*Prognosis*
<1.0	Up	1/12 (**8.5 %**)	Poor
	Down	5/11 (**45.5%**)	medium
1.0-1.4	Up	4/6 (**66.7 %**)	medium
	Down	5/6 (**83.3%**)	Good
>1.4	Not applicable	8/10 (**80%**)	Good

The prognosis in right CDH is more difficult to establish, given that hepatic herniation cannot be included in the algorithm used for left hernias. In general, a LHR of less than 1.0 and considerable hepatic herniation are considered signs of very poor prognosis.

PRENATAL MONITORING AND DELIVERY

Close sonographic monitoring should be done to rule out the appearance of polyhydramnios or hydrops, although these occur infrequently. Delivery should take place in a center with tertiary neonatal support and extracorporeal membrane oxygenation (ECMO) with experience in the management of diaphragmatic hernia, since this is associated with higher survival rates.[10] Elective cesarean delivery is not indicated. Programmed delivery is not necessary, as long as continuous availability of high level neonatal care is guaranteed. On the contrary, delivery as close as possible to 40 weeks might be desirable, since the best survival rates when ECMO is required have been recorded in fetuses with highest gestational age and birth weight.[10, 11]

IN UTERO THERAPY

Fetal therapy should only be offered in cases having a poor prognosis, as displayed in Table 3.3. In some clinical series these criteria have not been strictly met, and this has led to problems in the interpretation of the results.

Diaphragmatic hernia has been one of the classic targets for fetal therapy, given its condition of isolated defect with severe but potentially reversible consequences.[11] Experimental animal studies have demonstrated that it is possible to reverse pulmonary hypoplasia by prenatal repair of the defect with fetal surgery. Nevertheless, the use of open surgery for diaphragmatic hernia in humans was discontinued because of the elevated rate of associated complications and the considerable aggression to the mother and fetus.[12]

Since then, the strategies for prenatal treatment of CDH have been based on tracheal occlusion. As has been extensively proven in animal studies, tracheal occlusion accelerates pulmonary growth even exceeding the normal levels. Tracheal occlusion prevents tracheobronchial fluid from escaping the lungs and increases pressure of the lung fluid on the tracheobronchial tree and the pulmonary acini.

Stimulation of growth seems to operate by direct mechanical stimulation and through the secretion of growth factors in response to intraalveolar pressure. There is considerable evidence that tracheal occlusion reverses CDH-induced pulmonary hypoplasia in animal models. These findings have led to the design of strategies for the application of this approach in humans. *External* tracheal occlusion using tracheal clips placed by open surgery or endoscopy was attempted, but later discontinued because of its elevated aggressiveness.[12] More recently, advances in percutaneous fetoscopic techniques to achieve endotracheal occlusion by fetal tracheoscopy have resulted in a minimally invasive method with complication rates comparable to those associated with obstetric fetoscopy, thereby providing an acceptable alternative for fetal therapy.

Recently, the preliminary results of a multicenter clinical of fetoscopic traqueal occlusion (FETO) for CDH with an extremely poor prognosis (LHR<1.0 and hepatic herniation).[14] Therapy is performed at 26 to 28 weeks, when fetal tracheoscopy and intratracheal balloon insertion are carried out percutaneously (Figures 3.6 and 3.7). The balloon can be withdrawn at the time of delivery, by means of the EXIT procedure, or before, by means of ultrasound-guided puncture or a second fetoscopy.

Most recent clinical series suggest that the result of prenatal treatment is mainly dependent on the LHR before therapy. Thus, an LHR <0.6 seems to have a poor prognosis in spite of therapy (survival 10%, 1/10), 0.7 to 0.8 is associated with a 62% survival (15/21) and fetuses with LHR between 0.81 and 1.0 have a 85% survival (13/15).[15] The rate of PROM at less than 32 weeks in the last treated cases has been dramatically reduced to <15%. The0 mortality rate in contemporary groups of fetuses recruited in multicentre studies and meeting the criteria for FETO but declining therapy was 92%.[16] Therefore, there is strong evidence suggesting that fetoscopic intrauterine tracheal occlusion, which is minimally invasive, may significantly improve survival in severe CDH. Currently, randomized clinical trials are underway to evaluate this hypothesis.

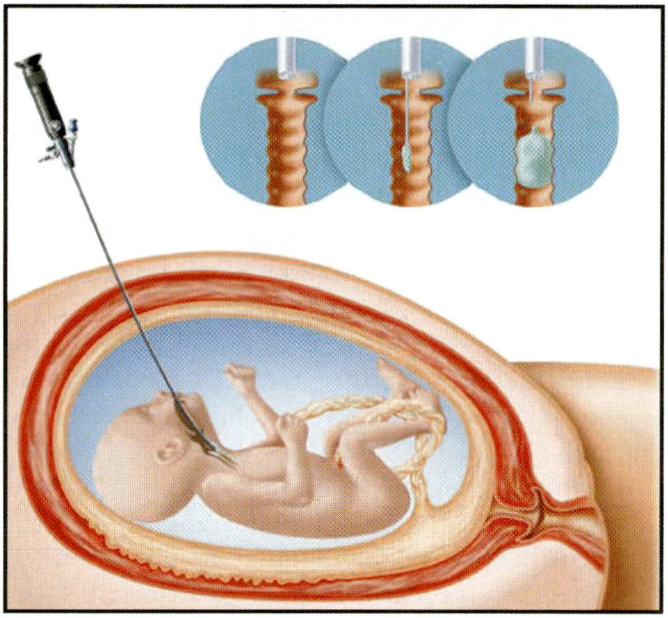

Figure 3.6: FETO procedure (© KULeuven, Belgium, reproduced with permission)

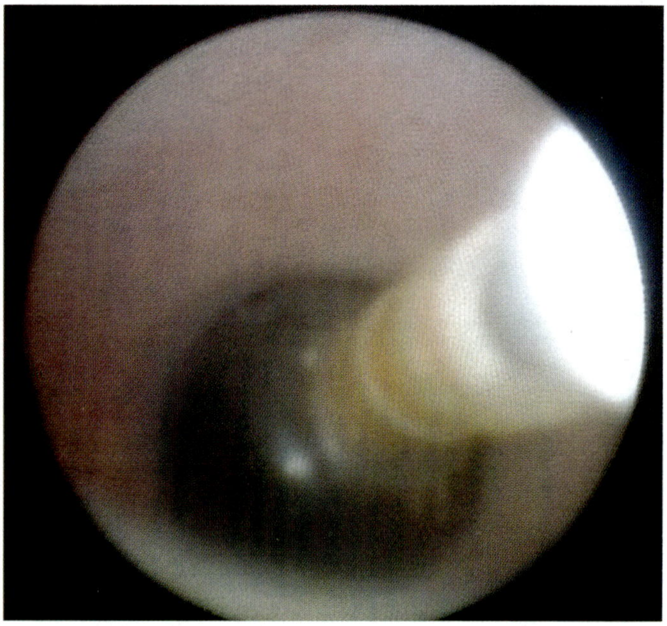

Figure 3.7: Endoscopic view of an endotracheal balloon after insertion

POSTNATAL MANAGEMENT AND LONG-TERM PROGNOSIS

Postnatal management is the same regardless of whether prenatal therapy has been done, and consists of intensive respiratory support and repair of the defect.[10] Current management strategies include gentle ventilation with tolerance to certain levels of hypercapnea, and liberal use of high-frequency oscillatory ventilation. The generally accepted attitude is to delay repair of the defect during the time necessary for ventilatory parameters to stabilize.[10] The application of ECMO varies considerably among centers, although it is usually indicated when the oxygenation index is below X. In contrast to reported data for other indications of ECMO, there is some controversy about the contribution of this technique to final survival in CDH, and this fact together with the rates of associated neurological sequelae has prompted some authors to advocate very selective use of this option in consensus with the family.[10]

The survival rates merit some comment, since the obstetric and pediatric literatures traditionally differ on this point. Reported neonatal survival rates in reference centers may be as high as 80% to 90%.[17] However, it must be stressed that these series have a case selection bias since they do not take into account the impact of prenatal diagnosis and elective termination, or those cases of immediate neonatal death, before transfer to a reference center is possible.

The quality of life of fetuses with diaphragmatic hernia varies substantially according to the series, but most authors agree that the large majority of survivors have an acceptable quality of life.[18] The most common sequela is, of course, respiratory insufficiency and particularly oxygen dependence, which may be present in up to 30% of cases, although generally with little or no clinical relevance.[18] The available series are not large enough to estimate quality of life according to the prenatal parameters of severity.

Except in the cases presenting within a syndrome, isolated CDH is almost always a sporadic malformation and therefore the risk of recurrence is extremely low.

REFERENCES

1. Moore KL. The developing human, clinically oriented embryology. 2004.
2. Torfs CP, Curry CJ, Bateson TF, Honore LH. A population-based study of congenital diaphragmatic hernia. Teratology 1992; 46(6):555-65.
3. Witters I, Legius E, Moerman P, Deprest J, Van Schoubroeck D, Timmerman D, et al. Associated malformations and chromosomal anomalies in 42 cases of prenatally diagnosed diaphragmatic hernia. Am J Med Genet 2001; 103(4):278-82.
4. Nobuhara KK, Wilson JM. Pathophysiology of congenital diaphragmatic hernia. Semin Pediatr Surg 1996; 5(4):234-42.
5. J Jani. Lung-to-head ratio and liver position to predict outcome in early diagnosed isolated left sided diaphragmatic hernia fetuses: a multicenter study. Am J Obstet Gynecol 2004.
6. Thilaganathan B. Routine ultrasound for the prenatal diagnosis of congenital diaphragmatic hernia: the 'isms'. Ultrasound Obstet Gynecol 2002; 19(4):327-8.
7. Song MS, Yoo SJ, Smallhorn JF, Mullen JB, Ryan G, Hornberger LK. Bilateral congenital diaphragmatic hernia: diagnostic clues at fetal sonography. Ultrasound Obstet Gynecol 2001; 17(3):255-8.
8. Lipshutz GS, Albanese CT, Feldstein VA, Jennings RW, Housley HT, Beech R, et al. Prospective analysis of lung-to-head ratio predicts survival for patients with prenatally diagnosed congenital diaphragmatic hernia. J Pediatr Surg 1997; 32(11):1634-6.
9. Mahieu-Caputo D, Sonigo P, Dommergues M, Fournet JC, Thalabard JC, Abarca C, et al. Fetal lung volume measurement by magnetic resonance imaging in congenital diaphragmatic hernia. BJOG 2001; 108(8):863-8.
10. Hedrick HL. Evaluation and management of congenital diaphragmatic hernia. Pediatr Case Rev 2001; 1(1):25-36.
11. Harrison MR, de Lorimier AA. Congenital diaphragmatic hernia. Surg Clin North Am 1981; 61(5):1023-35.
12. Sydorak RM, Harrison MR. Congenital diaphragmatic hernia: advances in prenatal therapy. World J Surg 2003; 27(1):68-76.
13. Flageole H, Evrard VA, Vandenberghe K, Lerut TE, Deprest JA. Tracheoscopic endotracheal occlusion in the ovine model: technique and pulmonary effects. J Pediatr Surg 1997; 32(9):1328-31.
14. Deprest J, Gratacos E, Nicolaides KH. Fetoscopic tracheal occlusion (FETO) for severe congenital diaphragmatic hernia: evolution of a technique and preliminary results. Ultrasound Obstet Gynecol 2004; 24(2):121-6.
15. Deprest J, Jani J, Cannie M, Debeer A, Vandevelde M, Done E, Gratacos E, Nicolaides. Prenatal intervention for isolated congenital diaphragmatic hernia. Curr Opin Obstet Gynecol. 2006;18:203-15.
16. Jani J, Keller RL, Benachi A, Nicolaides KH, Favre R, Gratacos E, Laudy J, Eisenberg V, Eggink A, Vaast P, Deprest J; Antenatal-CDH-Registry Group. Prenatal prediction of survival in isolated left-sided diaphragmatic hernia. Ultrasound Obstet Gynecol 2006; 27:18-22.
17. Javid PJ, Jaksic T, Skarsgard ED, Lee S. Survival rate in congenital diaphragmatic hernia: the experience of the Canadian Neonatal Network. J Pediatr Surg 2004; 39(5):657-60.
18. Poley MJ, Stolk EA, Tibboel D, Molenaar JC, Busschbach JJ. The cost-effectiveness of treatment for congenital diaphragmatic hernia. J Pediatr Surg 2002; 37(9):1245-52.

CHAPTER 4

Fetal Therapy: Other Possibilities

George Daskalakis

INTRODUCTION

Fetal medicine today focuses not only to the prenatal diagnosis, but also to the therapy of an affected fetus. Traditionally, either termination of pregnancy or selective termination of an affected fetus was the only option that was offered to the parents, following the diagnosis of a congenital anomaly. Because of our better understanding of fetal physiology and pathology, and the technological improvements during the last decade many experts in fetal medicine tried to correct the process of a developmental abnormality, early enough in order to prevent a permanent damage to the fetus. It is anticipated that fetal therapy will become a topic of great demand; therefore, research on this topic is markedly increased and the results of different trials are of paramount importance.

Due to the rarity of many conditions in which it is used, the application of fetal therapy is limited at present, and therefore a systematic review is not possible. However, an obvious benefit was noted following intervention in some conditions and promising results have been reported in many others. It is not only my opinion that the future of fetal medicine lies in the involvement of both researchers and clinicians alike, in the field of ultrasound, genetics, perinatology, neonatology, pediatrics and fetal surgery in an attempt to offer fetal therapy and improve the lives of fetuses with congenital anomalies which can be diagnosed prenatally. This chapter focuses on those conditions which are currently amenable fetal therapy, bearing in mind that the number of these conditions will be greatly increased in near future.

CLINICAL APPLICATIONS OF FETAL THERAPY

Fetal Anemia

Fetal blood transfusion is the only mode of treatment of fetal anemia, most commonly due to red cell alloimmunization. Intrauterine fetal blood transfusion was initially performed with intraperitoneal transfusion, in 1963 by Liley.[1] This method was in practice for approximately two decades, although it was associated with a poor survival rate, mainly because of the inadequate absorption of erythrocytes from the peritoneal cavity, especially in fetuses with hydrops.[2] Rodeck et al[3], described a technique of intravascular transfusion by needling the umbilical artery under direct fetoscopic vision. Although a survival rate of 84% was reported, the fetal loss rate was also high with this procedure. Direct intravascular transfusion under ultrasonographic guidance was then described by Bang et al.[4] The intrahepatic portion of the umbilical vein, the umbilical cord at the placental insertion and the fetal heart were the preferential targets of many groups that published their experience with survival rates ranging from 76 to 96%.

The umbilical vein is currently the first choice for intravascular access. The umbilical cord at its placental insertion is first determined. At this point the cord is anchored in a stable fashion, thus making dislodging of the needle difficult. Some prefer to use paralyzing agents in order to stop fetal movements and reduce maternal anxiety, but this is rarely needed. Then with a free-hand technique, a 20- to 22-gauge needle following surgical preparation is introduced into the umbilical vein under continuous ultrasonographic visualization. A sample of fetal blood is obtained to determine the pretransfusion hemoglobin concentration. Irradiated adult packed red cells are then transfused. The amount of blood infused depends on the gestational age, the pretransfusion hemoglobin concentration as well as on the hemoglobin concentration of the donor blood and the desired post-transfusion hemoglobin level. It can be calculated by applying mathematical formulae, usually automatically by computer programs. The blood is transfused at a rate of about 10 ml per minute. It is essential to monitor the turbulence caused by the injected blood in the vessel, so as to confirm proper needle placement. Needle displacement from the vessel can cause fatal tamponade of the vessel with little or no physical sensation by the operator who holds the needle. The fetal heart is periodically checked for the presence of bradycardia or heart enlargement as these are both indications to interrupt the procedure. At the end of the transfusion another fetal blood sample is taken to check the post-transfusion hemoglobin concentration.

The blood for the transfusion should be group O Rh(D) negative, collected during the last 24 hours and cross-matched against the maternal blood. Screening for hepatitis B and C, cytomegalovirus and human immunodeficiency virus (HIV) is necessary. Some centers use maternal blood in order to decrease the risk for sensitization to new red-cell antigens, but this has not been proved to be of any benefit.

Transfusions are repeated based on the post-transfusion fetal hemoglobin level and the observation that the mean fall in fetal hemoglobin following a transfusion is approximately 0.3 gm/dl per day and in fetal hematocrit 1% per day.[5,6] However, there is a wide variation in this, therefore additional criteria should be used to determine the time of the next transfusion. These include weekly ultrasound scans to detect early signs of anemia and middle cerebral artery Doppler to predict fetal hemoglobin concentration.[7] The last transfusion is planned at around 33 to 34 weeks and delivery is aimed at 34 to 38 weeks. The reported survival rate in red cell isoimmunized pregnancies treated with intrauterine intravascular transfusion is more than 84%.[8, 9]

Parvo-virus B19 infection is another usual cause of severe fetal anemia. Following viral infection an arrest of red blood cell precursors maturation and a decrease in the number of platelets can be caused. Heart failure due to myocarditis may also contribute to the development of fetal hydrops. Intensive fetal transfusions are indicated in this case, while if left untreated can lead to intrauterine death in severely affected fetuses.

Fetal Thrombocytopenia

This is a serious disorder, which is caused by maternal IgG antibodies directed against fetal platelet antigens mainly HPA-1a. It occurs in about 1 in 2000 pregnancies, an incidence surprising low considering that 2% of women are HPA-1a negative and that 98% of men are HPA-1a positive. Only 10% of HPA-1a negative women develop anti-HPA-1a. The clinical manifestations include purpura, hematuria and gastrointestinal hemorrhage. Approximately, 10 to 20% of affected neonates will develop intracranial hemorrhage (ICH), with 25 to 50% of these occurring prenatally.[10] It is of particular importance to note that the presence of platelet specific alloantibodies does not necessarily mean that there will be fetal or neonatal thrombocytopenia.

The first affected child is unexpected, and is an otherwise well neonate which has widespread purpura at or soon after birth. The first step is confirmation of isolated thrombocytopenia, and exclusion of other causes of neonatal thrombocytopenia, such as infection, disseminated intravascular coagulation, maternal autoimmune thrombcytopenia and conditions causing impaired neonatal megakaryocytopoiesis. Monitoring of maternal anti-HPA-1a antibodies has not proved to be useful in predicting fetal thrombocytopenia in subsequent pregnancies. The recurrence rate is more than 85% and the disease tends to become more severe. The only method to establish the diagnosis is fetal blood sampling (FBS), which also provides a means for transfusing HPA-1a negative platelets to severely affected fetuses. Women at risk include those with a previous history or those with a sister whose child died due to alloimmunization. Because of the risk of bleeding from the cord puncture site or obstruction of the cord circulation due to hematoma, platelet transfusion is usually given following FBS for suspected thrombocytopenia. The first procedure is performed at around 20 weeks for measurement of platelet count, determination of the platelet group and the detection of platelet-bound antibodies. FBS may be repeated at 28 to 32 weeks if the fetus is not seriously affected. The therapeutic options include maternal administration of intravascular immunoglobulin, corticosteroid therapy and fetal platelet transfusions. Early caesarean section alone is not considered to be effective in preventing antenatal or perinatal haemorrhage. A single pre-delivery transfusion may protect against bleeding at the time of delivery, but the fetus remains at risk of spontaneous intracranial haemorrhage earlier during pregnancy.

The severity of alloimmune thrombocytopenia is based on the previous history of affected pregnancies and the results of FBS. The disease is considered to be mild, moderate or severe if the neonatal platelet count in the previous pregnancy was $>100 \times 10^9/L$, 50 to $100 \times 10^9/L$ or $<50 \times 10^9/L$, respectively. When the disease is mild no intravascular immunoglobulin or steroids are given and FBS is performed at 30 weeks. Similarly no treatment is given for moderate disease but FBS is performed at 20 weeks. If the platelet count is $>100 \times 10^9/L$ a repeated FBS is performed in 10 weeks. If the platelet count is 50 to $100 \times 10^9/L$, then the mother should receive intravascular immunoglobulin and steroids weekly. Another FBS is arranged in 3 weeks. If the platelet count is $<50 \times 10^9/L$ platelet transfusions are given weekly until delivery, which is considered at 34 weeks. In case of a previous history of severe disease, steroids should be given from 16 weeks. All apparently successfully treated infants should have a cranial ultrasound or an MRI performed after birth, and developmental follow-up for at least two years to detect possible neurological impairment, due to occult ICH.

In summary, the development of the optimal antenatal management remains incomplete. Serial fetal platelet transfusions should be the treatment of choice for severely affected cases. Although the transfused platelet life span is about 4 to 5 days, several studies have shown the value of platelet transfusions in raising the platelet count,[11,12] and prevent ICH in severe cases.[13]

Treatment of Obstructive Uropathy

Fetal obstructive uropathies represent a heterogeneous group of developmental abnormalities that might result in significant morbidity and mortality due to progressive renal damage secondary to dysplasia of the kidneys and pulmonary hypoplasia caused by oligo- or anhydramnios. The most common etiologies involve posterior urethral valves, urethral atresia, or prune belly syndrome. Other etiologies may include anterior urethral valves, chromosomal defects, complex genetic syndromes such as megacystis/microcolon syndrome, or partial obstructions or strictures of the urethra.

The treatment of obstructive uropathies depends mainly on the underlying etiology. Intrauterine intervention would not be warranted if a fetus is afflicted with other life-threatening anomaly. Severe oligohydramnios, which persists from 25 weeks' gestation, is associated with neonatal mortality of more than 90%. Before any intervention sonographic evaluation of the fetus, karyotyping and renal function analysis are necessary. A detailed fetal sonographic survey is needed to rule out other anomalies, which would have an impact on the long-term prognosis. The main features of these fetuses include oligohydramnios or anhydramnios, bilateral hydroureters and hydronephrosis, and a thick-walled, enlarged bladder with the characteristic "keyhole" sign associated with proximal urethral distention. The normal bladder wall thickness should not exceed 3 mm. The bladder can become massive, filling the fetal pelvis and abdomen and when the obstruction is long standing there may be evidence of renal dysplasia. Long axis measurement of the kidneys is useful in the evaluation of hydronephrosis. A better prognosis is related to the presence of large for gestational age kidneys, which are less hyperechogenic, whereas the opposite is considered when the kidneys are hyperechogenic and small.[14,15] The presence of cortical cysts is associated with irreversible, advanced renal damage and had a 100% positive predictive value for renal dysplasia.[16] The presence of a severe pyelectasis in the absence of hydroureters may indicate an obstruction at the level of ureteropelvic junction. Female fetuses usually have complex developmental abnormalities of the cloaca, which have a poor prognosis. Therefore, intrauterine treatment is not indicated in these cases. Chromosomal anomalies usually trisomy 21, trisomy 18 and Klinefelter's syndrome, have been reported in 12% of cases of lower urinary tract obstruction[17] and need to be excluded before any intervention. Evaluation of the underlying renal function assists prognostication. Fetuses who demonstrate progressive hypertonicity on urine samples and have urinary sodium more than 100 mcg/L, chloride more than 90 mcg/L, osmolality more than 200 miliosmol/L and β_2 microglobulin more than 6 mg/L, have been shown to have a bad prognosis. Because of difference in these values depending on the gestational age it would be better to use gestationally referenced values. An algorithm which requires three sequential urine samples at 48 to 73 hr intervals has been proposed for better assessment of renal function.[18] Sequential urine sampling improves sensitivity of renal function prediction, but in practice this is only necessary if the first sample predicts poor outcome. However, the use of these markers is debatable, because they have not improved prediction of outcome or the selection of fetuses for fetal therapy.[19] Early diagnosis is crucial for salvage of renal function. Fetal therapy should be done early enough, before renal function become seriously impaired, but optimal criteria for timely intervention have not been established so far. High-field proton nuclear magnetic resonance spectroscopy to quantify low molecular weight metabolites, in fetal urine sample has been proposed,[20] but similarly to the biochemical urine analysis, has poor predictive value in the first half of pregnancy. Ultrasound-guided fetal renal biopsy has not also gained acceptance as a method of detection of renal dysplasia.[21] It can only be obtained in half of cases, and although can predict renal histology, it is not representative of the entire renal parenchyma, as renal dysplasia is distributed patchily.

The aim of intrauterine treatment is to decompress the renal tract, before irreversible damage occurs and to restore the amniotic fluid volume and thus preventing lung hypoplasia. A first approach to treat obstructive uropathy involved hysterotomy, exteriorization of the fetus and open fetal surgery, but this was abandoned because of the high rate of complications.[22] Modern management comprises vesicoamniotic shunting and fetal cystoscopy. The standard technique for shunting involves placing a shunt between the fetal bladder and amniotic cavity under continuous ultrasound guidance. The initial double J-stent[23] was subsequently modified by Rodeck et al into a double pigtail catheter.[24] Sometimes, amnioinfusion prior to the procedure is necessary to assist in sonographic visualization. The appropriate location for shunt placement is below the cord insertion in the midline or just lateral to it. Before entering the bladder color Doppler is used to avoid passage of the needle through the umbilical vessels which course laterally about the bladder. Positioning of the proximal and distal segments of the catheter as well as bladder drainage is confirmed sonographically. In some cases, the stent is placed too high within the bladder and following shrinkage of the bladder it is pulled within the fetal abdomen, resulting in massive urinary ascites. This can be treated ether with placement of a new shunt into the bladder, or with placement of a peritoneoamniotic shunt for continuous diversion of the urine into the amniotic cavity. The most frequent complications include shunt displacement (19%), preterm labor (12%), chorioamnionitis (5%), shunt obstruction, urinary ascites, iatrogenic gastroshisis, and limb contractures.[25,26] After adequate selection criteria an overall neonatal survival of 61% following the procedure, and an associated fetal loss rate of 4.8% were reported.[25,27] However, in the largest series reported so far examining the long-term outcome of fetuses following vesicoamniotic shunting only 54% of them had normal renal function at 2 years of age.[28]

An alternative to shunting technique for obstructive uropathy is percutaneous fetal cystoscopy. It can be used to confirm the diagnosis of posterior urethral valves which can be disrupted by laser.[29] Alternatively, gentler techniques like insertion of a guide wire or pressure saline injection have been described.[30] Laser treatment can also be used to treat other causes of obstruction such as large, prolapsing urethroceles, which if remained untreated may lead to bilateral renal damage. In conclusion, the efficacy of cystoscopy is not proven in humans. The method is limited by technical difficulty in negotiating the urethrovesical angle and it requires further evaluation when equipment modifications facilitate entry into the upper urethra.

Fetal Pleural Effusion

Fetal pleural effusion can be either unilateral or bilateral and may be an isolated finding or associated with fetal hydrops. The etiologies of pleural effusion include fetal aneuploidy, genetic diseases, viral infection, cardiovascular defects, lymphatic anomalies, and fetal anemia. Irrespective of the underlying cause, infants with pleural effusion usually present in the neonatal period with severe respiratory insufficiency due to pulmonary hypoplasia secondary to chronic intrathoracic compression. The natural history of this complication may include spontaneous resolution or progression to fetal hydrops, lung compression, swallowing restriction resulting in polyhydramnios, mediastinal shift of the fetal heart and great vessels and fetal death.

Poor prognostic factors are the presence of hydrops and an early gestational age at diagnosis.[31] The use of *in utero* therapy appears to improve the prognosis. The aim of the fetal therapy is to prolong pregnancy and prevent pulmonary hypoplasia. Thoracocentesis and thoracoamniotic shunting are the two forms of treatment. Fine needle thoracocentesis occasionally may solve the problem, but its main contribution is to establish whether or not the effusion is chylous. In rare cases the effusion will not recur, but in the majority of cases there is a rapid reaccumulation of the fluid and these cases will most likely benefit from continuous drainage through thoracoamniotic shunt placement. In isolated primary fetal pleural effusion a survival rate of 92% following thoraco-amniotic shunting has been reported compared to 50% in untreated cases.[32,33] In the largest single-center series published, 50% of the hydropic and 100% of the non-hydropic fetuses survived.[32] In a systematic review of the literature 99 cases of primary chylothorax were included. All fetuses had hydrops and the survival rate was 66% with shunting, compared to less than 25% without therapy.[34] Two recent studies reporting on thoraco-amniotic shunting for fetal pleural effusions the survival rate was 57% and 58% in the hydropic subgroup and 60% in the non-hydropic subgroup.[35,36]

Follow-up ultrasound evaluation is done 48 to 72 hours following shunt placement to confirm successful function of the catheter, re-expansion of the fetal lungs and restoration of normal mediastinal relationships. Then the patient is rescanned at weekly or longer intervals, depending on the sonographic findings. Complications of the procedure include shunt displacement, migration or obstruction, preterm premature rupture of membranes, and preterm labor, which can cause a poor outcome.

Fetal Drug Therapy

Several fetal pathological conditions have been shown to be amenable to prenatal pharmacologic therapy. The best example is the maternal administration of corticosteroids for the prevention of respiratory distress syndrome in preterm infants. Another example is the treatment of fetal cardiac arrhythmias by administering anti-arrhythmic drugs to the mother. Although temporary arrhythmias are not unusual in the second half of pregnancy, in 1 to 3% of cases are serious enough to jeopardize the outcome of the pregnancy. An exact diagnosis of the rhythm disorder should be made first and a detailed cardiac scan should exclude major fetal cardiac defects. The risks/benefits ratio of the therapy should be carefully calculated and explained to the parents. The mother in any case should stay in a specialized hospital, which can offer not only maternal-fetal monitoring but also postnatal assistance. Digoxin is the drug most commonly used, but in many cases of severe supraventricular tachycardias sotalol and flecainide have been proved more effective. Although the maternal transplacental approach is the most common modality of the drug administration, direct administration to the fetus by intramuscular injection, or by introduction of the drug into the amniotic fluid have been extremely useful.[37]

Fetal hypothyroidism may have severe fetal and neonatal consequences, and it is another condition which can be treated *in utero*. Fetal hypothyroidism can be diagnosed by measuring the levels of free T4, total T4, free T3, total T3 and TSH, following cordocentesis. Intra-amniotic administration of thyroxin at a dose of 10 mg/kg, is the recommended treatment.[38] Congenital adrenal hyperplasia is a group of autosomal recessive disorder which is characterized by enzyme deficiency and increased androgen levels in the fetus. This can cause masculinization in a female fetus. Prenatal diagnosis of the disease can be made by chorionic villus sampling or amniocentesis. Maternal dexamethasone administration can suppress the fetal adrenal glands, thus preventing fetal female genital birth defects.[39]

Sealing of Membranes in Previable Premature Rupture of Membranes

Perinatal mortality of previable preterm premature rupture of membranes (PPROM) is approximately 60%.[40] The main complications include pulmonary hypoplasia and chronic lung disease, cerebral palsy and blindness. Management of cases of spontaneous preterm rupture of membranes before 23 weeks' gestation usually only consists of induction of labor, for the fear of infection and the low likelihood of neonatal survival. However, some cases of preterm premature rupture of membranes can be treated with intra-amniotic injection of platelets and cryoprecipitate. Quintero et al first described a technique for successful treatment of iatrogenic PPROM, which was called "amniopatch".[41] The rationale for the technique was to allow platelets to identify the area of injury and stabilize the clot with cryoprecipitate. Knowledge of the exact location of the defect is not required for the "amniopatch". Platelets and cryoprecipitate are injected under ultrasound guidance in a free pocket of amniotic fluid. The appropriate dose of platelets and cryoprecipitate needs to be established.[42] Preliminary experience with this technique showed that it can seal a defect ranging from 0.72 to 3.8 mm, following iatrogenic PPROM and that the pregnancy can continue uneventfully thereafter. However, initial experience with the use of "amniopatch" in patients who had spontaneous PPROM was unsuccessful.[43] The investigators concluded that the etiology and the clinical behavior of iatrogenic PPROM are different than spontaneous PPROM and this is the reason for the different therapeutic response to the "amniopatch".

In Utero Stem Cell Transplantation

In utero stem cell transplantation is a new approach to the treatment of genetic disorders in the fetus. There are some inherited hematological, immunological, neuromuscular or metabolic disorders, in which transplantation of allogenic stem cells *in utero* could help to reverse pathology and maintain integrity of organs before irreversible damage occurs.

The fetal immune system at an early stage is unable to distinguish between self and non-self antigens. At this stage an HLA-matched donor is not needed for a transplantation. With the maturation of T-cells, a process of negative selection takes place in the thymus. The prenatal exposure to donor antigens during this "window of opportunity" induces tolerance, and their recognition as "self" allowing postnatal cellular therapy from the same donor. It is logical that hematological disorders may be treated with hematopoietic stem cells, abnormal liver function and protein production may be treated by hepatocytes and muscular disorders may be amenable to myoblast therapy. There are some prerequisites for institution of fetal therapy:

A. Known pathophysiology of the disease.
B. Ability to perform prenatal diagnosis in the first trimester.
C. Incomplete amelioration of the disease by postnatal treatment.

So far, *in utero* therapy has been achieved in the group of severe combined immunodeficiencies (SCID).[44] The identification of the relevant cells, as well as the preservation of their function *in vivo* so as to sustain engraftment for a wide range of genetic diseases remains a challenge.

Gene Therapy

Gene therapy is the transfer of an exogeneous normal gene into somatic cells of a patient in an attempt to treat a genetic disease. The success of this treatment has been limited mainly due to low efficiency of gene transfer into the target cells and poor expression of the gene once transferred. Prenatal gene therapy may be more effective than therapy in children and adults. In early pregnancy the fetus seems to be largely tolerant of foreign antigens. Gene transfer to the fetus at this period may induce permanent immune tolerance against vector and the therapeutic gene. Moreover, early treatment could allow the correction of genetic diseases before the appearance of any clinical manifestations. Cystic fibrosis, hemophilia and Duchene muscular dystrophy are some examples of genetic diseases which could be amenable to *in utero* treatment. Currently, termination of pregnancy is offered to parents following prenatal diagnosis of inherited diseases. Prenatal gene therapy would give another choice to the couples of affected fetuses. Many ethical, social and safety concerns are being raised on the use of this treatment. Gene therapy would be an option only if a life-threatening incurable disease is to be cured. Parents must be informed about the procedure, the potential benefits and what types of side effects could be expected. The procedure should be available to everybody, therefore its cost should be low. Currently research focuses on cystic fibrosis, α-thalassemia, hemophilia B, Duchene muscular dystrophy and immunodeficiency disorders.[45,46]

REFERENCES

1. Liley AW. Intrauterine transfusion of fetus in haemolytic disease. BMJ 1963;2:1107-9.
2. Lewis M, Bowman JM, Pollock J, Lowen B. Absorption of red cells from the peritoneal cavity of a hydropic twin. Transfusion 1973;13:37-40.
3. Rodeck CH, Holman CA, Karnicki J, et al. Direct intravascular fetal blood transfusion by fetoscopy in severe rhesus isoimmunisation. Lancet 1981;1:625-7.
4. Bang J, Bock JE, Trolle D. Ultrasound-guided fetal intravascular transfusion for severe rhesus haemolytic disease. BMJ 1982;284:373-4.
5. Nicolini U, Rodeck CH. A proposal scheme for planning intrauterine transfusion in patients with severe Rh-immunization. J Obstet Gynecol 1988;9:162-3.
6. Ronkin S, Chayen B, Wapner RI, et al. Intravascular exchange and bolus transfusion in the severely isoimmunized fetus. Am J Obstet Gynecol 1989;160:407-11.
7. Abdel-Fattah SA, Soothill PW, Carroll SG, Kyle PM. Non-invasive diagnosis of anemia in hydrops fetalis with the use of middle cerebral artery Doppler velocity. Am J Obstet Gynecol 2001;185:1411-5.
8. Queenan JT. Rh-disease: a perinatal success story. Obstet Gynecol 2002;100:405-6.
9. Mesogitis S, Daskalakis G, Pilalis A, Papantoniou N, Antsaklis A. Fetal intravascular transfusion for hydropic disease due to rhesus isoimmunization. Fetal Diagn Ther 2005;20:431-6.
10. Sharif U, Kuban K. Prenatal intracranial hemorrhage and neurologic complications in alloimmune thrompocytopenia. J Child Neurol 2001;16:838-42.
11. Nicolini U, Rodeck CH, Kochenour NK, et al. In utero platelet transfusion for alloimmune thrombocytopenia. Lancet 1988;2:506.
12. Murphy MF, Waters AH, Doughty HA, et al. Antenatal management of fetomaternal alloimmune thrombocytopenia-report of 15 affected pregnancies. Transfusion Med 1994;4:281-92.
13. Murphy MF, Pullon HWH, Metcalfe P, et al. Management of fetal alloimmune thrombocytopenia by weekly *in utero* platelet transfusions. Vox Sang 1990;58:45-9.

14. Mahony BS, Callen PW, Filly RA. Fetal urethral obstruction: US evaluation. Radiology 1985;157:221-4.
15. Crombelholme TM, Harrison MR, Golbus MS, et al. Fetal intervention in obstructive uropathy: prognostic indicators and efficacy of interventions. Am J Obstet Gynecol 1990;162:1239-44.
16. Mahony BS. Fetal renal dysplasia: sonographic evaluation. Radiology 1984;152:143-6.
17. Cusick EL, Didier F, DroullP, Schmitt M. Mortality after an antenatal diagnosis of foetal uropathy. J Pediatr Surg 1995;30:463-6.
18. Johnson MP, Bukowski TP, Reitleman C, Isada NB, Pryde PG, Evans MI. In utero surgical treatment of fetal obstructive uropathy: a new comprehensive approach to identify appropriate candidates for vesicoamniotic shunt therapy. Am J Obstet Gynecol 1994;170:1770-6.
19. Guez S, Assael BM, Melzi ML, Tassis B, Nicolini U. Shortcomings in predicting postnatal renal function using prenatal urine biochemistry in fetuses with congenital hydronephrosis. J Pediatr Surg 1996;31:1401-4.
20. Eugene M, Muller F, Dommergues M, Le Moyec L, Dumez Y. Evaluation of postnatal renal function in fetuses with bilateral obstructive uropathies by proton nuclear magnetic resonance spectroscopy. Am J Obstet Gynecol 1994;170:595-602.
21. Bunduki V, Saldanha LB, Sadeki L, Miguelez J, Miyadahira S, Zugaib M. Fetal renal biopsies in obstructive uropathy: feasibility and clinical correlations-preliminary results. Prenat Diagn 1998;18:101-9.
22. Harrison MR, Golbus MS, Filly RA, et al. Management of the fetus with congenital hydronephrosis. J Pediatr Surg 1982;17:728-42.
23. Golbus MS, Harrison MR, Filly RA, Callen PW, Katz M. In utero treatment of urinary tract obstruction. Am J Obstet Gynecol 1982;142:383-8.
24. Rodeck CH, Fisk NM, Fraser DI, Nicolini U. Long-term in utero drainage of fetal hydrothorax. N Engl J Med 1988;319:1135-8.
25. Elder JS, Duckett Jr JW, Synder HM. Intervention for fetal obstructive uropathy: has it been effective? Lancet 1987;2:1007-10.
26. Chan FY, Borzi P, Cincotta R, Burke J, Tudehope D. Limb constriction as a complication of intra-uterine vesico-amniotic shunt: fetoscopic release. Fetal Diagn Ther 2002;17:315-20.
27. Freedman AL, Bukowski TP, Smith CA, et al. Fetal therapy for obstructive uropathy: diagnosis specific outcomes. J Urol 1996;156:720-4.
28. Freedman AL, Johnson MP, Smith CA, Gonzalez R, Evans MI. Long-term outcome in children after antenatal intervention for obstructive uropathies. Lancet 1999;354:374-7.
29. Quintero RA, Hume R, Smith C, et al. Percutaneous fetal cystoscopy and endoscopic fulguration of posterior urethral valves. Am J Obstet Gynecol 1995;172:206-9.
30. Agarwal SK. Fisk NM. In utero therapy for lower urinary tract obstruction. Prenat Diagn 2001;21:970-6.
31. Weber A, Philipson E. Fetal pleural effusion: A review and meta-analysis for prognostic indicators. Obstet Gynecol 1992;79:281-6.
32. Nicolaides KH, Azar GB. Thoraco-amniotic shunting. Fetal Diagn Ther 1990;5:153-64.
33. Hagay Z, Reece A, Roberts A, Hobbins JC. Isolated fetal pleural effusion: a prenatal management dilemma. Obstet Gynecol 1993;81:147-52.
34. Aubard Y, Derouineau I, Aubard V, Chalifour V, Preux PM. Primary fetal hydrothorax: A literature review and proposed antenatal clinical strategy. Fetal Diagn Ther 1998;13:325-33.
35. Picone O, Benachi A, Mandelbrot L, et al. Thoracoamniotic shunting for fetal pleural effusions with hydrops. Am J Obstet Gynecol 2004;191:2047-50.
36. Smith RP, Illanes S, Denbow ML, Soothill PW. Outcome of fetal pleural effusions treated by thoracoamniotic shunting. Ultrasound Obstet Gynecol 2005;26:63-6.
37. Hansmann M, Gembruch U, Bald R, Manz M, Redel DA. Fetal tachyarrhythmias: transplacental and direct treatment of the fetus: a report of 60 cases. Ultrasound Obstet Gynecol 1991;1:162-70.
38. Hadi HA, Strickland RT. In utero treatment of fetal goitrus hypothyroidism caused by maternal Graves' disease. Am J Perinatol 1995;12:455-8.
39. Pang S, Pollack MS, Marshall RN, Immken L. Prenatal treatment of congenital adrenal hyperplasia due to 21-hydroxylase deficiency. N Engl J Med 1990;322:111-5.
40. Bengston JM, VanMarter LJ, Barss VA, Greene MF, Tuomala RE, Epstein MF. Pregnancy outcome after premature rupture of the membranes at or before 26 weeks' gestation. Obstet Gynecol 1989;73:921-7.
41. Quintero RA, Romero R, Dzieczkowski J, Mammen E, Evans MI. Sealing of ruptured amniotic membranes with intra-amniotic platelet-cryoprecipitate plug. Lancet 1996;347:1117.
42. Quintero R, Morales W, Allen M, Bornick P, Arroyo J, LeParc G. Treatment of iatrogenic previable premature rupture of membranes with intra-amniotic injection of platelets and cryoprecipitate (amniopatch):Preliminary experience. Am J Obstet Gynecol 1999;181:744-9.
43. Quintero R, Morales W, Kalter C, et al. Treatment of preterm premature rupture of membranes with an "amniopatch": preliminary experience. Am J Obstet Gynecol 1998;178:S197.
44. Flake AW, Zanjani ED. In utero hematopoietic stem cell transplantation: ontogenic opportunities and biologic barriers. Blood 1999;94:2179-91.
45. Staff AC. An introduction to gene therapy and its potential prenatal use. Acta Obstet Gynecol Scand 2001;80:485-91.
46. David AL, Themis M, Waddington SN, et al. The current status and future direction of fetal gene therapy. Gene Therapy and Molecular Biology 2003;7:181-209.

CHAPTER 5

Fetoscopy: Current Status

George Daskalakis

INTRODUCTION

Prenatal diagnosis has become increasingly sophisticated as diagnostic capabilities and invasive therapies have been developed since the pathophysiologic understanding of structural abnormalities. The aims of prenatal diagnosis are fourfold:[1]

- The identification at an early gestation of abnormalities incompatible with survival, or likely to result in severe handicap, in order to prepare the parents.
- The identification of conditions which may influence the timing, site or mode of delivery.
- The identification of fetuses who would benefit from early pediatric intervention.
- The identification of fetuses who may benefit from *in utero* treatment.

The last aim was rare due to limitations largely related to the primitive optics and instrumentation. In the modern era of minimally invasive surgery, minimally invasive fetal surgery is feasible due to technological advances. The small uterine puncture sites required for fetoscopic surgery would, in theory, obviate the morbidity of a large hysterotomy used in open fetal surgery. Specifically, the fetoscopic approach could reduce the risk of preterm labor, hemorrhage, amniotic fluid leakage, and uterine rupture, as well as eliminating the need for cesarean delivery after fetal surgery.[2]

DIAGNOSTIC EMBRYO-FETOSCOPY

Embryoscopy and fetoscopy are invasive techniques for direct transuterine visualization of the embryo and the fetus. The first attempt to visualize the fetus with a panendoscope was performed in 1954. Both procedures were developed in the 1970s. Embryoscopy is a term that is appropriate only before 12 weeks of gestation while fetoscopy may be used for procedures at a later gestational age.[3] Embryoscopy was first performed via the transcervical approach in order to obtain a phenotypic diagnosis. Later, percutaneous techniques were developed in order to introduce the fetoscope in the amniotic cavity transabdominally.[2] A diagnostic embryo-fetoscopy can be performed in combination to amniocentesis to add a phenotypic evaluation to the karyotype result. However, the obvious procedure related risks, restrict this approach to families with possible recurrence of genetic conditions associated with external fetal abnormalities, in order to confirm a diagnosis suspected through noninvasive means.[4, 5]

Fetal Muscle Biopsies

Duchenne muscular dystrophy (DMT) is a progressive, degenerative muscle disease, inherited in an X-linked recessive way. Its incidence is estimated to be 1 in 3,500 live-born male infants and is caused by a dystrophin deficiency protein component of muscle tissue. By isolation of the dystrophin gene and its normal protein product, diagnosis can now be achieved on a molecular basis. However, because of the tremendous size of the DMT gene and variation in molecular abnormalities, the underlying gene defect, usually a deletion has been able to be identified in only 65% of the affected individuals. In such a case, female carriers can be identified with molecular testing and future male pregnancies can be tested for that specific families gene defect. In 1991, the first case of *in utero* fetal muscle biopsy for DMD diagnosis was described in a family in which the carrier status of the mother could not be determined. Using a renal biopsy device directed into the fetal buttock by ultrasound guidance, a skeletal muscle biopsy was obtained for analysis and was shown to contain normal amount of dystrophin protein. The pregnancy continued and delivered at term, and the infant was confirmed to have normal dystrophin postnatally. Since then, more pregnancies have undergone *in utero* diagnosis using fetal muscle biopsy. Several procedures have been performed under combined ultrasound and fetoscopic guidance. Nevertheless, the benefits of fetoscopic over ultrasound-guided muscle biopsy remain unproven, and most procedures are now performed with ultrasound alone.[2]

THERAPEUTIC FETOSCOPY

Diaphragmatic Hernia

Congenital diaphragmatic hernia (CDH) is a simple anatomic defect in the diaphragm. Severe CDH has high associated morbidity and mortality rates because of pulmonary hypoplasia and secondary pulmonary hypertension, due to herniation of the abdominal contents into the thoracic cavity. Despite advances in neonatal therapy, little impact on mortality rates has been observed among severely affected infants as no postnatal treatment modality, at the present time can specifically address or reverse the underlying pathogenesis of pulmonary hypoplasia. The rationale for prenatal therapy is to prevent or reverse pulmonary hypoplasia and to restore adequate lung growth for neonatal survival.[6] This technique has been tested in animal models successfully[7] so the Children's Hospital of Philadelphia published recently outcomes from a prospective study examining only the results of open tracheal occlusion. This study showed that in high risk fetuses with a 90% predicted mortality, *in utero* treatment resulted in impressive lung growth, although out of 13 patients there were only 5 long term survivors due to pulmonary function abnormalities and as consequence of prematurity.[6] The University of California at San Francisco (UCSF) group published also recently results from a retrospective study[8] showing that endoscopic techniques were effective at enlarging the hypoplastic lungs, reducing the viscera into the abdomen, and improving lung function and survival.

Nevertheless, complications regarding tracheal dissection, recurrent herniation and problems associated with preterm labor and preterm rupture of membranes necessitated development of the endoluminal balloon tracheal occlusion techique.[9] Using simultaneous realtime ultrasonography and fetal bronchoscopy through a single port, they placed a detachable balloon in the trachea of 2 fetuses with severe CDH. In both fetuses, the fetal lung subsequently enlarged, allowing survival after birth. This technique is being evaluated in an NIH-sponsored prospective randomized clinical trial comparing fetoscopic endoluminal balloon/ FETENDO clip tracheal occlusion to conventional postnatal therapy.[2] Tracheal occlusion increases the pressure in the tracheobronchial tree, accelerating pulmonary growth. It is performed in cases with a poor prognosis, and involves the percutaneous insertion of a balloon into the fetal trachea, with direct tracheoscopy. The balloon is then withdrawn either before, or at the time of the delivery.

Sacrococcygeal Teratoma

Sacrococcygeal teratoma (SCT) is the most common tumor in newborns occurring approximately in 1 in 35,000 live births. Although the actual rate is unknown due to the high rate of fetal loss from spontaneous demise or elective termination, the true incidence is estimated to be as high as 1 in 10,000 pregnancies with a striking female to male ratio of approximately 4:1.[10] SCT is usually benign and the primary cause of the rare deaths in postnatal cases results from malignant invasion. In contrast, prenatal SCT cases develop complications due to prematurity and exsanguinating tumor hemorrhage at delivery.[2]

Routine prenatal ultrasound has improved the diagnosis of SCT based on recognition of a characteristic sacral or intrapelvic mass. The most common indication is for a uterus large for gestational age secondary to polyhydramnios or rapid tumor enlargement. Recently, MRI has been also used for diagnosis and assessment of fetal SCT with no proven benefit over the sonographic approach.[11] Mintz et al reported the first fetal intervention for SCT in 1983 as needle aspiration of a large cystic mass. This intervention was performed to reduce the risk of dystocia at birth and was not indicated by the presence of fetal hydrops. Langer et al reported the first prenatal resection for fetal salvage and hydrops in 1989 with unfavorable outcome. Azdick et al reported the first successful fetal resection for SCT and hydrops in 1997. A 25 weeks' gestation fetus was identified as having a large SCT, hydrops, and placentomegaly. Additionally, the mother demonstrated signs of impeding mirror syndrome. Maternal laparotomy and hysterotomy was performed and the tumor was resected with a 90 mm surgical stapler. Fetal hydrops resolved and mother and fetus did well until 29 weeks' gestation when preterm labor mandated early cesarean section. The infant did well and underwent a second operation to fully resect the mass and coccyx.[12] Hescher et al reported minimally invasive fetoscopic treatment in 1996. This pregnancy was complicated by polyhydramnios and despite two attempts at 20 and 26 weeks' gestation, the tumor feeding vessels were ablated unsuccessfully. The fetus was delivered by elective cesarean section at 37 weeks' gestation and did well with postnatal resection.[12]

Radiofrequency ablation (RFA) has been used to coagulate feeding vessels to the SCT, in order to reverse the high-output state, under ultrasound guidance. The power of the RFA could not be accurately controlled and the fetus suffered soft tissue injury (necrosis of the anus, vagina, bladder), with damage to the sciatic nerve.[13] Finally, thermo-coagulation of fetal sacrococcygeal teratoma in order to disrupt blood flow to the tumor has been reported as an alternative minimally invasive technique by Lam et al in 2002. Unfortunately, the fetal outcome was unfavorable.[14]

In conclusion, minimally invasive techniques can potentially reduce the risk of premature rupture of membranes and premature labor, so future studies are required. Safer application of RFA and/or fetoscopic resection of fetal SCT with hydrops could be anticipated.

Amniotic Band Syndrome

Amniotic band syndrome (ABS) is a sporadic condition that occurs in approximately 1 in 1.200 to 1 in 15.000 live births. Although the exact cause is unknown, early rupture of the amnion resulting in bands that insert on the body of the fetus is considered the most accepted view. The bands may lead to amputations, constrictions and other fetal deformities.[15] The earliest that amniotic bands have been diagnosed is 12 gestational weeks by transvaginal ultrasound, although ABS is more often diagnosed by the effect of the bands on fetal anatomy such as absent digits, or portion of the limbs, a swollen distal arm or leg.[16] In such a case, fetoscopic lysis of amniotic bands can be lifesaving.

Quintero et al reported two cases of fetuses with ABS associated limb constriction in which the amniotic band was surgically interrupted to avoid spontaneous amputation of the extremity. Adequate blood flow distal to the obstruction was preserved and significant functional improvement of the extremity occurred in both cases, preserving the limbs.[15] Few more cases have been reported, establishing the fetoscopic feasibility releasing amniotic bands involving the extremities and umbilical cord.

Myelomeningocele

Myelomeningocele is the most common congenital malformation of the central nervous system. It results from a defect in the process of neurulation. During the fourth gestational week, the neural placode folds around itself to form the neural tube. In myelomeningocele this process fails resulting in a defect of the skin and the dorsal spinal elements associated with a central sac containing cerebrospinal fluid and a dysmorphic spinal cord and its associated nerve roots. Patients with myelomeningocele, suffer from some degree of lower extremity or bladder and sphincteric weakness and sensory deficits. In addition, hydrocephalus and Chiari type II malformation are noted.[17]

Despite reductions in the incidence of the disease based on the widespread use of folic acid supplementation, the treatment timing remains critical. It was noted that exposure of the already malformed spinal cord tissue to the intrauterine environment might lead to secondary neurological damage. Keeping this in mind, a group from Vanderbilt University attempted an open intrauterine myelomeningocele repair (IUMR). The uterus was exteriorized and three fetoscopic ports were placed, one for the fetoscope and two operative ports. A maternal split-thickness skin graft was placed over the myelomeningocele defect using Surgicel and fibrin glue in four patients between 22 and 24 weeks of gestation.[18] Despite the initial disappointing results, a collaborative study[19] comparing 104 patients who had undergone intrauterine myelomeningocele repair and 189 conventionally treated patients concluded that the IUMR reduces the incidence of shunt-dependent hydrocephalus in properly selected patients and that Chiari malformation patients appear improved. As the above mentioned conclusion was based in comparison with a historic control, organization of an RCT was thought appropriate to determine the potential benefit of prenatal over conventional treatment. The National Institute of Child Health and Human development designed and funded the above mentioned RCT named Management of Myelomeningocele Study (MOMs)[20] that began early in 2003. If the RCT proves the benefit of intrauterine repair, future effort will be expected to focus on the refinement of the technique. Robot-assisted surgery holds a promising position toward this direction.

Fetoscopic Treatment in Twin-twin Transfusion Syndrome

The most common cause of severe polyhydramnios in twins is twin-twin transfusion syndrome (TTTS). In this case excessive amniotic fluid volume is observed in one of the twins, while severe oligohydramnios is found in the other. TTTS is the major complication of monochorionic (MC) twin pregnancy, which has an extremely high perinatal mortality and morbidity if left untreated. TTTS complicates up to 20% of diamniotic MC twin pregnancies and accounts for 15 to 20% of perinatal mortality in twins.

The presumed mechanism is blood shunting from one fetus (the donor) to the other (recipient) via placental anastomoses. The woman presents with acute polyhydramnios in a MC twin pregnancy during the mid-to-late second trimester. This acute polyhydramnios leads to preterm labor, premature rupture of the membranes, and high perinatal mortality if no action is taken.[21] The donor twin is characterized by oliguria, oligohydramnios or anhydramnios, growth restriction and abnormal umbilical artery Doppler velocimetry. The recipient, on the other hand, is characterized by polyuria, polyhydramnios, abnormal venous Dopplers, cardiac enlargement/failure, and eventually hydrops.

Sonographic criteria suggestive of TTTS include:

1. Monochorionicity.

2. Discrepancy in amniotic fluid between the amniotic sacs with polyhydramnios of one twin (largest vertical pocket > than 8 cm) and oligohydramnios of the other (largest vertical pocket < than 2 cm).
3. Small or no bladder visualized in twin with oligohydramnios.
4. Large bladder visualized in twin with polyhydramnios.
5. Discrepancy in size of the umbilical cords.
6. Presence of cardiac dysfunction in the polyhydramniotic twin.
7. Characteristically abnormal umbilical artery or ductus venosus Doppler velocimetry.
8. Less specifically, significant growth discordance (often >20%).

Additionally to the common sonographic criteria for TTTS, Quintero et al proposed a staging system.[22]

Stage I: The bladder of the donor twin is still visible.

Stage II: The bladder of the donor twin is no longer visible (in >60 min of observation). This fetus is in renal failure.

Stage III: Critically abnormal Doppler studies characterized by absent or reverse end-diastolic velocity in the umbilical artery, or pulsatile umbilical venous flow, or reverse flow in the ductus venosus in either twin.

Stage IV: Hydrops of one or both fetuses.

Stage V: Demise of one or both fetuses.

Treatment of TTTS has always been controversial. Expectant management has been associated with almost 100% perinatal mortality.[23] In stage I patients, expectant management is possible as long as the degree of polyhydramnios is not too large (maximum vertical pocket around 8-9 cm) and the cervical length is adequate (2.5 cm).

Amnioreduction

Amnioreduction was first used as a mean to control polyhydramnios and prolong the pregnancy. The goal of serial amniocentesis is to decrease the likelihood of miscarriage or preterm labor by reducing the amniotic fluid volume in the sac of the recipient twin. In addition, amnioreduction improves uteroplacental blood flow, likely by reduction of pressure from the amniotic fluid. Moise et al in a review paper dating from 1930s, found an overall survival of 49%.[24] Clearly the survival rate varies directly proportional to the severity of TTTS. The earlier in gestation TTTS presents, the worse the prognosis; conversely, the later in gestational age TTTS presents, the better the prognosis.[25] Mari et al found that patients presenting with advanced TTTS prior to 22 weeks' gestation and absent end-diastolic flow in the recipient umbilical artery had a survival of both twins with aggressive amnioreduction of only 13% and with absent end-diastolic flow in the donor umbilical artery, survival was 33%.[25]

Septostomy

Iatrogenic disruption of the dividing membrane (septostomy) is performed in an attempt to equilibrate the pressure between the two amniotic cavities. Saade et al reported the results of a prospective multicenter randomized clinical trial comparing amnioreduction to septostomy.[26] The survival in each arm of the study was 65% consistent with the notion that the effect of amnioreduction may be inadvertent septostomy. However, this theory has not been proved and many arguments to this practice have been made.[27]

Umbilical Cord Occlusion

Umbilical cord occlusion technique stops blood exchange between the fetuses at the level of the umbilical cord of one of the twins. This can be accomplished by ligating the umbilical cord endoscopically, under ultrasound guidance, or by using bipolar electrocautery under ultrasound guidance. This procedure is reserved for severe cases in which spontaneous fetal death of one of the twins is likely to happen, particularly with the presence of hydrops.[27]

Laser Treatment

Fetoscopic laser treatment was used to eliminate blood exchange between the fetuses, allowing each fetus to continue the pregnancy on its own. De Lia et al reported a survival rate of 53% in 26 patients.[28] Although survival was not significantly better compared to amnioreduction, 96% of survivors had a normal neurologic outcome. Ville et al reported a 53% survival with a nonselective laser technique, with an improved neurological outcome in comparison to serial amnioreduction.[29]

In 1998, selective laser photocoagulation of communicating vessels (SLPCV) was described by Quintero et al.[30] According to the described technique, each placental artery is followed to its terminal end in the placenta (arteries cross over veins). A returning vein from that cotyledon should normally drain back to the same twin. If blood is drained to the other twin, deep arteriovenous anastomoses (AV) are present. Arterio-arterial or veno-venous anastomoses are identified easily by noting lack of a terminal end for an artery or a vein, respectively. SLPCV is associated with an 85% success rate (likelihood that at least one fetus survives) and a 3 to 5% risk of cerebral palsy. Additionally, it compares favorably with the previous nonselective technique, resulting in lower rate of dual fetal demise (5.6% versus 22% respectively). The advantages of laser coagulation lie in the prospect of a causal therapy through a single intervention, and the rate of survival appears higher and the handicap rate lower than after amniodrainage alone.

The Eurofoetus consortium conducted a study investigating the efficacy of laser coagulation of anastomoses and serial amniodrainage as a primary therapy for severe, mid-gestational twin-to-twin transfusion syndrome. Study results have been presented at the 24th Annual Meeting of the Society for Maternal Fetal Medicine in New Orleans.[31] Among a total of 142 patients enrolled in the study, 6-month survival rate of at least one of the twins was significantly higher in the laser group (76.4%) than in the amniodrainage group (51.4%). A higher median gestational age at birth and birth weight were observed in the laser group (33.3 vs 29.0 weeks and 1,757 gm vs 1,359 gm respectively). Periventricular leukomalacia was less frequent (5.6% vs 14.5%), and survival rate without major neurological morbidity at 6 months was found to be higher in the laser group as well (50% vs 29.8%). The study concluded that endoscopic laser coagulation of chorionic plate vascular anastomoses is a more effective first-line treatment of severe twin to twin transfusion syndrome before 26 weeks' than serial amniodrainage improving survival and neurologic outcome at six months of life.[32]

These findings suggest a stage tailored treatment scheme for TTTS. Stage I and possibly stage II patients (>22 weeks) could be treated by serial amniocentesis, whereas stage III and stage IV patients are probably best treated with SLPCV.[33] In any case, individualized management of a TTTS case is required considering every aspect of the presentation including gestational age, stage, Doppler findings, echocardiographic findings, concomitant placental insufficiency, and maternal risk factors. A judicious application of invasive procedures should be employed in order to optimize the risk-benefit ratio for mother and fetus.

REFERENCES

1. Magowan B. Obstetrics and Gynaecology (2nd edition). Churchill Livingstone, 2002;2.
2. Crombleholme T, Johnson M. Fetoscopic Surgery. Clin Obstet Gynecol 2003;46:76-91.
3. Ville Y, Dumez Y. Endoscopy in fetal medicine. Ville Y, Barki G, Bui TH, Hecher K, Dumez Y, Nicilini U (Eds). The EUROFETUS Group, 2002, Chapter 1: 7-8.
4. Ville Y. Diagnostic embryoscopy and fetoscopy in the first trimester of pregnancy. Prenat Diagn 1997; 17:1237-46.
5. Miliou-Paouleskou D, Antsaklis A, Papantoniou N, et al. First trimester transabdominal embryo fetoscopy. Early Pregn 2001;5(1):36-7.
6. Flake A, Crombleholme T, Jonshon M, et al. Treatment of severe congenital diaphragmatic hernia by fetal tracheal occlusion: clinical experience with fifteen cases. Am J Obstet Gynecol 2000;183:1059-66.
7. DiFiore JW, Fauza DO, Slavin R, et al. Experimental fetal tracheal ligation reverses the structural and physiological effects of pulmonary hypoplasia in congenital diaphragmatic hernia. J Pediatr Surg 1994;29:248
8. Harrison MR, Mychaliska GB, Albanese CT, et al. Correction of congenital diaphragmatic hernia in utero. IX. Fetuses with poor prognosis (liver herniation and low lung-to-head ratio) can be saved by fetoscopic temporary tracheal ocllusion. J Pediatr Surg 1998;33:1017-22.
9. Harrison MR, Albanese CT, Hawgood SB, et al. Fetoscopic temporary tracheal occlusion by means of detachable ballon for congenital diaphragmatic hernia. Am J Obstet Gynecol 2001;185:730-3.

10. Tuladhar R, Patole SK, Whitehall JS. Sacrococcygeal teratoma in the perinatal period. Postgrad Med J 2000;76:754-9.
11. Avni FE, Guibaud L, Robert Y, et al. MR imaging of fetal sacrococcygeal teratoma: diagnosis and assessment. AJR Am J Roentgenol 2002;178:179-83.
12. Hirose S, Farmer D. Fetal surgery for sacrococcygeal teratoma. Clin Perinatol 2003;30:493-506.
13. Paek BW, Jennings RW, Harrison MR, et al. Radiofrequency ablation of human fetal sacrococcygeal teratoma. Am J Obstet Gynecol 2001;184;503-7.
14. Lam YH, Tang MH, Shek TW. Thermocoagulation of fetal sacrococcygeal teratoma. Prenat Diagn 2002;22:99-100.
15. Quintero R, Morales W, Philips J, et al. In utero lysis of amniotic bands. Ultrasound Obstet Gynecol 1997;10:316-20
16. Lockwood C, Ghidini A, Romero R, et al. ABS: reevaluation of its pathogenesis. Am J Obstet Gynecol 1989;160:1030-3.
17. Tulipan N. Intrauterine myelomeningocele repair. Clin Perinatol 2003;30:521-30.
18. Bruner JP, Richards WO, Tulipan N, et al. Endoscopic coverage of fetal myelomeningocele in utero. Am J Obstet Gynecol 1999;180:153-8.
19. Tulipan N, Sutton LN, Bruner JP, et al. The effect of intrauterine myelomeningocele repair on the incidence of shunt-dependent hydrocephalus. Pediatr Neurosurg 2003;38(1):27-33.
20. National Institute of Child Health and Human Development. Management of myelomeningocele study. 2003. www.spinabifidamoms.com
21. Cincota RB, Fisk NM. Current thoughts on twin-twin transfusion syndrome. Clin Obstet Gynecol 1997;20(2):290-302.
22. Quintero R, Morales W, Allen M, et al. Staging of twin-twin transfusion syndrome. J Perinatol 1999;19:550-5.
23. Weir P, Ratten G, Beischner N. Acute Polyhydramnios: a complication of monozygous twin pregnancy. Br J Obstet Gynecol 1979;86:849-53.
24. Moise KJ Jr. Polyhydramnios: problems and treatment. Semin perinatol 1993;17:197-209.
25. Mari G, Roberts A, Detti L, et al. Perinatal morbidity and mortality rates in severe twin-twin transfusion syndrome: results of the International Registry. Am J Obstet Gynecol 2001;185:708-15.
26. Saade G, Moise K, Dorman K, et al. A randomized trial of septostomy versus amnioreduction an the treatment of twin oligohydramnios polyhydramnios sequence (TOPS). Am J Obstet Gynecol 2003;SMFM Abstracts:187(6).
27. Quintero R. Twin-twin transfusion syndrome. Clin Perinatol 2003; 30:591-600.
28. De Lia JE, Kuhlmann RS, Harstad RW, Cruikshank DP. Fetoscopic laser ablation of placental vessels in severe twin-twin transfusion syndrome. Am J Obstet Gynecol 1995;172:1202-11.
29. Ville Y, Hyett J, Hecher K, Nicollaides KH. Preliminary experience with endoscopic laser surgery for severe twin-twin transfusion syndrome. N Engl J Med 1995;332:224-7.
30. Quintero R, Morales W, Mendoza G, et al. Selective photocoagulation of placental vessels in twin-twin transfusion syndrome: evolution of a surgical technique. Obstet Gynecol Surv 1998;53:s97-103.
31. Senat MV, Deprest J, Boulvain M. Fetoscopic laser surgery versus serial amniodrainage in the management of severe twin-to-twin transfusion syndrome at midgestation. A randomized controlled trial. Am J Obstet Gynecol 2003;SMFM Abstracts:S56.
32. Senat MV, Deprest J, Boulvain M. Endoscopic laser surgery versus serial amniodrainage for severe twin-to-twin transfusion syndrome. N Engl J Med 2004;351:136-44.
33. Quintero R, Dickinson J, Morales W, et al. Stage-based treatment of twin-twin transfusion syndrome. Am J Obstet Gynecol 2003;188:1333-40.

CHAPTER

6

Celocentesis: An Alternative Technique for Prenatal Diagnosis

George Makrydimas

INTRODUCTION

First trimester invasive prenatal diagnosis can be performed by chorionic villous sampling (CVS) or early amniocentesis. However, the risk of limb reduction syndrome and oromandibular hypoplasia associated with very early CVS and the higher risk of miscarriage and talipes, when early amniocentesis is performed, have limited their use after 10 and 15 weeks respectively (Firth et al 1994, Nicolaides et al 1994).

The need for earlier diagnosis essentially centers around two issues. Firstly, earlier reassurance of parents that the fetus is normal and safer termination in cases of affected fetuses. Termination can now be performed successfully in over 90% of the cases with the use of misoprostol when it is administered prior to the ninth week of gestation (Singh et al 2003). Secondly, the potential for intrauterine corrective therapy, such as stem cell transplantation, because after 11 weeks the fetus becomes immunologically intolerant.

In the first 10 weeks of pregnancy celomic fluid surrounds the amniotic sac. Celocentesis is a new technique, which involves the ultrasound guided insertion of a needle into the extra-amniotic cavity through the vagina, from as early as six weeks gestation (Jurcovic et al 1993). Several studies have reported successful transvaginal aspiration of celomic fluid and proved the feasibility of the use of this fluid in prenatal diagnosis. Moreover, this technique may be safer than CVS or amniocentesis because it does not necessitate puncture of the placenta or the amniotic sac.

Numerous studies during the last 15 years examined the early fetal physiology, the potential of prenatal diagnosis and the safety of celocentesis. This chapter reviews the main findings of these studies focusing in prenatal diagnosis.

EMBRYOLOGY

At days 11 and 12 post-conception, a new population of cells appears between the inner surface of the cytotrophoblast and the membrane which lines the primary yolk sac (Heuser's membrane). These cells, which are derived from the yolk sac, form a fine, loose connective tissue, the extraembryonic mesoderm, which eventually fills all the space between the trophoblast externally and the amnion and Heuser's membrane internally. The celomic or extraembryonic cavity develops during the fourth week of gestation, within the extraembryonic mesoderm which surrounds the bilaminar embryonic disk. The developing celomic cavity splits the extraembryonic mesoderm in two layers the somatic and splanchnic mesoderm.

At 13 days post-conception, cells from the hypoblast (small cuboidal cells adjacent to the primary yolk sac) migrate along Heauser's membrane, proliferate, and gradually form the secondary yolk sac. During the formation of the secondary yolk sac, large portions of the cavity of the primary sac are pinched off and they can be found in the celomic cavity as exocelomic cysts. The embryo is suspended in the celomic cavity by means of the connecting stalk (which, with development of blood vessels, becomes the umbilical cord). During the first nine weeks of gestation, the celomic cavity is the largest space inside the gestational sac (Figure 6.1).

The use of high resolution transvaginal ultrasound probes allowed a more accurate examination of the early pregnancy. The visualization of the membranes separating the amniotic and celomic cavity made possible the selective aspiration of celomic fluid from as early as five weeks gestation.

CELOCENTESIS

The patient is placed in lithotomy position. The external genitalia and the vagina are carefully cleansed with an antiseptic solution. Subsequently, transvaginal sonography, with a 5 MHz ultrasound transducer covered with a sterile rubber, was performed. The fetal crown-rump length and fetal heart rate are measured, and the amniotic membrane, celomic space and yolk sac are identified. A 20 G needle is then introduced transvaginally into the celomic cavity, through a guide attached to the transducer and fluid is aspirated (Figure 6.2). Celocentesis is performed immediately prior to surgical termination of pregnancy under general anesthesia. When the safety of the technique is examined no local or general anesthesia is used and patients feel only minimal discomfort. The first sample of 0.2 ml is discarded to avoid contamination with maternal tissue and a new syringe is then used to aspirate 1 to 2 ml which was used for analysis.

STUDIES ON PHYSIOLOGY

Numerous studies have shown that the celomic fluid is essentially an ultrafiltrate of the maternal plasma, with the addition of substances derived by the trophoblast, the membranes, the yolk sac and the

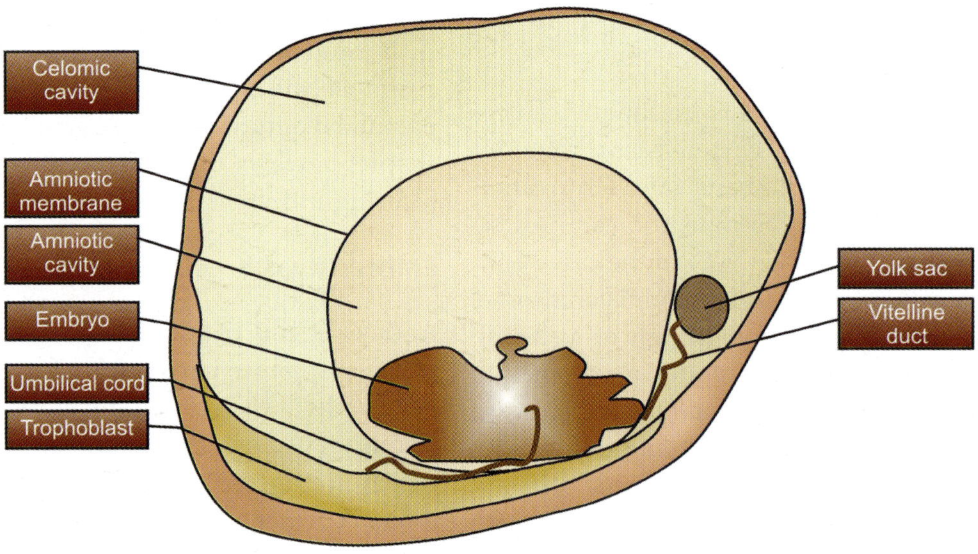

Figure 6.1: Schematic representation of human pregnancy at seven weeks' gestation

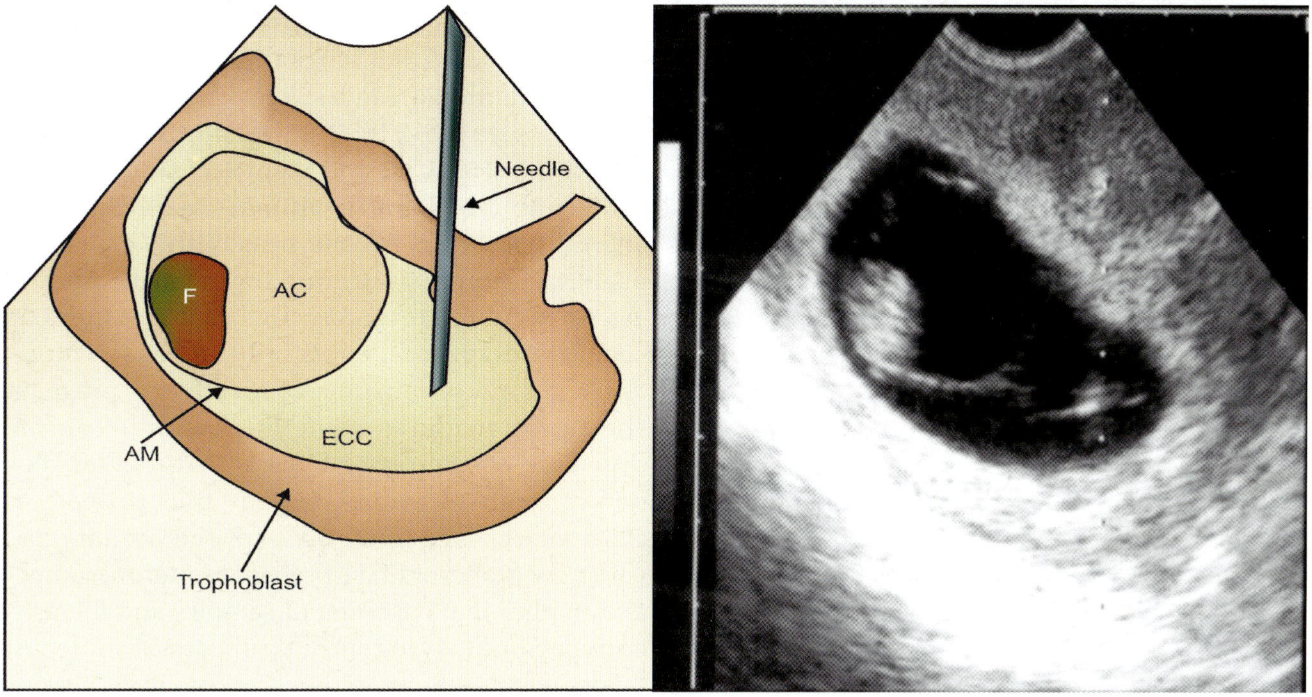

Figure 6.2: Schematic representation and ultrasound image of celocentesis. F = fetus, AC = amniotic cavity, EAC = extra-amniotic cavity, T = trophoblast, AM = amniotic membrane, N = needle

embryo (Jauniaux and Gulbis 2000). Cells from the trophoblast, the membranes, the yolk sac and probably the embryo itself are shed in the celomic cavity and can be found in the celomic fluid.

The celomic cavity is in direct contact with the villous trophoblast, with no anatomical barrier between them, and substances produced in the trophoblast (especially the villous trophoblast) appear in markedly higher concentrations in the celomic fluid that in the maternal serum. There is also transportation of substances between the celomic cavity and yolk sac, with the yolk sac mainly absorbing molecules from the celomic fluid and transferring them to the fetus. Celomic fluid can thus be the optimal medium for measurement of placental products in early pregnancy.

The transfer of substances between the celomic fluid and the embryo appears to take place principally at the level of the yolk sac. The main flux of molecules occurs from outside the yolk sac (i.e. from the celomic cavity) in the direction to the lumen and subsequently to the embryonic gut and circulation. The direct (i.e. through the amniotic membrane) transfer of molecules between the celomic and the amniotic cavity is restricted according to the molecular weight of each substance. The concentration of larger molecules such as proteins is higher in the celomic than in the amniotic fluid (from 2 to 50 times, depending on the molecular weight of each protein investigated), while small molecules such as urea have similar levels in the two compartments (Gulbis et al 1992).

The concentration of placental products (e.g. hCG, hPL activin-A, etc) is higher in the celomic fluid than in both the maternal serum and amniotic fluid. This is explained by the close anatomical relationship between the trophoblast and the amniotic fluid.

Celocentesis was also used to study the pathophysiology of early pregnancy failure. For example leptin was measured in the celomic fluid amniotic fluid and maternal serum in pregnancies undergoing termination for phychological reasons and missed miscarriages (Makrydimas et al 2005). In the pregnancies with missed miscarriage the median celomic fluid leptin concentration was increased. This finding suggests that embryonic death was presumably preceded by placenta hypoxia-related increased production of leptin. Previous studies have reported that in pregnancies with severe pre-eclampsia maternal serum levels of leptin are increased and placental expression of leptin mRNA is markedly augmented. This has been attributed to the associated impaired uteroplacental perfusion and consequent hypoxia, which augments leptin gene expression. The same mechanism may also be true in at least some pregnancies resulting in early embryonic death.

PRENATAL DIAGNOSIS FROM CELOMIC CELLS

Several studies reported on the feasibility of prenatal diagnosis using celomic cells. In terms of standard cytogenetic cultures, although initial reports have been disappointing (Jurkovic et al 1993), Cruger et al (1996) reported successful culture and cytogenetic analysis of 9 out of 10 samples of celomic fluid. However, these results were never reproduced by another study. Recently, a study in baboons reported successful karyotyping using the standard techniques in five out of nine cases at 36 to 42 days of gestation (Santolaya Forgas et al 2005). The authors of this study concluded that at this stage of pregnancy there are living cells in the celomic cavity and improvements in the cytogenetic techniques may increase the success rates in karyotyping.

In fact the results of the first published study, from the group of Nicolaides in London (Jurcovic et al 1993) have shown that although the standard cytogenetic techniques for fetal karyotyping cannot be used successfully, the fetal sex can be determined using FISH or PCR. In all 20 fetuses examined, the results were concordant between celomic cells and trophoblast. However, Pandya et al (1995) used FISH to determine the fetal sex in 32 samples of celomic fluid. Although fetal sex was always concordant between celomic fluid and trophoblast, the determination was not possible in four (12.5%) of the celomic samples. Lau et al (1998) used PCR for determination of fetal sex and found that the concordance between the celomic and fetal samples in 35 cases was 91%. Nevertheless, a recent study (Chatzimeletiou et al 2005) examining 12 celomic fluid samples demonstrated successful analysis of 11 chromosomes using FISH in uncultured cells (Figure 6.3). The fact that interphase molecular cytogenetics can accurately identify numerical chromosomal aberrations opens up the possibility of analysing prenatal samples without the need to undergo extensive culture protocols. This enables a quick and accurate diagnosis, especially in cases where a decision for a termination of an affected pregnancy should be made as soon as possible. The only drawback of interphase FISH is that it is unable to detect translocations when the probes are centromeric. The latter stresses the limitations of using centromeric FISH probes in interphase nuclei and implies that culturing of samples and the use of conventional cytogenetics or other molecular cytogenetic techniques like comparative genomic hybridization (CGH) or microarrays might be mandatory for accurate diagnosis. CGH and microarrays do not require cells in metaphase and can screen the whole genome for global gains and losses. CGH has been successfully applied on chorionic villus samples and amniocytes (Lestou et al 2000; Tabet et al 2001) and in the future both CGH and microarrays may be used for the analysis of celomic samples.

Jauniaux et al (2003) employed quantitative fluorescence PCR in 17 samples of celomic fluid. They used several markers for chromosomes X, Y, 21, 18 and 13. Prenatal detection of the fatal sex was successful in all cases. Moreover, in one case with trisomy 13 the results from the celomic fluid were concordant to those of the placenta. Seven samples contained only fetal DNA, while in the remaining eight there were also small amounts of maternal DNA that did not interfere with the QF PCR analysis. It appears that QF PCR, which requires very small amounts of DNA may be useful in aneuploidy screening in celomic fluid samples.

Amplification of DNA extracted from celomic cells has been successfully used to identify single gene disorders, such as sickle cell anemia (Jurkovic et al 1995, Makrydimas et al 2004), β-thalassemia

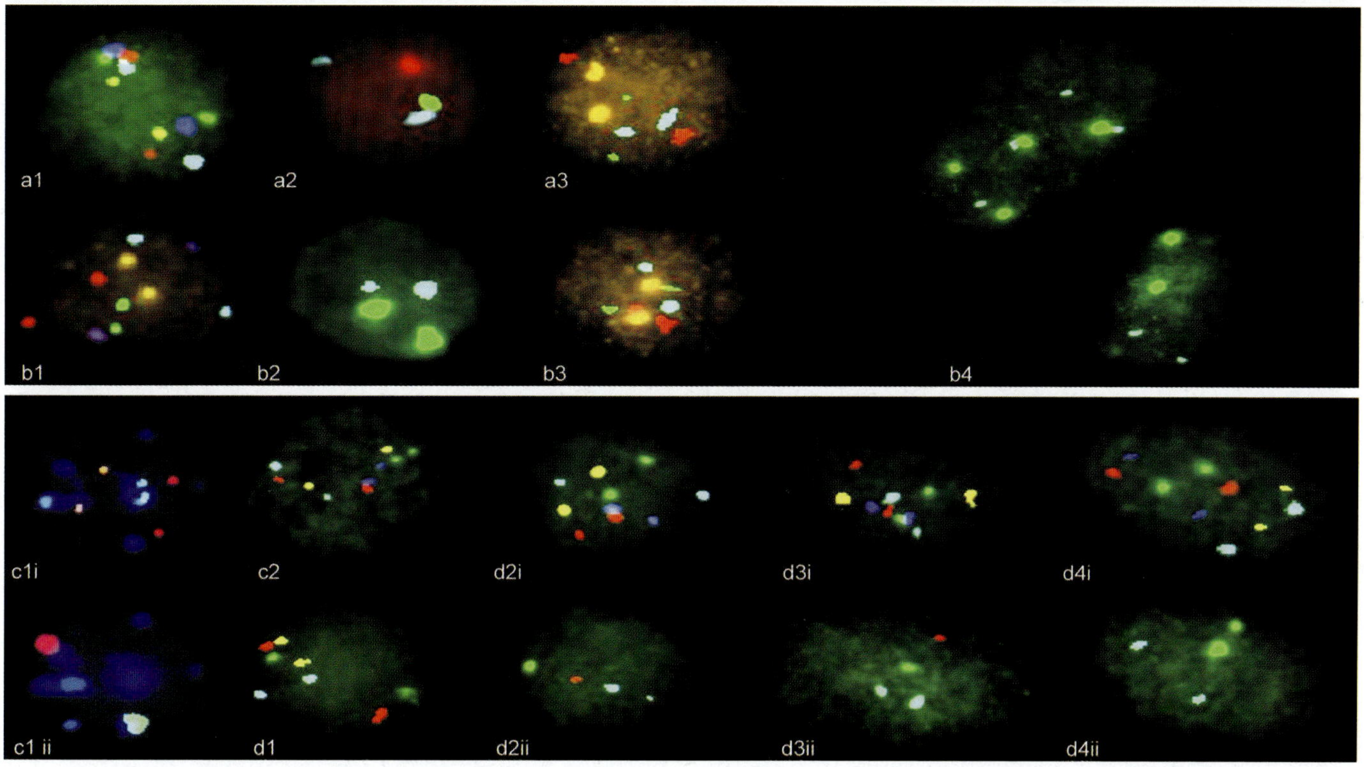

Figure 6.3: Photomicrographs showing fluorescence *in situ* hybridization on celomic fluid samples and placental tissue

(Makrydimas et al 1997, Makrydimas et al 2004), and Marfan syndrome (Makrydimas et al 2004). In addition DNA analysis of the TPO and Apo B loci was used for paternity testing in 20 samples of celomic fluid. There was concordance between the results of the celomic fluid and the placental samples; in 2 of 20 cases the polymorphisms were not conclusively informative (Makrydimas et al 2004).

STUDIES ON SAFETY

The most likely mechanisms by which coelocentesis or any other invasive technique could affect the fetus causing fetal demise or fetal abnormalities are hypovolemia due to hemorrhage, hypoxia due to uterine contractions and the direct action on the heart and the blood vessels of vasoactive substances in response to the intrauterine trauma. It is hypothesized that these mechanisms are responsible for the oromandibular hypoplasia and limb abnormalities observed in fetuses after early CVS (Firth et al 1994). However, we have shown previously that the concentration of maternal serum AFP and the fetal heart rate were not altered following celocentesis demonstrating that this procedure is not associated with a significant degree of fetomaternal hemorrhage and does not affect the fetal cardiovascular system (Makrydimas et al 1997 a, b).

Moreover, in another study, from our group, (Makrydimas et al 2002) examining the short-term safety of celocentesis, involving 107 women that have had celocentesis and 337 controls, it was suggested that the risk of fetal death between 7 and 9 weeks of gestation is about 2%. However, the number of cases that were examined was small and to demonstrate that the excess rate of fetal loss from coeloentesis is about 2% it is necessary to undertake a comparative study involving a minimum of 250 patients. If the rate of fetal loss that could be attributed to celocentesis is about 2%, this would be similar to the excess fetal loss following CVS over the background rate in pregnancies that did not have prenatal diagnosis. For example, in the European study of CVS, where the mean maternal age was 37.8 years and the gestation at CVS was 9.6 weeks, the rate of fetal loss was 14%; in the ultrasound screening study for women at 30 to 39 years of age and live fetuses at 10 weeks the subsequent risk of fetal death was about 9%.

Another study, examining the safety of celocentesisin baboons (Santolaya Forgas et al 1998) reported that this procedure may be safe for the pregnancy, if it is performed at about 40 days of gestation using a 20 G needle and less than 3 ml of celomic fluid is aspirated. They performed celocentesis in nine cases and in the only one that miscarried they used a 17 G needle, aspirating 5 ml of fluid. None of the remaining eight cases miscarried, where they used thinner needles and aspirated ≤ 3 ml of celomic fluid. In contrast to the findings of these studies, Ross et al (1997) reported a 25% fetal loss rate within 2 to 3 days following celocentesis. Their study design was similar to ours, however the number of patients enrolled in their study was less than one-fifth used in our study. Moreover, they did not mention the name of the operator and his experience in this procedure. For example, in CVS the risk of miscarriage is much greater with a less experienced operator. In our study, none of the last 42 cases miscarried and although this is probably a coincidence, the increased experience of the operator may have played a role.

The ultrasonographic appearance of the miscarriages described by Ross et al, with the gestational sac filled with echogenic material so that the fetal pole was not visible, a probable consequence of hemorrhage, was also differenent from our findings. In our study, a missed abortion with a well recognizable fetal pole and no cardiac activity was diagnosed in all cases.

More recently (Makrydimas et al 2004) we have reported our results in continuing pregnancies undergoing celocentesis for prenatal diagnosis. Celocentesis was performed in nine pregnant women, at 7 to 8 weeks of gestation at the department of Obstetrics and Gynecology in Ioannina University Hospital. Six of them presented requesting prenatal diagnosis for β thalassemia or sickle cell anemia. In all six cases, both parents were carriers of the β thalassemia or sickle cell trait. In two cases celocentesis was performed for paternity testing and in one for Marfan's syndrome. In two cases, pregnancy termination was performed, one because the fetus was found to have sickle cell anemia and the second after paternity testing demonstrated that the father was not the husband. In both cases the results were confirmed from the placental samples collected after the pregnancy termination. In all continuing pregnancies, an amniocentesis was performed at the second trimester and the results were in concordance with the results from the DNA extracted from the celomic fluid. In all cases, ultrasound scans were done every three weeks showing normal anatomy and growth. Although, the short-term risks of miscarriage from celocentesis may be similar to those of other diagnostic techniques, the long-term risks both in terms of fetal death and possible structural abnormalities, remain to be assessed. Only twelve human pregnancies continued following celocentesis and all babies were born without any abnormality. Similarly, no structural abnormalities were observed in the baboons.

CONCLUSION

Celocentesis is a useful technique for the investigation of early fetal physiology and pathophysiology. Moreover, it offers the possibility for very early prenatal diagnosis, from at least seven weeks gestation. However, there are three main limitations to the introduction of celocentesis as an alternative to amniocentesis or chorionic villus sampling, for fetal karyotyping. Firstly, the number of studies examining the safety of the technique is small. Secondly, conventional cytogenetic analysis is not a realistic approach because of the difficulty in culturing celomic cells. Thirdly, screening for chromosomal defects has shifted from the traditional approach of maternal age to fetal nuchal translucency and first or second trimester biochemistry. Therefore, further, larger studies are needed to prove the safety of the technique, comparative genomic hybridization or microarrays could be used to examine the fetal karyotype and new ultrasound or biochemical markers for chromosomal abnormalities should be identified in the early first trimester. Nevertheless, for the diagnosis of conditions, such as β thalassemia where the risk for an affected fetus is 25%, celocentesis may be a realistic alternative.

BIBLIOGRAPHY

1. Chatzimeletiou K, Makrydimas G, Sotiriadis A, Paraskevaidis E, Nicolaides KH. Aneuploidy screening in celomic samples using fluorescence in situ Hybridisation (FISH). Prenat Diagn 2005:25: 919-26.
2. Cruger DG, Bruun-Petersen G, Kolvraa S. Early prenatal diagnosis: standard cytogenetic analysis of celomic cells obtained by coelocentesis. Prenat Diagn 1996; 16:945-9.
3. Firth HV, Boyd PA, Chamberlain PF, MacKenzie IZ, Morriss-Kay GM, Huson SM. Analysis of limb reduction defects in babies exposed to chorion villus sampling. Lancet 1994;343:1069-71.
4. Gublis B, Jauniaux E, Jurkovic D, Thiry P, Campbell S, Ooms HA. Determination of protein pattern in embryonic cavities of human early pregnancies: a means to understand materno-embryonic exchanges. Hum. Reprod. 1992; 7: 886-9.
5. Jauniaux E, Cirigliano V, Adinolfi M. Very early prenatal diagnosis on celomic cells using quantitative fluorescent polymerase chain reaction. Reprod Biomed Online 2003;6:494-8.
6. Jauniaux E, Gublis B. Fluid compartments of the embryonic environment. Hum Reprod Update 2000:6: 268-78.
7. Jurcovic D, Jauniaux E, Campbell S, Pandya P, Cardy DL, Nicolaides KH. Coelocentesis: a new technique for early prenatal diagnosis. Lancet 1993;341:1623-4.
8. Jurkovic D, Jauniaux E, Campbell S, Mitchell M, Lees C, Layton M. Detection of sickle gene by coelocentesis in early pregnancy: a new approach to prenatal diagnosis of single gene disorders. Hum Reprod. 1995;10:1287-9.
9. Lau TK, Fung TY, Wong YF, Fung HY. A study of fetal sex determination in celomic fluid. Gynecol Obstet Invest. 1998:45:16-8.
10. Lestou VS, Desilets V, Lomax BL, Barrett IJ, Wilson RD, Langlois S, Kalousek DK. Comparative genomic hybridization: a new approach to screening for intrauterine complete or mosaic aneuploidy. Am J Med Genet 2000 92: 281-4.
11. Makrydimas G, Georgiou I, Bouba I, Lolis D, Nicolaides KH. Early prenatal diagnosis by coelocentesis. Ultrasound Obstet Gynecol 2004;23:482-5.
12. Makrydimas G, Georgiou I, Kranas V, Kaponis A, Lolis D. Prenatal paternity testing using DNA extracted from celomic cells. Fetal Diagn Ther 2004; 19: 75-7.
13. Makrydimas G, Georgiou I, Kranas V, Zikopoulos K, Lolis D. Prenatal diagnosis of β thalassaemia by coelocentesis. Mol Hum Reprod 1997;3:729-31.
14. Makrydimas G, Kaponis A, Skendou C, Lolis D. Short-term safety of celocentesis for the mother and the fetus. Ultrasound Obstet Gynecol 2002;19:243-5.
15. Makrydimas G, Lolis D, Georgiou I, Navrozoglou I, Nicolaides KH. Fetomaternal bleeding following coelocentesis. Hum. Reprod 1997a;12:845-6.
16. Makrydimas G, Lolis D, Georgiou I, Skendou C, Nicolaides KH. Fetal heart rate following coelocentesis. J Matern Fetal Med 1997b;6:314-6.
17. Makrydimas G, Vandecruys H, Sotiriadis A, Lakasing L, Spencer K, Nicolaides KH. Celomic fluid leptin concentration in normal first trimester pregnancies and missed miscarriages. Fetal Diagn Ther 2005; 20: 406-9
18. Nicolaides K, Brizot Mde L, Patel F, Snijders R. Comparison of chorionic villus sampling and amniocentesis for fetal karyotyping at 10-13 weeks' gestation. Lancet 1994; 344:435-9.
19. Pandya PP, Cardy DL, Jauniaux E, Campbell S, Nicolaides KH. Rapid determination of fetal sex in celomic and amniotic fluid by fluorescence in situ hybridisation. Fetal Diagn Ther. 1995; 10:66-70.
20. Ross JA, Jurkovic D, Nicolaides K. Coelocentesis: a study of short-term safety. Prenat Diagn. 1997;17:913-7.
21. Santolaya Forgas J, De Leon Luis J, Shen Z, McCorquodale M. Chromosomal studies on 2 ml of celomic fluid obtained during the fifth week of development in the timed-pregnant baboon model. J Reprod Med 2005;50:692-6.
22. Santolaya-Forgas J, Vengalil S, Kushwaha A, Bieniarz A, Fortman J. Assesment of risk for fetal loss after the coelocentesis procedure using a baboon model. Fetal Diagn Ther 1998; 13: 257-60.
23. Singh K, Fong YF, Dong F. A viable alternative to surgical vacuum aspiration: repeated doses of intravaginal misoprostol over 9 hours for medical termination of pregnancies up to eight weeks. BJOG 2003;110:175-80.
24. Tabet AC, Aboura A, Dauge MC, Audibert F, Coulomb A, Batallan A, Couturier-Turpin MH, Feldmann G, Tachdjian G. Cytogenetic analysis of trophoblasts by comparative genomic hybridization in embryo-fetal development anomalies. Prenat Diagn 2001; 21:613-8.

CHAPTER 7

Celocentesis for in Utero Gene Therapy in Functionally Immunoincompetent Embryos: An Alternative Technique for Prenatal Diagnosis

Juan De León-Luis, Joaquin Santolaya-Forgas

THE CELOCENTESIS TECHNIQUE

Ultrasound-guided celocentesis are performed using the most simple needle itinerary and avoiding the amnion and the yolk sac (Figure 7.1). The needle used for sampling depends on the transmaternal route of access—in our time pregnant non-human primate research model we use 20 G needles for trans-abdominal celocentesis and 18 G needles for trans-vaginal celocentesis. All our studies have been performed under sterile conditions, in sedated animals and under approved research protocols.

Celocentesis can be performed by a single operator—with one hand the transducer is kept in place while with the other the needle tip is placed in the target and then an assistant removes the stilet from the needle, fixes the syringe, and aspirates or injects from or into the celomic cavity—or, with the two-operator method in which one individual controls the ultrasound image to provide continuous guidance, while the other inserts the needle and aspirates or injects from or into the celomic cavity. The embryonic heart rate should be recorded frequently throughout the procedure. The main risks of celocentesis are bleeding from the uterine wall into the celomic cavity, infection, and pregnancy loss. The procedure related pregnancy loss rate within three days of celocentesis ranges between 3% and 20% using the transvaginal approach in humans.[1-3] In the nonhuman primate model, the risk of pregnancy loss ranges from a 3 to 10%.[4]

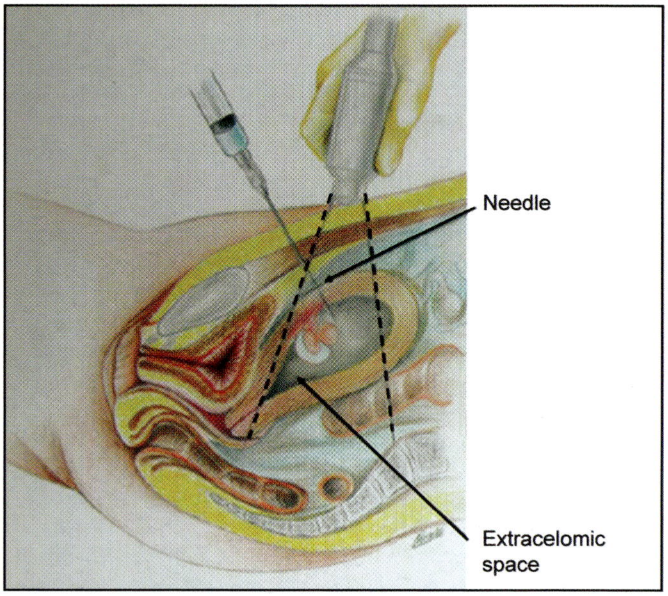

Figure 7.1: Ultrasound-guided transabdominal celocentesis

PRENATAL DIAGNOSIS OF GENETIC DISORDERS VIA CELOCENTESIS PRIOR TO STEM CELL THERAPY

Atkinson and associates,[5] from St. James University Hospital in Leeds, were the first to report on a 65% rate of success in cytogenetic analyses using human extracelomic fluid samples obtained between the 7th and 9th weeks of gestation. Gruger et al[6] then reported a 90% success in cytogenetic analyses after culturing celomic cells in a cocktail that contained used fibroblast culture media. More recently, the same group reported on the use of direct interphase FISH analysis of chromosomes 18, 13/21, X and Y.[7, 8] Makrydimas and collegues[9] have diagnosed β-thalassemia at 7 weeks of gestation and excluded maternal contamination by confirming the expected allelic distribution of the parental apolipoprotein B (ApoB) gene in analyzed cells. This group has also performed paternity testing by analyzing the segregation of parental alleles for trombopoietin (TPO) and ApoB genes in extracelomic cells.[10] Lau et al[11] have reported a 91% success for determining fetal sex using PCR amplification of a specific Y chromosome DNA sequence extracelomic fluid samples. We have confirmed the existence of viable cells in the baboon's extracelomic fluid and argued that studies should be undertaken to improve on the conditions necessary to enhance the extracelomic cells *in vitro* proliferation for cytogenetic studies.[12]

THE BABOON ANIMAL MODEL AS A SURROGATE TO HUMAN PREGNANCY FOR CELOCENTESIS

The gestational sac compartments of humans and baboons are ultrasonographically very similar between the 17th and 23rd Carnegie's stages of embryonic development which is equivalent to 56 days of development in humans and 40 days in baboons.[13] This ultrasonographic similarity validates the baboon animal model as a surrogate to human pregnancy for ultrasound-guided celocentesis. Moreover, since the biochemical composition of the human[14, 15] and baboon celomic fluid are also very similar,[16] results obtained from this animal model can be extrapolated to human pregnancies. Indeed, the baboon animal model can be used for *in utero* stem cell therapy via celocentesis because recent reports have suggested that human hematopoietic stem cells can survive *in vitro* in baboon extracelomic fluid.[17] Furthermore, the baboon extracelomic fluid can be partially exchanged *in vivo* with hematopoietic stem cell culture medium without causing abortion.[17, 18] These observations suggest that stem cell proliferation could be enhanced *in vivo* following the celocentesis procedure by adding specific culture medium and that this methodological change could improve the odds of achieving a cellular chimerism within the yolk sac and embryo proper.

IN UTERO HEMATOPOIETIC STEM CELL THERAPY VIA CELOCENTESIS IN FUNCTIONALLY IMMUNO-INCOMPETENT EMBRYOS

During development, hematopoiesis is multifocal and multilinear as a response to local production of hematopoietic growth factors and cytokines.[19] Hematopoietic stem cells, therefore, can colonize target tissues. In cattle, spontaneous hematopoietic allo-transplantations were reported decades ago within non-identical twins which opened the door to the possibility of *in utero* stem cell therapy.[20-22] Based on these findings, *in utero* stem cell therapy could potentially be used for a variety of conditions that can be diagnosed prenatally (Table 7.1). However, as it happens with other medical treatments, *in utero* stem cell treatment will have advantages and disadvantages that need to be considered and discussed with the patient prior to clinical application (Table 7.2).

Since the year 1986, *in utero* stem cell transplantations have been attempted for a variety of inherited disorders in fifty human fetuses. However, these procedures have been therapeutically effective in only a few cases affected with X-linked severe combined immunodeficiency (Table 7.3 summarizes reported cases).[23-40] The reason for lack of success in cases in which the fetus was not affected with an immune deficiency may relate to diminish proliferative advantage of donor's cells when

Table 7.1: Example of diseases that could be susceptible to *in utero* stem cell therapy

Entity	*Inheritance*	*Genetic map*
Sickle cell disease	AR	11 (11p15.5)
α Thalassemia	AR	X (Xq13)
α Thalassemia	AD	11 (11p15.5)
Chronic granulomatous disease	AR or X-linked	X-linked (50-65%) y X (Xp21-1)
Kostmann syndrome	AR	19 (19p13.3)
Chediak-Higashi syndrome	AR	1 (1q42.1-q42.2)
Glanzmann disease	AR	17 (17q21.32-17q21.32).
Mucolipidosis type I	AR	6 (6p21.3)
Adrenoleucodystrophy	AR or X-linked	X (Xq-28).
Hurler disease type I	AR	4 (4p16.3)
Hurler disease type II	X-linked	28 (28 q)).
Sanfilippo syndrome	AR	17 (17q25.3)
Morquio disease	AR	16 (16q24.3)
Sly syndrome	AR	7 (7q21.11).
Mucolipidosis type IV	AR	19 (19p13.3-p13.2)
Mucolipidosis type II	AR	X (Xq28)
Maroteaux-Lamy syndrome	AR	5 (5q11-q13)
Metachromatic leucodystrophy	AR	22 (22q13.31-qter)
Fucosidosis	AR	1 (1p34)
Fabry disease	X-linked	X (Xq22.1).
Pompe disease	AR	17 (17q25.2-q25.3).
Niemann-Pick disease type A&D	AR	11 (11p15)
Gaucher disease	AR	1 (1q21).
Krabbe disease	AR	14 (14q31)
Wiskott Aldrich	X-linked	Xp11.23-p11.22

AR= autosomal recessive; AD = autosomal dominant

Table 7.2: Advantages and disadvantages of *in utero* hematopoietic stem cell therapy

Advantages	*Disadvantages*
Possible prevention of the phenotypic alterations	It requires prenatal diagnosis Risk of iatrogenic miscarriages.
Decreased risk of rejection due to immature immune system	The appropriate dose of hematopoietic stem cells is not known nor is the proliferative potential of donor cells
Possibility to induce specific immunotolerance to the donor's cells with serial transplants	High failure prior of engraftment
Free space available in the stroma	Ethical concerns
Sterile intrauterine environment	Still in experimental stages

compared to host cells in these clinical scenarios. Due to lack of optimal results with mid-pregnancy *in utero* stem cell therapy and because of the enhanced understanding of the biological roles of the first trimester gestational sac compartments, a number of researchers are becoming interested in creating therapeutic cellular chimeras in "pre-immune" embryonic states.

Gestational age at the time of celocentesis is a major advantage for *in utero* stem cell therapy because: (i) prior to 12 weeks gestation the embryo does not have a completely functional immune system, and (ii) hematopoietic stem cells have not completely colonized all their niches. These two factors support the possibility of attempting direct donor stem cells transplantation in embryos that have inherited a metabolic disorder with very uncertain post-partum treatment. Moreover, donor stem cells injected into the gestational sac during the *pre-functional immunologic window* may prolong, or allow for permanent, state of tolerance to the donor's cells and therefore permit serial transplantations of the same donor cell population during pregnancy or after delivery of the newborn to achieve a complete clinical reconstitution without myeloablative or immunosupresive therapy.[40, 41]

Animal models have been developed for *in utero* stem cell therapy (reviewed in Table 7.4).[20, 41-58] In one of these studies performed by Noia and collaborators it was reported that hematopoietic stem cells injected via celocentesis in pregnant sheep can migrate from the extraembryonic celomic cavity and engraft in the embryo.[57] However, the placenta and extraembryonic celome of sheep are different from that of primates, which questions the feasibility of this route in humans. One other issue of concern when animal experimentation is used for development of *in utero* stem cell therapy procedures relates to the degree of clinical matching, that is, are developmental stages of the fetuses in research animal models equivalent to that of humans in potential clinical trials? We have proposed that Carnegie's developmental stages could be used to achieve this purpose. Briefly, the Carnegie Institute for Advancement in Science has a collection of vertebrate embryos in which three-dimensional developmental landmarks can be identified and used to match the time at which different vertebrates reach a particular developmental stage. We believe that this information can be used to standardize interspecies developmental stages.

Table 7.3: Examples of hematopoietic stem cell transplantations performed during human development

Indication	*GA (weeks)*	*Donor cell source*	*Chimera*	*Survival*	*Ref.*
Rh(D) alloimmunization	17,12	Maternal bone marrow	No	Yes	23, 28
Nude lymphocyte syndrome	30	Fetal thymus and liver	Yes	Yes	24
Severe Combined immunodeficiency	28	Fetal liver	Yes	Yes	25
Severe Combined immunodeficiency	20	Maternal bone marrow	No	VIP	26
α Thalassemia	18	Maternal bone marrow	Yes	VIP	
Chediak-Higashi disease	19	Maternal bone marrow	No	Yes	
β Thalassemia	18, 25	Brother's bone marrow	No	Yes	27
β Thalassemia	18	Fetal liver	Uncertain	No	
Metachromatic leucodytrophy	23, 37	Paternal bone marrow	No	Yes	
β Thalassemia	14	Fetal liver	Uncertain	No	29
Hurler syndrome	14	Fetal liver	No	Yes	
α Thalassemia	15, 31	Fetal liver	No	Yes	30
β Thalassemia	18	Fetal liver	No	Yes	
Sickle cell anemia	13	Fetal liver	No	Yes	
Severe X-linked combined immunodeficiency	14	Fetal liver	Yes	Yes	
Severe X-linked combined immunodeficiency	16, 17.5, 18.5, 21, 22	Paternal bone marrow	Yes	Yes	31, 32, 33
Severe combined immunodeficiency	23, 24	Paternal bone marrow	Yes	Yes	
Chronic granulomatous disease	17, 21	Fetal liver	Uncertain	No	34
Chediak-Higashi disease	19	Maternal bone marrow	No	Yes	35
Globoid cell leukodystrophy	14	Paternal bone marrow	Yes	No	36
β Thalassemia	13, 19 , 24	Paternal bone marrow	Yes	Yes	37
β Thalassemia		Paternal bone marrow	No	Yes	38
Globoid cell leukodystrophy	13, 13	Paternal bone marrow	No	Yes	39
Severe X-linked combined immunodeficiency	14	Fetal liver	Yes	Yes	40

VIP = voluntary interruption of the pregnancy; GA: gestational age at attempted *in utero* transplantation; Surv = survival; UC = Uncertain.

Currently, there are two major complications that need to be minimized during *in utero* hematopoietic stem cell therapy: (i) rejection of donor cells by the fetus, and (ii) graft versus host disease. Transplantation during the preimmune embryonic status could avoid rejection of the donor cells. Moreover, engraftment can be enhanced by the administration of doses greater than 2×10^6 hematopoietic stem cells per kg of recipient's weight[44] and by the mixture of a small number of T cells (CD3+) with the hematopoietic precursors—several authors have performed successful *in utero* allogenic hematopoietic stem cells transplanations in primates by including 10^6 to 10^7 T cells per kg of estimated fetal weight. However, these same authors that a small number of T cells have also raised concenrns for increased risk for *hydrops fetalis* secondary to massive lymphocytic infiltration if more than 10^8 T cells per kg are transfused.[45] Therefore, to avoid graft versus host disease injected hematopoietic stem cells-CD34+, Lin- cells collected from umbilical cord blood or bone marrow, expanded or not *ex vivo,*[46] need to purged from most of the T cells and from the *natural killer cell* population that may be present in the sample (NK) (CD3+CD56+).[59] Evidence supporting this last statement comes from: (i) NK cells are known to be present in the embryonic liver from the 6th week of gestation and these cells represent 35 and 75% of the liverworts CD45+ cells during the second trimester of pregnancy,[47] (ii) NK cells constitute 29% of

Table 7.4: Example of animal models for *in utero* hematopoietic *xeno*-trasplantation

Models	*Human hematopoietic cells source*	*Percentage of cases with successful implant*	*Chimerism percentage quantification*	*Authors*	*Years*	*Refs*
Sheep	ABM	43%	6% PB	Srour et al	1992	42
Sheep	FHC	40%	13–33% PB	Srour et al	1992	43
Sheep	ABM	33%	ND	Zanjani et al	1993	20
Rat	FHC	29%	ND	Pixley et al	1994	44
Sheep	FHC + HGF	40%	ND	Flake et al	1995	45
Baboon	Fetal liver	33%	1,5% PB/BM	Shields et al	1995	46
Sheep	FL-*in utero* after previous xenochimerism	33%	ND	Zanjani et al	1995	20
Sheep	AMS	28%	ND	Almeida et al	1996	47
Sheep	ABM	49%	ND	Kawashima et al	1996	48
Sheep	ABM	60%	1- 0,0001% PB	Bernstein et al	1997	49
Rat	ABM	29% SP, 4,12% BM 7,14% thymus	0,1-2,93% PB	Pixley et al	1998	50
Rat	FBM Fetal liver	12% MO, 10% liver 86,6% spleen	ND	Turner et al	1998	51
Dog	ABM/RETROVIRUS	100% PB/BM	PB 38% to 0,05% BM 20% to 0,05% 10-44 weeks	Omori et al	1999	52
Macacca	APB	100%	0,1-1,7% PB	Tarantal et al	2000	53
Sheep	AMS	80%	ND	Liechty et al	2000	54
Sheep	ABM y AMS	43%	ND	Porada et al	2000	41
Goat	Umbilical cord	1-3%	ND	Huang et al	2002	55
Sheep	ABM y AMS	40%	ND	MacKenzie et al	2002	56
Sheep	Umbilical cord	100%	6-32% PB/BM	Noia G et al	2003	57
Pig	Umbilical cord	66%	0,1-2% PB	Fujiki Y et al	2003	58

ABM: adult bone marrow; FBM: fetal bone marrow; FHC: Fetal haematopoietic cells; HGF: Haematopoietic grows factors; AMS: Adult medullar stroma; APB: adult peripheral blood; PB: peripheral blood; BM: bone marrow; ND: not described

circulating fetal lymphocytes at 13 weeks gestation and 6% at term, which suggests that they are a first line of defense during development,[48] (iii) *in vitro* studies have demonstrated that NK cells have greater immunocompetent capacity than T cell lymphocytes prior to the presence of antigens or IL-2/IL-12 cytokines,[49] and (iv) we have observed in our baboon model that cases that ended in fetal loss after *in utero* transplanatation xeno-transplantation that the number of NK cells present in the donor sample was 3 to 8 times higher than in cases that survived the *in utero* procedure.[60]

CONCLUSION

During a relatively short period of time, first trimester screening and diagnosis is surfacing to increase the options available to patients. The new challenge is to develop techniques that can be used during the first trimester of pregnancy to avoid or reduce the phenotypic expression of inherited inborn errors of metabolism. For this reason, experimental *in-vivo* ultrasound-guided stem cell transplantations have been performed during very early intrauterine development. One of the approches for *in utero* stem cell treatment is the celocentesis procedure. Indeed, celocentesis has already brought new insights into the composition of celomic fluid in humans and primates and some of the biological roles of celomic fluid in primates are beginning to be elucidated,[61] prenatal diagnosis of genetic disorders is feasible, and maternal tolerance to xeno-transplantations via celocentesis at 40 days from fertilization has been proven in the baboon animal model.[60] Finally, very recently, it has been reported that the celomic fluid can be partially replaced *in vivo* by stem cell culture medium opening the doors to transforming the celomic fluid into a "bio-reactor" that would prolong the survival and permit the expansion of the limited number of stem cells that can be injected into the celomic cavity.[18]

REFERENCES

1. Ross JA, Jurkovic D, Nicolaides K. Coelocentesis: a study of short-term safety. Prenat Diagn 1997;17(10):913-7.
2. Makrydimas G, Lolis D, Georgiou I, Navrozoglou I, Nicolaides KH. Feto-maternal bleeding following coelocentesis. Hum Reprod 1997;12(4):845-6.
3. Makrydimas G, Kaponis A, Skentou C, Lolis D. Short-term safety of celocentesis for the mother and the fetus. Ultrasound Obstet Gynecol 2002;19(3):243-5.
4. Santolaya-Forgas J, Vengalil S, Kushwaha A, Bieniarz A, Fortman J. Assessment of the risk of fetal loss after the coelocentesis procedure using a baboon model. Fetal Diagn Ther 1998;13(4):257-60.
5. Atkinson G, Rane V, Linton G, Campbell J. Early prenatal diagnosis of fetal aneuploidy using coelomic fluid. Early Hum Dev 1996;47 (Suppl):S103-4.
6. Gruger DG, Bruun-Petersen G, Kolvraa S. Early prenatal diagnosis: standard cytogenetic analysis of coelomic cells obtained by coelocentesis. Prenat Diagn 1996;16(10):945-9.
7. Gruger DG, Bruun-Petersen G, Kolvraa S. Turner's syndrome 45,X found by coelocentesis. Prenat Diagn 1997;17(6):588-9.
8. Gruger DG, Bruun-Petersen G, Kolvraa S. Quantitative evaluation of fluorescence in situ hybridization (FISH) signals in uncultured coelomic cells. Prenat Diagn 1997;17(7):635-42.
9. Makrydimas G, Georgiou I, Kranas V, Zikopoulos K, Lolis D. Prenatal diagnosis of beta-thalassaemia by coelocentesis. Mol Hum Reprod 1997;3(8):729-31.
10. Makrydimas G, Georgiou I, Kranas V, Kaponis A, Lolis D. Prenatal paternity testing using DNA extracted from coelomic cells. Fetal Diagn Ther 2004;19(1):75-7.
11. Lau TK, Fung TY, Wong YF, Fung HY. A study of fetal sex determination in coelomic fluid. Gynecol Obstet Invest 1998;45(1):16-8.
12. Santolaya-Forgas J, De Leon-Luis J, Shen Z, McCorquodale M. Chromosomal studies on 2 mL of celomic fluid obtained during the fifth week of development in the timed-pregnant baboon model. J Reprod Med 2005;50(9):692-6.
13. Deleon-Luis J, Santolaya-Forgas J. Ultrasonographic development of human and baboons according to the Carnegie stages of embryonic development: applications for in utero gene therapy in pre-immune embryos. Ultrasound Obstet Gynecol 2004;24 (3):280-1.
14. Santolaya-Forgas J, De Leon-Luis J, Espinoza J, Goncalves LF, Romero R. Solutes in maternal circulation and gestational sac compartments during early human development. Fetal Diagn Ther 2006;21(3):287-92.
15. De Leon-Luis J, Santolaya-Forgas J. Catalog of solutes measured in paired extraembryonic celomic fluid and maternal serum samples. J Reprod Med 2006;51(4):311-6.
16. Santolaya-Forgas J, Duval J, Prespin C, Vengalil S, Kushwaha A, Wilson L, et al. Extracoelomic fluid osmometry and electrolyte composition during early gestation in the baboon. Am J Obstet Gynecol 1998;179(5):1124-7.
17. Santolaya-Forgas J, Galan I, Deleon-Luis J, Roman W. A study to determine if human umbilical cord hematopoietic stem cells can survive in baboon extra-embryonic celomic fluid: a prerequisite for determining the feasibility of in-utero stem cell xeno-transplantation via celocentesis. Fetal Diagn Ther 2006;in press.
18. Santolaya-Forgas J, Deleon-Luis J, Galan I. Can extra-embryonic celomic fluid be partially replaced with stem-cell culture medium? Ultrasound Obstet Gynecol 2006;28(2):232-3.
19. Galan I, Deleon-Luis J, Diaz L, Khalek N, Munoz M, Santolaya-Forgas J. Effect of a bone marrow microenvironment on the ex-vivo expansion of umbilical cord blood progenitor cells. Clin Lab Haematol 2006;in press.
20. Zanjani ED, Anderson WF. Prospects for in utero human gene therapy. Science 1999;285(5436):2084-8.
21. Anderson WF. Human gene therapy. Nature 1998;392(6679 Suppl):25-30.
22. Douar AM, Themis M, Coutelle C. Fetal somatic gene therapy. Mol Hum Reprod 1996;2(9):633-41.
23. Yong KL, Fahey A, Pahal G, Linch DC, Pizzey A, Thomas NS, et al. Fetal haemopoietic cells display enhanced migration across endothelium. Br J Haematol 2002;116(2):392-400.
24. Touraine JL, Raudrant D, Royo C, Rebaud A, Roncarolo MG, Souillet G, et al. In-utero transplantation of stem cells in bare lymphocyte syndrome. Lancet 1989;1(8651):1382.
25. Touraine JL. In utero transplantation of fetal liver stem cells in humans. Blood Cells 1991;17(2):379-87.
26. Diukman R, Golbus MS. In utero stem cell therapy. J Reprod Med 1992;37(6):515-20.
27. Slavin S, Naparstek E, Ziegler M, Lewin A. Clinical application of intrauterine bone marrow transplantation for treatment of genetic diseases—feasibility studies. Bone Marrow Transplant 1992;9 (Suppl 1):189-90.

28. Thilaganthan B, Nicolaides KH, Morgan G. Intrauterine bone-marrow transplantation at 12 weeks' gestation. Lancet 1993;342(8865):243.
29. Hajdu K, Tanigawara S, McLean LK, Cowan MJ, Golbus MS. In utero allogeneic hematopoietic stem cell transplantation to induce tolerance. Fetal Diagn Ther 1996;11(4):241-8.
30. Westgren M, Ringden O, Eik-Nes S, Ek S, Anvret M, Brubakk AM, et al. Lack of evidence of permanent engraftment after in utero fetal stem cell transplantation in congenital hemoglobinopathies. Transplantation 1996;61(8):1176-9.
31. Flake AW, Roncarolo MG, Puck JM, Almeida-Porada G, Evans MI, Johnson MP, et al. Treatment of X-linked severe combined immunodeficiency by in utero transplantation of paternal bone marrow. N Engl J Med 1996;335(24):1806-10.
32. Lau AS, Sigaroudinia M, Yeung MC, Kohl S. Interleukin-12 induces interferon-gamma expression and natural killer cytotoxicity in cord blood mononuclear cells. Pediatr Res 1996;39(1):150-5.
33. Wengler GS, Lanfranchi A, Frusca T, Verardi R, Neva A, Brugnoni D, et al. In-utero transplantation of parental CD34 haematopoietic progenitor cells in a patient with X-linked severe combined immunodeficiency (SCIDXI). Lancet 1996;348(9040):1484-7.
34. Touraine JL. In utero transplantation of fetal liver stem cells into human fetuses. J Hematother 1996;5(2):195-9.
35. Flake AW, Zanjani ED. In utero hematopoietic stem cell transplantation. A status report. JAMA 1997;278(11):932-7.
36. Bambach BJ, Moser HW, Blakemore K, Corson VL, Griffin CA, Noga SJ, et al. Engraftment following in utero bone marrow transplantation for globoid cell leukodystrophy. Bone Marrow Transplant 1997;19(4):399-402.
37. Hayward A, Ambruso D, Battaglia F, Donlon T, Eddelman K, Giller R, et al. Microchimerism and tolerance following intrauterine transplantation and transfusion for alpha-thalassemia-1. Fetal Diagn Ther 1998;13(1):8-14.
38. Dufour P, de Bievre P, Vinatier D, Tordjeman N, Da Lage B, Vanhove J, et al. Varicella and pregnancy. Eur J Obstet Gynecol Reprod Biol 1996;66(2):119-23.
39. Leung W, Blakemore K, Jones RJ, Moser HW, Mukherjee G, Griffin CA, et al. A human-murine chimera model for in utero human hematopoietic stem cell transplantation. Biol Blood Marrow Transplant 1999;5(1):1-7.
40. Westgren M, Ringden O, Bartmann P, Bui TH, Lindton B, Mattsson J, et al. Prenatal T-cell reconstitution after in utero transplantation with fetal liver cells in a patient with X-linked severe combined immunodeficiency. Am J Obstet Gynecol 2002;187(2):475-82.
41. Porada CD, Park P, Almeida-Porada G, Zanjani ED. The sheep model of in utero gene therapy. Fetal Diagn Ther 2004;19(1):23-30.
42. Srour EF, Hoffman R, Zanjani D. Animal models for human hematopoiesis. J Hematother 1992;1(2):143-53.
43. Srour EF, Zanjani ED, Brandt JE, Leemhuis T, Briddell RA, Heerema NA, et al. Sustained human hematopoiesis in sheep transplanted in utero during early gestation with fractionated adult human bone marrow cells. Blood 1992;79(6):1404-12.
44. Pixley JS, Tavassoli M, Zanjani ED, Shaft DM, Futamachi KJ, Sauter T, et al. Transplantation in utero of fetal human hematopoietic stem cells into mice results in hematopoietic chimerism. Pathobiology 1994;62(5-6):238-44.
45. Flake AW, Hendrick MH, Rice HE, Tavassoli M, Zanjani ED. Enhancement of human hematopoiesis by mast cell growth factor in human-sheep chimeras created by the in utero transplantation of human fetal hematopoietic cells. Exp Hematol 1995;23(3):252-7.
46. Shields LE, Gaur LK, Gough M, Potter J, Sieverkropp A, Andrews RG. In utero hematopoietic stem cell transplantation in nonhuman primates: the role of T cells. Stem Cells 2003;21(3):304-14.
47. Almeida-Porada GD, Hoffman R, Manalo P, Gianni AM, Zanjani ED. Detection of human cells in human/sheep chimeric lambs with in vitro human stroma-forming potential. Exp Hematol 1996;24(3):482-7.
48. Kawashima I, Zanjani ED, Almaida-Porada G, Flake AW, Zeng H, Ogawa M. CD34+ human marrow cells that express low levels of Kit protein are enriched for long-term marrow-engrafting cells. Blood 1996;87(10):4136-42.
49. Bernstein J, Boyle DW, Srour EF, Cooper R, Jacobs C, Freie B, et al. Variation in long-term engraftment of a large consecutive series of lambs transplanted in utero with human hematopoietic cells. Biol Blood Marrow Transplant 1997;3(5):247-54.
50. Pixley JS, Zanjani ED, Shaft DM, Porada C, Mackintosh FR. Prolonged hematopoietic chimerism in normal mice transplanted in utero with human hematopoietic stem cells. Pathobiology 1998;66(5):230-9.
51. Turner CW, Archer DR, Wong J, Yeager AM, Fleming WH. In utero transplantation of human fetal haemopoietic cells in NOD/SCID mice. Br J Haematol 1998;103(2):326-34.
52. Omori F, Lutzko C, Abrams-Ogg A, Lau K, Gartley C, Dobson H, et al. Adoptive transfer of genetically modified human hematopoietic stem cells into preimmune canine fetuses. Exp Hematol 1999;27(2):242-9.
53. Tarantal AF, Goldstein O, Barley F, Cowan MJ. Transplantation of human peripheral blood stem cells into fetal rhesus monkeys (Macaca mulatta). Transplantation 2000;69(9):1818-23.
54. Liechty KW, MacKenzie TC, Shaaban AF, Radu A, Moseley AM, Deans R, et al. Human mesenchymal stem cells engraft and demonstrate site-specific differentiation after in utero transplantation in sheep. Nat Med 2000;6(11):1282-6.
55. Huang S, Zeng F, Gong Z, Lu J, Huang W, Hu W, et al. [A study of the engraftment, expansion and differentiation of human hematopoietic stem cells in goats]. Zhonghua Yi Xue Za Zhi 2002;82(2):86-9.
56. Mackenzie TC, Flake AW. Multilineage differentiation of human MSC after in utero transplantation. Cytotherapy 2001;3(5):403-5.

57. Noia G, Pierelli L, Bonanno G, Monego G, Perillo A, Rutella S, et al. A novel route of transplantation of human cord blood stem cells in preimmune fetal sheep: the intracelomic cavity. Stem Cells 2003;21(6):638-46.
58. Fujiki Y, Fukawa K, Kameyama K, Kudo O, Onodera M, Nakamura Y, et al. Successful multilineage engraftment of human cord blood cells in pigs after in utero transplantation. Transplantation 2003;75(7):916-22.
59. Zanjani ED, Srour EF, Hoffman R. Retention of long-term repopulating ability of xenogeneic transplanted purified adult human bone marrow hematopoietic stem cells in sheep. J Lab Clin Med 1995;126(1):24-8.
60. Deleon-Luis J, Galan I, Noble V, Gooch J, Santolaya-Forgas J. Feasibility of human hematopoietic stem cell injection via celocentesis in pre-immune baboon fetus. In: Genetics ACGMACoM, editor. Orlando, Florida; 2004.
61. Santolaya-Forgas J, Roman W, Edwin S, Pitt A, Nien J. Concentration of soluble VEGF-R1 and VEGF-R2 in extraembryonic celomic fluid in primates. In. Miami; 2006.

CHAPTER
8

Fetal Biopsy Procedures in Prenatal Diagnosis

Juan M Troyano, M Alvarez de la Rosa, I Martinez-Wallin

INTRODUCTION

Since the early eighties a varied amount of experiences and trials of fetal puncture (fine needle aspiration) have been carried out with diagnostic aims.[1-5] At the beginning, the only possible way to enter the fetal evironment was with the support of a fetoscope but the spectacular development of the already well known ultrasonography has permited the invasion of the intrauterine enviroment with tools that are more and more harmless in the use, especially in the gradually tighter sections and the evolution of certain characteristics of the new needles that are now being incorporated into the new biopsy techniques.[3,6,7]

Fetal puncture with diagnostic aims is technically possible, provided it is done by adequatelly trained hands, but the essential problem lies in establishing the correct indications which are not yet quite defined.[8]

TECHNIQUE GENERALIZATION

Whatever the location of the fetal puncture may be, a certain number of requirements are imperative.

1. The operator must have sufficient working experience in invasive echography.
2. The room should have surgical consideration or rank, it is necessary to have an aseptic room for echographic intervention. A sterile wrap is recommended for the ultrasound probe. We use a surgical glove for an airtight seal.
3. The characteristics of the surgical equipment or the obtaining of the sample.
   As the tendency is to obtain samples with the maximum diagnostic guarantee and a minimal risk to the integrity of the pregnancy, it is of capital importance, with few exceptions, to use sectio needles no smaller than 18 G.
   It is clear that depending on the tissue sample we are aiming to obtain, it is not always possible to use innocuous tools. A clear example are the devices used to date for skin biopsies to diagnose some types of *genodermatosis*, which consist on clipper forceps measuring 2.5 mm.
   These methods in many cases require the use of an anesthetic, including in some, general anesthesia, previous to proceeding to the incision in the maternal abdomen, with a scalpel, and the introduction of a trocar sheath enquivalent in sectio to a Verre's needle that serves as a guide vehicle for the mentioned system or method.
   The complications derived from the use of 2.5 mm sectio needles and the transabdomen forceps method are closer to those of the fetoscope, added

to the fact that the great flexibility in many cases of the method itself, having the availability of a great variety of needles of relatively small calibre (18 G standard), obtaining very good biopsies, including in skin samples and visceral solid areas (Figure 8.1).[2,7]

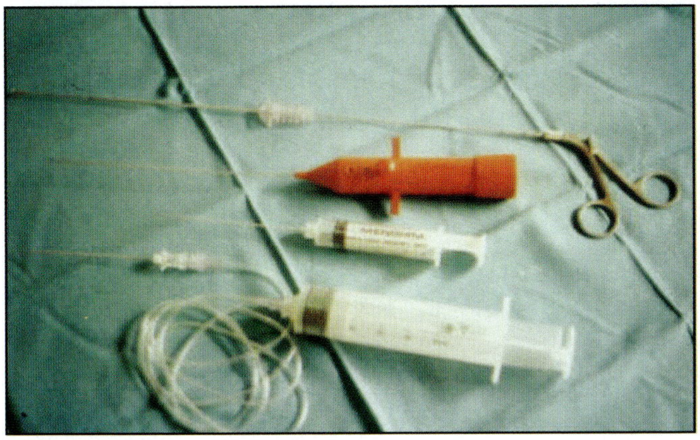

Figure 8.1: Different types of needles and system for fetal biopsy

Within the organs that are intrauterinally reachable. With worthy guarantees, the one that follows in difficulties after the skin sampling, is the kidney, fundamentally due to its histological parenchymal stratum constitution.[9]

We can only consider satisfactory the samples or cylinders that include corticomedular stratum. The fetal availability in respect of its intrauterine position, the distance and the interposed tissue to the kidney (skin, muscle) as well as perirenal fat and the very capsule, are the elements that obstruct the obtaining of valid samples.

The use in these cases of a catheter of 14 to 16 G calibre with isometric aspiration techniques with constant vacuum, allow to obtain valid samples, between 69 and 80%, while the use of 18 to 20 G caliber catheter obtains the very best specimens between 25 and 30%. This means that isometric (fine needle) puncture-aspiration techniques do not always offer the results hoped for on solid organs, fundamentally the kidney, unless wider catheters are used, that are far from the "harmless philosophy" that should prevail in these processes. For these cases and others that are similar that could present themselves, depending on the tissue characteristics, the use of methods such as the *aspiration biopsy set* that includes an 18 G bisided trocar syringe in all its circumference, acting as a circular blade, and a conical sheath with vacuum suction embolous contriving through its interior which allows to obtain cylinders of 2 to 5 mm in maximum length, with optimal safety conditions and histological quality, similar to those of the *tru-cut* method.

Of all the viscus solid organs within reach, the one that offers the least problem is the liver, its spongy tissue constitution and its great size and volume in the fetal abdomen allows optimal accessability and consequently offers samples in practically 100% of all cases, using a conventional fine needle of 18 to 20 G.

The obtention of muscle tissue samples offers one of the main difficulties due to the topographic and anatomical characteristics of the skeleton, also the important motorous innervation. For this reason it is necessary to correctly select the spot and the muscular area least suspectible to provoke indelible functional lessions.

The most accessible topographic areas are the external face of either thigh, but it is technically more attainable the vastus externus muscle (Figure 8.2); it is a zone covered by the subtrochanteric fascia lata in an oblicular direction descending towards the fetal femur, The use of the *sure cut* systems 18 G with incorporated vacuum aspiration allows a sucess rate over 75%. Conventional spinal needles with complementary aspiration by 50 cc syringe vacuum allows to obtain sample with great difficulties.

When the puncture area has liquid characteristics, the echographic view is wide ranged, allowing a large field of action.

4. In general, technically it is precise to choose the most direct route, avoiding any interpositing obstacles, being also of interest to avoid the placenta, if, at all, possible.
5. Once the crucial point to puncture has been determined, the needle should be introduced within the field of view of the probe, frame by frame until reaching the fetus.
6. It is recommended to approximate the puncture point without making direct contact with it in the first instance, until quite certain of the needles angle to the chosen spot, being of capital importance to enter with only one *sudden jab* to avoid sudden fetal jolts or movements.

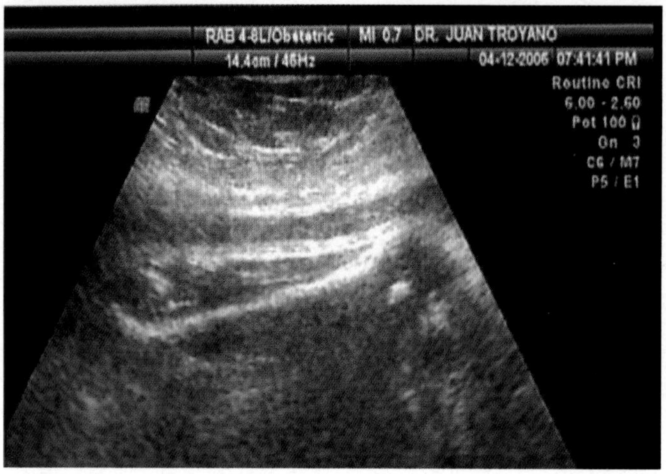

Figure 8.2: Subtrochanteric muscle biopsy: echographic monitoring. The arrow indicates the puncture position obliquely to the fetal femur

7. It is advisable in all *free-hand* fetal punctures carried out, that the operator should take into account the dynamic variations of fetal positions.
8. For better manipulation, an assistant should be in charge of carrying out the isometric aspiration process at a prudential distance, approximately a meter away from the surgical table, interplacing a serum of the same length between the needle and the syringe.
9. Except in exceptional circumstances such as pericardiac and pleural overflow that need an operating time of about 15 to 30 minutes, it is absolutely feasible to carry out without any anesthetic procedures.

Aspiration in cystic disorders will fundamentally orientate the diagnosis. Aspiration on ovarian cysts is only indicated in complex cases derived from its dynamic volume or due to rare structural types with therapeutic aims more than to diagnostic ones.

We collect suspicious chylous collections, where the presence of high lymphocyte concentrations practically give a sure diagnosis also the fact that it allows a genetic study in very few days, justifies this type of procedures (Figure 8.3).

The puncture of pericardic discharges has also the same diagnostic aims as well as being therapeutic.

Concerning brain punctures, the most representative, the *ventriculocentesis*, also allows us to accomplish serological marker studies in RCL, independent to any derived therapeutic attitude, although in this last case the efficiency of the derivative procedures in hydrocephalia is uncertain (Figure 8.4).

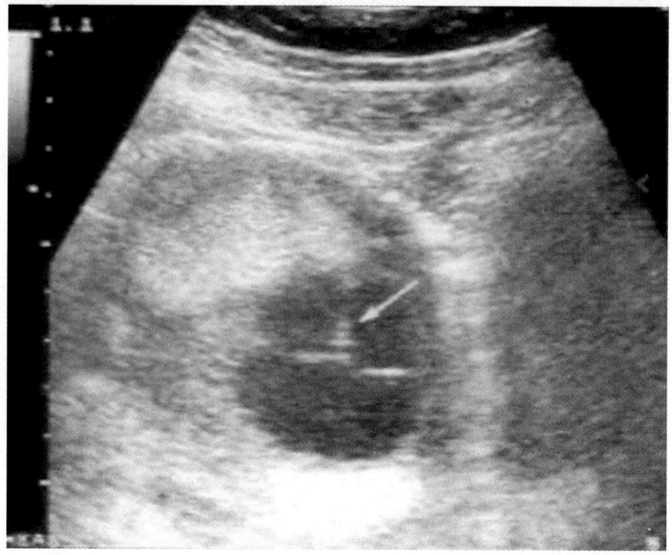

Figure 8.3: Cystic lymphangioma: percutaneous puncture determines qualitative and genetic characteristics (lymphocytes)

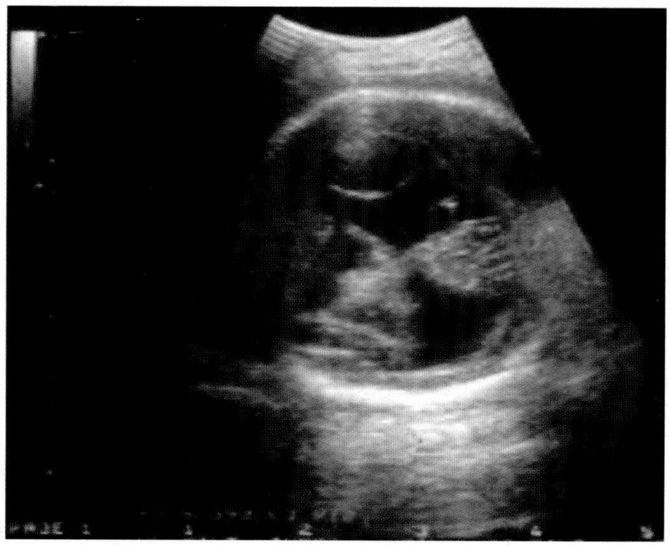

Figure 8.4: Ventriculocentesis: obtaining cephalorhachidian liquid determines the presence of viral bodies by polymerase chain reaction

Of all the structurally cystic processes, the obtention of fetal urine in dilated urological pathology represents the greatest and highest interest for diagnosis value. The biochemical analysis of the fetal urine allows us to detect irreversible tubular lessions from those which have a normal renal function.

There is no doubt that the incorporation of biological molecular techniques and DNA studies allow to establish in many of the cases, the alterations of any determined genetic locus.[10-13]

Ocassionally, we may find that we do not have enough material due to the lack of family records of desceased relations, in these cases the absence of this previous information constitutes a serious inconvenience in order to establish a prenatal diagnosis, as this is based only on a small chorionic-villi, funicular or amniotic sample.[11,14]

This situation is where sampling directly from the fetal tissue is of special relevance for the diagnose of one or the other, or in order to rule out any pathological suspicion of family inheritance that are being submitted to any particular study.

"The taking of fetal samples by biopsy techniques is justified only in cases when the prenatal diagnosis of any specific pathological illness is not possible, or is frankly difficult, using any of the existing conventional techniques."

LIVER BIOPSY

Technique

Fetal transabdominal aspiration-puncture using 18 G needles with conic catheter or spinal needles of the same sectio with isometric vacuum aspiration using a 50 cc syringe and serum system. Once introduced into the fetal kidney, soft brief *inward outward* movements should be made in the same direction as the puncture.

Firstly, the aspiration system should be extracted and last of all the needle, to avoid contaminating any other tissue. The spot to be puntured should be situated between the belly bottom and the border of the rib. This fate is helped by the physiological hepatomegalia, introducing the needle aproximately one centimetre under strict echographic monitoring. Preferably the external third of the right lobe, should be chosen, as it offers a minor principal vascularization, if not, the suprahepatic vessels should be avoided (Figure 8.5).

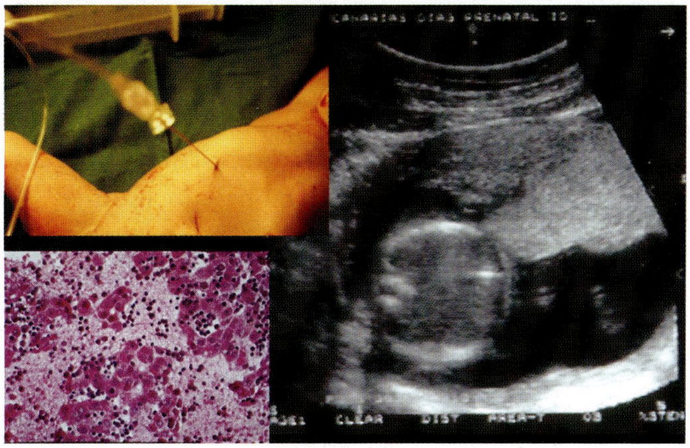

Figure 8.5: Liver biopsy: echographic monitoring and histological samples of fetal liver (19 weeks). Extramedullary hematopoietic foci can be detected

If the diagnosis being sought for is histological, the cylinder should be conserved in formaldehyde if on the contrary it is enzymatic, it should then be airtight sealed in carbonic snow.

The gestational age recommended should be around 20 weeks, provided that the hepatic metabolism and main enzymatic processes are well, or practically established.

Indications

Prenatal diagnosis, fundamentally of enzymatic alterations and of lethal metabolic characteristics.[15,16]

Ornitil Transcarbamylase Deficiencies (OTC)

This mitochondrial enzyme of the urea cycle is synthesized in the liver or the intestines. Sex-linked disorders tied to the sex, are shown on the screening data of mothers who have urine excretion of orotic acid.

Primary Hyperoxaliuria (PH)

This is severe, charted renal insuffiency of rapid evolution, that is characterized by the presence of calcic oxalate deposits in the renal tubule, microlithiasis and interstitial fibrosis. The hepatic level is accompanied by a total absence of alanine, inactivity of the catalitic gliosilate aminotranferase and immunoreactive proteins. This is incompatible with life.

For diagnosis it is fundamental to have the previous family clinical history available.

Carbamoyl Phosphate Synthetase Deficiency

This is an enzymatic defects of the urea cycle with recesive autosomic inheritance.

Other autosomic recesive disorders may be detected by means of hepatic biopsy, including:

- Non-ketotic hyperglycinemia
- Prenatal diagnosis of infantile neuronal ceroid-lipofuscinosis
- Biliary atresia (type I cysts)
- Long-chain 3-hydroxyacyl-CoA dehydrogenase.[17-20]

Complications

The prenatal liver biopsy has few risks on a tissular level, due to its own visceral characteristics. Those risks are derived from the main vascular tears which will have great bleeding resulting in fetal death. In our experience (7 prenatal punctures), we have observed no complications (Table 8.1).

Table 8.1: Experience with seven prenatal punctures for liver biopsy

Reasons for biopsy	Number of cases
OTC diseases in the same family	4
Previous affected brother	1
Mitochondrial respiratory deficit	1
Non-ketotic hyperglycinemia	1
Results	
Prenatally confirmed diagnosis of OTC deficiency	2
Prenatally non-confirmed diagnosis with neonatal exitus by hyperammonemia	1
Prenatally confirmed as non-affected fetuses	4

FETAL PUNCTURE IN THE EVALUATION OF RENAL STATUS

The correction of a theoretic renal obstruction problem is possible, in spite of the difficulties and risks that it holds, even if in the majority of cases it is not necessary. We should start by stating that an ultrasound echography diagnosis of the obstructed renal pathology does not necessarilly imply an irrevesible function alteration. In this sense the amniotic volume can be used as an indirect marker of the actual renal function, but this does have the inconvenience that it includes the possible measuring of the intrinsic clearance function.

When taking into account the possibility of practising an intrauterine derived therapy, this can only be justificable in those fetuses in whose kidneys there has been no irreversable damage. However, this makes it essential to establish a precise evaluation of the renal function, in order to adequately select those fetuses that will benefit from prenatal therapy.

The most conflictive situation is the renal dysplasia. In the latter coexist tissular phenomena that are characterized by fibrosis, dysplasia, cartilagenosis, frequently associated to corticomedular cysts, although not always so (Figure 8.6).

Aproximately 90% of all kidney dysplasias is associated to dilated or obstructive disorders. In these cases it can be remarked that any derived therapeutic action is unnecessary.

The high resolution echography has turned into the unquestionable kidney evaluation processes, however, it does have a few diagnostic limitations: (Table 8.2).

Table 8.2: Fetal neuropathy: echographic prediction

Tissue markers	*Sensibility*	*Specificity*
Hyperechongenicity	60%	90%
Hydronephrosis	75%	70%
Hydronephrosis + cysts	90%	100%

In our experience the obstruction of a kidney without objectible cysts or hyperechoes does not, however, exclude dysplasia. This quite alarming fact occurs approximately in 25 to 30% of all cases.[8-21]

From this we can deduce that the echography on its own does not diagnose all renal dysplasias, and for this reason fetuses with pelvic dilation are subsidiary of derived drainage.

A biochemical study of fetal urine is capital data in the managing of these fetuses. The composition of the fetal urine stays constant, practically throghout the pregnancy and with hypotonic characteristics. This fact has automatically demonstrated an optimal and reliable renal function and on the contrary and iso or hypertonic urine, a defficiency in renal function with an infastous prediction.

The biochemical markers that have close relation with a renal function are defined by the Na^+, Cl^- and osmotic urine.

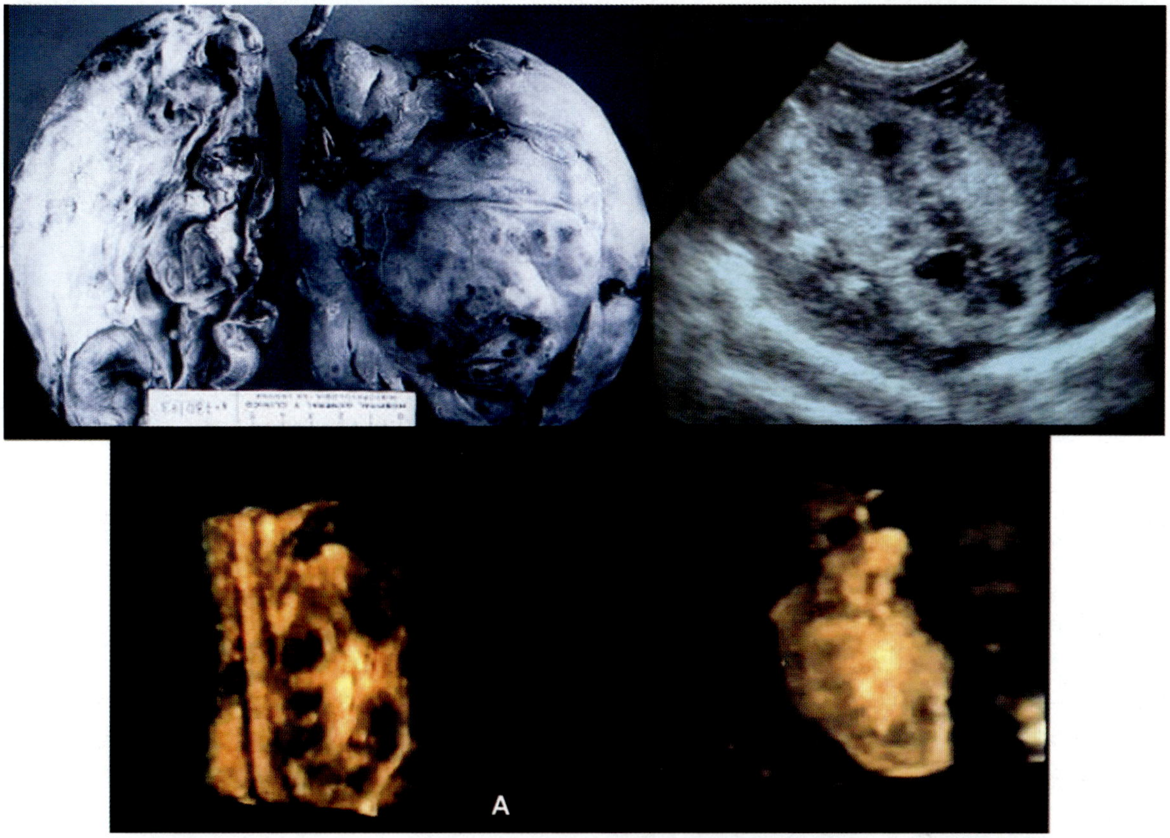

Figure 8.6: Fibrocortical dysplasia associated with corticomedullary cyst and renomegalia (A) Polycystic kidney by 3D US scan

Another determining factor in the normal renal clearance function derived from the near high reabsorvative tubular activity, is the establishing of specific proximal tubular lession selective markers.

These markers correspond to lysosomal proteins exclusive of the proximate tubular structure and become expressed by NAG (N-acetyle D-glucosaminidase). Low molecular weight proteins filtered by the glomerular system and reabsorbed practically in their totality by the proximal tube, if it is present in fetal urine and in the amniotic fluid in large quantities (higher than 8 U/L), it is indicative of tubular tissue destruction.

The detection of β-2 microglobulin would be considered in the same manner (Figures 8.7 to 8.8) (Corresponden a los dos esquemas de la nefrona).

We found that the levels of biochemical markers are sensibly low in the physiological urine in comparison with the cases affected with irreversible renal disorder. The same outcome occurs with the tissular markers, NAG and microglobulin (Table 8.3).

Table 8.3: Fetal urinary aspiration: pathological biochemical markers

	Pathological urine values		
	Weeks		
	18-20	*20-30*	*>32*
Na^+ (mEq/ml)	120.0	126.44±11.50	139.60
Cl^- (mEq/ml)	119.0	132.50±7.18	141.00
Osm (mOsm)	240	261.50±24.20	281.00
NAG (U/L)	18.0	25.83±0.85	25.73
G (ml/L)	26.0	38.97±1.30	38.72
K^+ (mEq/mL)	3.1	3.41±0.66	3.90
Creatinine (ml/L)	1.2	2.54±0.83	3.70

When we compare the relationship between the ionic concentrations and the osmolarity (Na^+ and Cl) of the fetal urine, and those of the amniotic liquid, we do not find significant differences between fetuses with conserving and fetuses with patological functionalities. But comparing the levels of NAG and β2-microglobulin, a significantly greater concentrations of the two markers in the amniotic liquid of the affected fetuses have been observed (Tables 8.4 and 8.5).

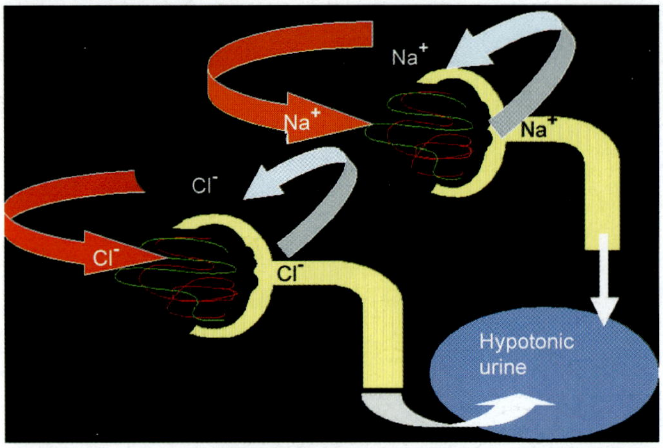

Figure 8.7: Biochemical markers that have close relation with a renal function are defined by the NA$^+$, Cl$^-$ and osmotic urine derived from the near high reabsorptive tubular activity. Fetal urine stays constant, practically through the pregnancy and with hypotonic characteristics

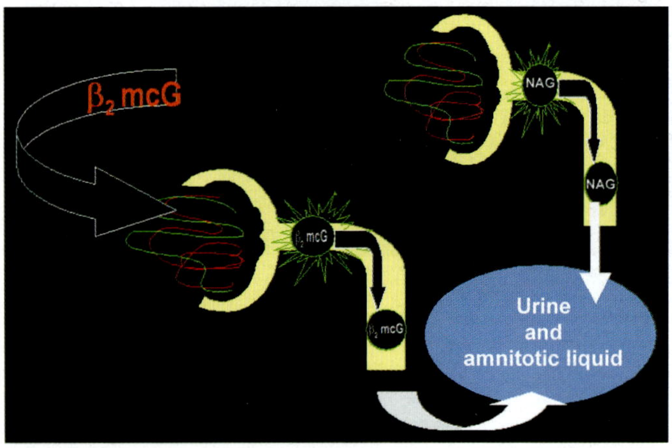

Figure 8.8: Another determinating factors in the normal renal cleareance function correspond to lysosomal proteins exclusive of the proximate tubular structure (NAG), if it is present in fetal urine and amniotic fluid in large quantities, it is indicative of tubular tissue destruction. Beta-2 microglobulin would be considered in the same manner

Table 8.4: Physiological values: urine vs. amniotic liquid

	Weeks		
Urine/amn. liquid	*18-20*	*20-30*	*>32*
Na$^+$ (mEq/ml)	42/137	42/140	47/140
Cl$^-$ (mEq/ml)	23/109	47/109	41/108
OsM (mOsm)	98/267	102/273	102/271
NAG (U/L)	2.0/3.6	2.7/3.62	2.0/4.69
G (ml/L)	4.7/4.5	5.1/5.0	5.3/5.8
K$^+$ (mEq/ml)		41/140	
Creatinine (ml/L)		1.9/.6	

Table 8.5: Pathological values: urine vs. amniotic liquid

	Weeks		
Urine/amn. liquid	*18-20*	*20-30*	*>32*
Na$^+$ (mEq/ml)	120/132	126.4/140	139.6/140
Cl$^-$ (mEq/ml)	119/107	132.5/149	141/158
OsM (mOsm)	240/267	261.5/273	281/296
NAG (U/L)	18/16.9	25.83/20.34	25.73/20.8
G (ml/L)	26/22.3	38.9/28.74	38.72/30.0
K$^+$ (mEq/mL)	3.1/138	3.4/140.6	3.9/148
Creatinine (ml/L)	1.2/0.7	2.54/0.82	3.7/0.9

The increase in concentration of NAG and β_2 microglobulin increase possibly due to the cumulative effect of the amniotic clearance mechanism.

This opens the field of study of nephrouropathies through the determination of these and other parameters in the amniotic liquid, without the need for invasive study of the fetal urine.[21]

The K$^+$ and creatinine concentrations are different in their predictive evaluation as there exists a great clearance effect in the placenta and great variability in its ionic charge, that makes the potasium filtration very disperse, in the other hand 90% of the K$^+$ concentration are intracellular.[8,21]

Summarizing, we can adventure a prediction of renal viability in relation to those parametres expressed. In Table 8.6 taking into account that these values are applicable to any gestational age.

Table 8.6: Fetal urine: biochemical markers applicable to any gestational age and echographic image and amniotic liquid volume to determine a renal function status

Prediction	*Bad*	*Good*
Echographic image	hyperechog + Cyst.	Normal echography
Amniotic liquid	Oligoamnios	Normal
	Fetal urine	
Na$^+$	>100 mEq/ml	<100 mEq/ml
Cl$^-$	>90 mEq/ml	<90 mEq/ml
Osmolarity	>210	<210
NAG	>8 U/L	<8 U/L
β-2 microglob	>4 mg/L	<4 mg/L
K$^+$	Indifferent	Indifferent
Creatinine	Indifferent	Indifferent

The intrauterine determination of the characteristics of fetal urine offers absolute diagnostic possibilities about the normal renal clearance function.

Urine aspiration puncture with diagnostic aims is technically feasable, using conventional spinal needles of 18 G having an aspiration system connected to a 20 cc syringe.

The way to aproach this depends on the fetal position available.

If at the posterior back position we would not find any great inconveniences in punctioning the bladder whilst for a lateral or anterior back where a nephrostomic aspiration is chosen (Figure 8.9).

In neither one nor the other, can any noticeable complications be found, at least in our experience.[8,21]

The nephrostomy aspiration allows us firstly to re-evaluate the echostructural characteristics of the expanded kidney parenchyma, and secondly, as long as we use the 16 G *sure cut* aspiration system, to carry out at the same time a renal biopsy without any technical difficulties.

For this, once the nephrostomy urine aspiration has been done, without taking the needle out move it towards the renal parenchyma and carry out the aspiration with a *swing* movement over the corticomedullary area.

The obtaining of samples of 2 mm in length is enough for the detection of the histological characteristics that define a kidney dysplasia.[8,9,21-23]

But the use of 16 G catheters *aspiration biopsy set*, once the technical problems of involving tissues have been solved, allowes to obtain samples in the 65% of the cases. If conventional 18 G catheters are used but inocuous, only 30% of the cases are obtained. (J. Troyano, Ian Donald, School Interuniversity of Medical Ultrasound, Dubrovnik August 1996, unpublished observations).

SKIN BIOPSY

As already stated in the generalization section about fetal biopsies, the skin biopsy entails the most serious difficulties in the obtaining of adequate or sufficient samples that would allow correct histopathological diagnosis or prediction.

The most important aspect is the obtention of valid samples, for this we need at least 1 mm strips of skin and no smaller in surface area and that also include a thickness of the epithelial stratum, and comprising of conjunctive areas and basal membrane. Only by this can an acceptable reading be obtained.[24]

The second aspect to be taken into account is the surgical biopsy material. We have already exposed previously that the use of section 2.5 mm clipping tongs (forceps/clippers) introduced into the amniotic eviroment by trocar, will allow the obtention of skin

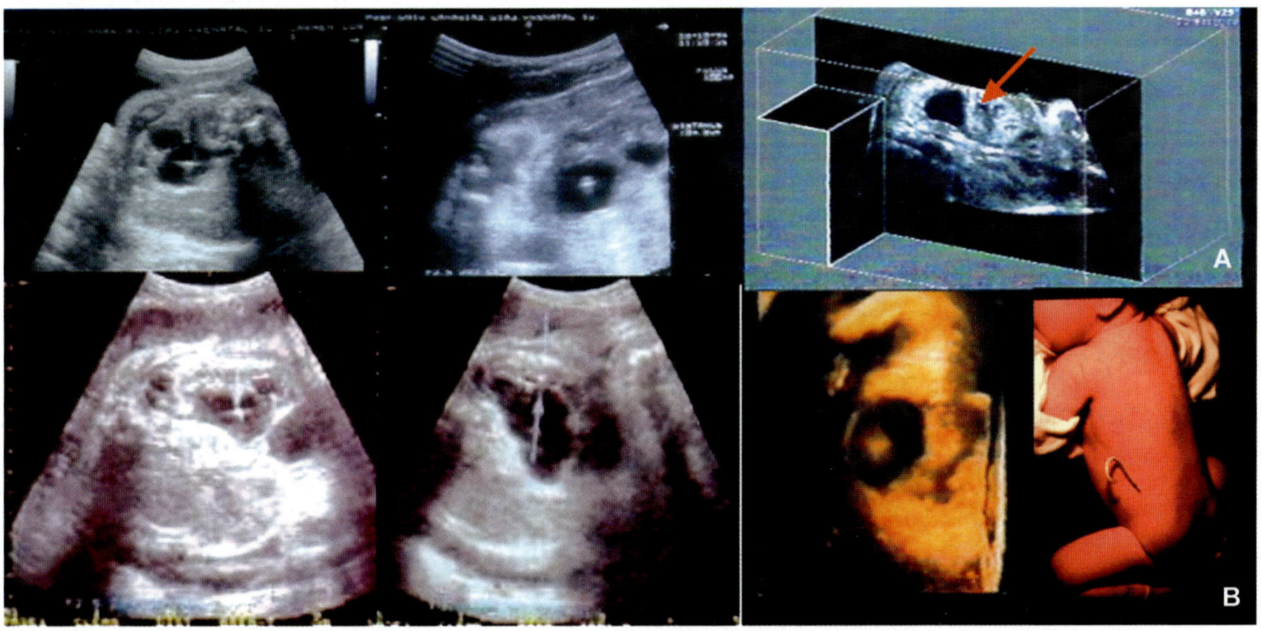

Figure 8.9: Aspirative nephrostomy: echographic monitoring; A. Niche mode, B. Ultrasound 3-D monitoring

samples in 100% of all cases, and it is true that the residual skin lesions and any pregnancy complications there maybe, will not render any noticeable benefits in relation to the diagnostic data.

The use of conventional needles and isometric aspiration practising the *slice* technique, that consists in inserting the needle sidelongly over the skin and make *scratching* or *scraping* movements, as this will allow us to obtain skin strips of optimum quality with minimum damage to the integrity of the pregnancy (Figure 8.10).[25-28]

The third aspect to consider is the place selected to proceed for the taking of the sample, as depending on the disorder that we aim to diagnose prenatally, the biopsy area would be different. Not always the same area of the fetal skin wrap will be valid, or will suit the purpose of the biopsy.

Technique

Skin samples should, if possible, be taken from different areas of the fetus.

The pregnancy stage recommended for this is around 20 weeks, as after this time, the pilose folicles and keratinization mechanisms begin to develop. The study of the elements involved in the keratinization (keratohyalin and tonofibers), initially give suspicions of the disorder.

On the other hand, at this stage in the pregnancy the dermoepidermical junction has definitively been established, and the gradual rise of intercellular desmosomes, is a great help for the diagnosis of different forms of epidermolysis.

The sequence should follow the following steps:

- Echographic monitoring
- If it is possible, the placenta must be avoided
- Take into consideration the fetal position as on some ocassions it will be necessary to obtain samples from different skin areas
- Rigorous sterilization
- Optional local anesthesia, depending on the surgical timing
- Oblique needle incidence in the thickness and surface of the skin, making a scraping or scratching movement without pulling back
- Try to obtain at least 1 mm strips. The use of the vacuum needles allow the collection of various fragments from the interior without the need of withdrawing the needle
- Immediately proceed to swim the samples in saline serum for their histological staining and fixing process or for electronic microscopy analysis.

Indications

They are most frequently based on the diagnosis of some types of genodermatosis or congenital dermoepidermic disorders, of dominating autosomic transmission as well as recesive types, the majority being lethal in short- or medium- terms.

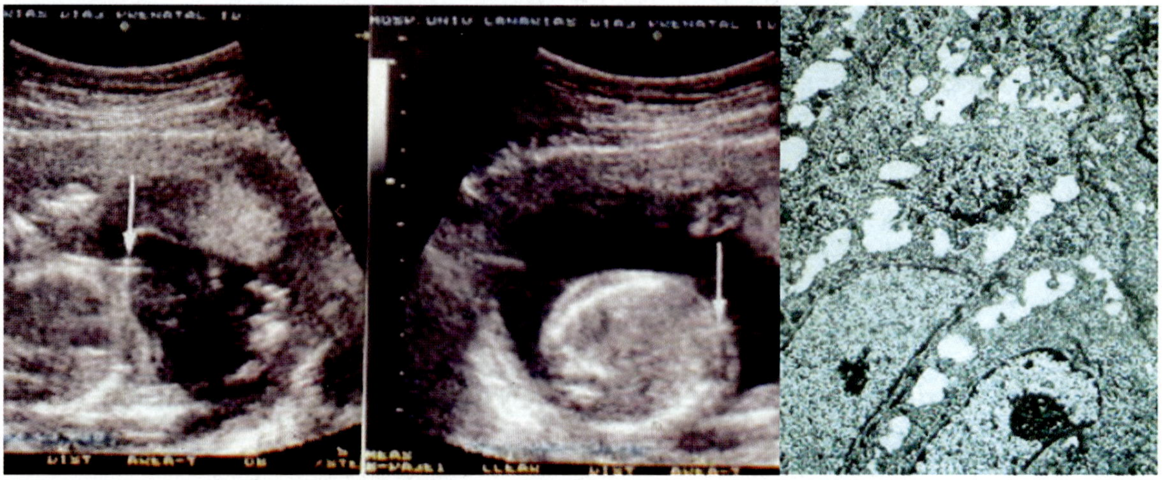

Figure 8.10: Left: skin biopsy in fetal abdomen, sidelongly scratching. Right: mature histological cutaneous samples where keratohyalin and hemidesmosomes are detected

These disorders can be classified as follows:

- *Bullous epidermolysis:* Fetuses with large scale blistered areas that once the blisters break, set off intensive erosive zones with a fast loss of electrolytes are affected.[6,10,29,30]
- *Anhidrotic ectodermic dysplasias:* Recessive disorder linked to the sex. The fetuses are born without pilose follicles, without any hair or sudoriparous glands. They develop hyperthermic affectation by disregulation and general dryness syndromes.[31]
- *Keratinization disorders:* Also called Colodion baby syndrome, characterized by the appearance of reptile skin due to epidermic membranes that are of quick shedding. Severe and lethal dehydrating disorders.[32,33]
- *Pigmentary atopies:* Ocular syndromes with severe intolerance to light and early or premature development of skin cancers.[31,34,35]

The diagnostic problems faced with these dermatosis are due to the development of the lesion has different topographic origins, so the need to select the punture spot has to be in accordance to the illness that one is traying to detect.

The diagnostic possibilities of skin biopsies are summarized in Table 8.7.

Table 8.7: Diagnoses possible in fetal skin biopsies

- Keratinization disorders:
  - o Harlequin fetus
  - o Colodion baby
  - o Sjögren-Larsson syndrome
  - o Congenital icthyosis

The puncture spot is in trunks and buttocks (Figure 8.11)

- Ampollous diseases:
  - o Herlitz ampollous junctional disease
  - o Hallopeau-Siemens ampollous dermolytic disease
  - o Inverse dystrophic ampollous disease
  - o Cockayne-Touraine dystrophic ampollous disease

The puncture spot is in waist, skin folds, abdomen and buttocks (Figure 8.12)

- Pigmentary disorders:
  - o Negative tyrosinase oculocutaneus albinism
  - o Chediak-Higashi disease
  - o Anhidrotic ectodermic disease

The puncture spot in the skin-head (scalp) (Figure 8.13)

It is fundamental to have objective family history in order to determine the biopsy spot.[34,36,37]

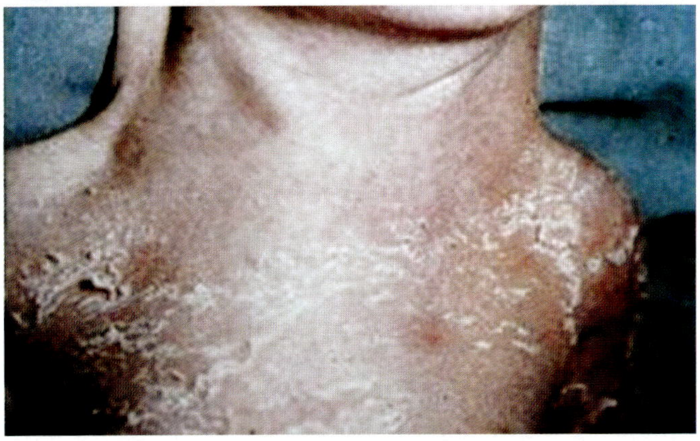

Figure 8.11: Keratinization disorder

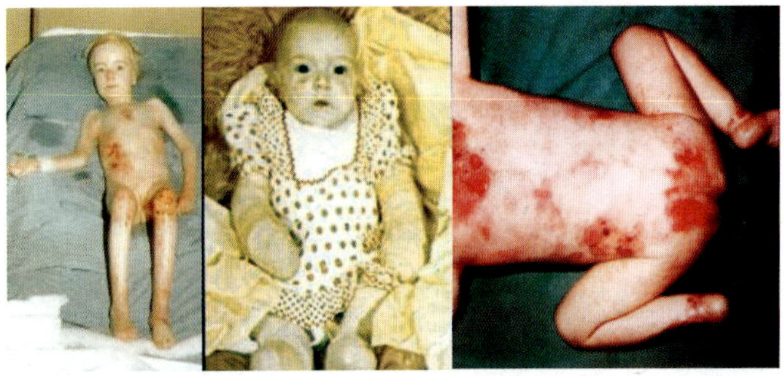

Figure 8.12: Ampollous disease

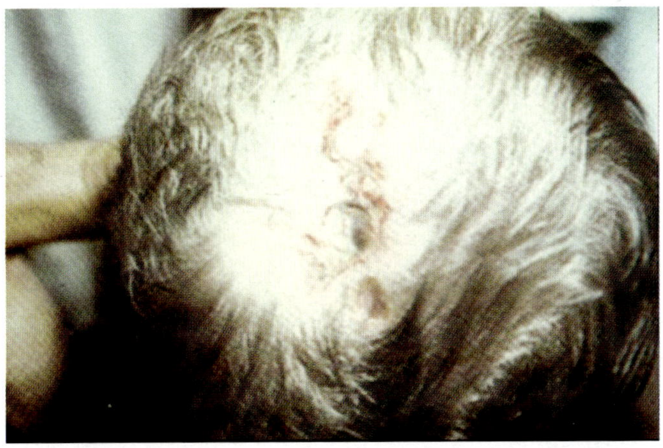

Figure 8.13: Pigmentary disorder (scalp lesions)

Complementary Requirements

The study of the samples will be based on the ultrastructural features stated beforehand. A great deal of experience in fetal dermatology using electronic microscopy is required to make the diagnosis.

It is fundamental to have objective family history knowledge in order to determine the prenatal dermoepidermic structural markers.

It is recommended to have kept previous samples in order to be used as a *study bank*.

Complications

Now the tendency is to propose minimally invasive techniques by the use of conventional needles 7.[38]

The use of conventional needles does not withhold more risks than the amniocentesis. On the other hand, the trocar techniques and the 2.5 mm section biopsy provoke around 5% of miscarriages due to iatrogenic amniorhexis, although similarly some indelible fetal skin lesions have been described (Figure 8.14). This does not occur in cases where the *scalp* technique is carried out with the use of conventional needles.

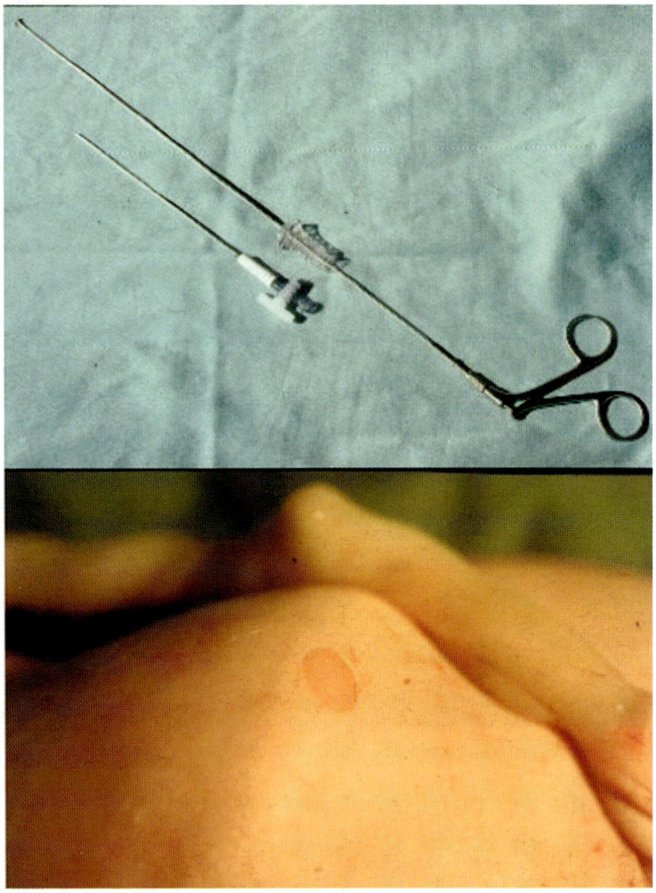

Figure 8.14: Residual cutaneous lesion after biopsy with clipper system

MUSCLE BIOPSY

This is carried out preferably for the prenatal diagnosis of Duchenne's muscular dystrophy (DMD), although it is also possible to detect other heredetary myopathies as long as there is some clinical family history of these disorders.[11,38,39]

For the diagnosis of Duchenne's muscular dystrophy, it is usual for the DNA analysis to be used. When the recombinations within the DMD gene or the DNA analysis are not sufficiently informative, or if from the family history it is not clear if there are possible carriers, so the direct examination of the muscle and its analysis is the only way to give the basis of an objective prenatal diagnosis.

The marker used is the dystrophine, its determination by means of immunofluorescence allows to differenciate the features of affected muscles from those of the healthy ones. The absence of this protein from the skeleton muscles is practically pathognomonic of DMD[11,14,39,40] (Figure 8.15).

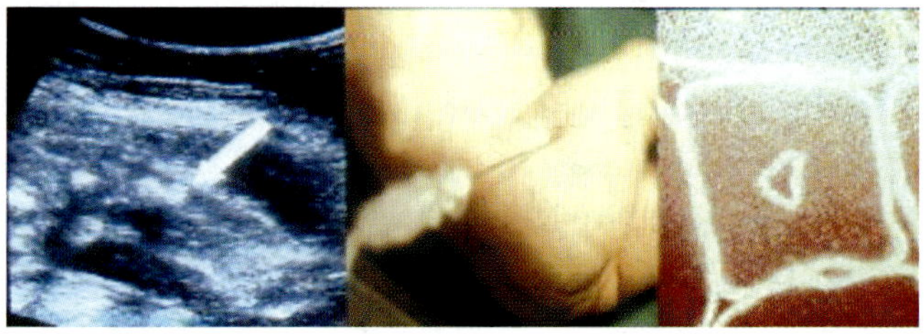

Figure 8.15: Subtrochanteric muscle biopsy; the detection of dystrophin by immunofluorescence determines healthy muscle

Some other times the prenatal diagnosis of DMD may be impossible when there is only one previously affected male in the family, and there is no identificable delection.

The absence of dystrophine in a skeleton muscle, is worth in itself the determination of the screening of the DMD. Nevertheless, this diagnosis can be reinforced by detecting a rise in phosphocreatine–kinase of more than 10 times its normal value in fetal blood.

Within the possibilities that can reinforce a prenatal DMD diagnosis or prediction we have:

- Sex linked
- High values of fosfocreatinkinase
- Absence of dystrophine
- Degenerated muscle
- Fat infiltration
- Connective infiltration
- Nuclear and cellular morphological alterations (Figure 8.16).

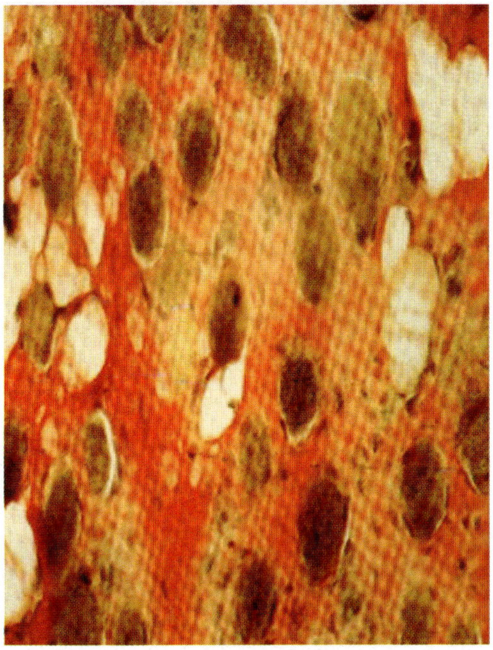

Figure 8.16: Duchenne´s muscular dystrophy; degenerated muscle as an associated sign: fat and connective infiltration, and morphological cellular alterations and leucocytes infiltration

Technique

Any muscular skeleton area is good, preferably of the external face of any of the thighs or nuckle areas, avoiding topographic places with inervation or vital vascularization, in this manner indelible functional lessions will not be provoked. Preferably using 18 G conventional needles or even better, the *sure cut* method that have already been described[8,38,41-43] (see Figure 8.2).

Carrying out subtrochanteric punctures in a descending obliquest manner as possible, orientated towards the fetal femur (see Figure 8.2).

The puncture success rate is of 75%.

It is essential to determine muscle dystrophy by immunofluorescence, being advisable but not determining the detection of phosphocreatinekinase and the study of the muscular structure at a morphological muscular level, fat and connective infiltration.

No complications are described.

The fetus is susceptible to being studied by invasive techniques. These techniques are only justified by the seriousness of a possible inherited illness, or by any other disorder detected during pregnancy; in the latter the need for biopsy diagnosis is exceptional, as the thoracocentesis, pericardiocentesis and punctures of other thoracoabdominal, primary seek a therapeutic attitude, using the extracted material for studying its analytical components.

Other punctures on fetal tumor formations (sacrococcygeal teratomas, solid cervical teratomas, etc.), or liquid collections, such as pericardiocentesis, do not have an acceptable justification from a therapeutic or diagnostic point of view, as the echographic evaluation and the present application of biophysical methods (color Doppler amongst them) give an acceptable identification of their vascularization and origin, including those of suspicious neoplasm.[44,45] (A. Kurjak, In: Ian Donald., University School of Medical Ultrasound 16th Course, - Granada, Spain, June 14th-16th 1993, Unpublished)

In agreement with our conduct, we wolud like to express this thought: ***The fetus has been endowed by nature to surpass several inconveniences provided by its forty weeks of developing. It is a "Real Titan" front any adversity and, its adaptability is exceptional.***

Don´t we disturb it!

Don´t we invade its privacy agressively!

Let´s observe it minutelly and, only when it need us, which generaly happens in few occations, it will advise us, then, let´s help it.

JM Troyano-Luque (1993)

REFERENCES

1. Bahado-Singh RO, Morotti R, PirhorenJ, Lopez JA, Mahoney MJ. Invasive techniques for prenatal diagnosis: current concepts. J Assoc Acad Minor-Phys 1995;6:28-33.
2. Cadrin C, Golbus MS. Fetal tissue sampling indications, techniques, complications and experience with sampling of fetal skin, liver and muscle. West J Med 1993;159:269-72.
3. Golbus MS, Sagebield RW, Filly RA, et al. Prenatal diagnosis of congenital icthyosiform erythroderma (epidermolytic hyperkeratosis) by fetal skin biopsy. N Engl J Med 1980;302:93.
4. KouseffBG, Matsouca LY, Stenn RS, et al. Prenatal diagnosis of Sjögren-Larsson syndrome. J Pediatr 1082;101:998.
5. Robjn AJ, David B, Gardner A, Rodeck CH. Prenatal diagnosis of oculocutaneous albinism by electron microscopy of fetal skin. J Invest Dermatol 1983;80:210-2.

6. Dolan CR, Smith LT, Syber UP. Prenatal detection of epidermolysis bullosa fetalis with pyloric atresia in a fetus by abnormal ultrasound and elevated alphafetoprotein. Am J Genet 1993;47: 395-400.
7. Rodeck CH. Fetoscopy guided by real time ultrasound for pure fetal samples, fetal skin samples and examination of the fetus in utero. Br J Obstet Gynaecol 1980;87:449-56.
8. Troyano JM, Padron E, Clavijo M. Fetal biopsy and puncture. Actual status. Balkan Ohrid's School of Ultrasound. Advanced Ultrasound II, Vol. 9. Ohrid, Macedonia: Dobri S. Filipche, 1996:51-61.
9. Campbell WA, Yamase HT, Salafia CA, Vintilizeos AM, Rodis JF. Fetal renal biopsy: technique development. Fetal Diagn Ther 1993; 8:135- 43.
10. Dunnill MG, Rodeck CH, Richards AJ et al. Use oftype VII collagen gene (COL7A1) markers in prenatal diagnosis of recessive dystrophic epidermolysis bullosa. J Med Genet 1995;32: 749-50.
11. Evans MI, Farrell SA, Greb A, Ray P, Johnson MP, Hoffman EP. In utero fetal muscle biopsy for the diagnosis of Duchenne musçular dystrophy in a female fetus' suddenly at risk'. Am J Med Genet 1993;46:309-12.
12. Fox J, Hack AM, Fenton WA, et al. Prenatal diagnosis of ornithine transcarbamylase deficiency with the use of DNA polymorphisms. N Engl J Med 1986;315:1205.
13. Matilla 1, Corral J, Miranda M, et al. Prenatal diagnosis of Werdnig-Woffmann disease: DNA analysis of a mummified umbilical cord using closely linked microsatellite markers. Prenat Diagn 1994;14:219-22.
14. Kuller JA, Hoffman EP, Fries MH, Golbus MS. Prenatal diagnosis of Duchenne muscular dystrophy by fetal muscle biopsy. Hum Genet 1992;90:34-40.
15. Illum N, Lavard L, Danpure ZJ, Aerenlund Jensen H, Skovby F. Primary hyperoxaluria type 1: clinical manifestation in infancy and prenatal diagnosis. Child Nephrol Urol 1992;12:225-7.
16. Rodeck CH, Patrick AD, Pembrey ME, Tzannatos C, Whitfield AE. Fetal liver biopsy for prenatal diagnosis of ornithine carbamyl transferase deficiency. Lancet 1982;1: 297-9.
17. Goebel HH, Vesa J, Reiter B, et al. Prenatal diagnosis of infantile neuronal ceroidlipofuscinosis: a combined electron microscopic and molecular genetic approach. Brain Dey 1995;17:83-8.
18. Murotsuki J, Vehara 5, Okamura K, Yajima A, Oura 1, Miyabayashi 5. Fetal liver biopsy for prenatal diagnosis of carbamoyl phosphate synthetase deficiency. Am J Perinatol 1994;11: 160-2.
19. Tsushida Y, Kawarasaki H, Iwanaka T, Uchida H, Nakanishi H, Uno K. Antenatal diagnosis of biliary atresia (type 1 cyst) at 19 weeks gestation: differential diagnosis and etiologic implications. J Pediatr Surg 1995;30:607-9.
20. Von Dobeln V, Venizelos N, Westgren M, Hagenfeldt L. Long chain 3-hydroxylacyl-CoA dehydrogenase in chorionic villi, fetal liver, and fibroblasts and prenatal diagnosis of 3-hydroxylacyl-CoA dehydrogenase. J Inherit Metab Dis 1994;17:185-8.
21. Troyano JM, de la Fuente P, eds. Prenatal features of fetal kidney physiopathology and their intra and extrauterine treatment. A multidisciplinary problem. Santa Cruz de Tenerife: University Hospital of the Canary Islands, 1993:35-9.
22. Greco P, Loverro G, Carusso G, Clement R, Selvaggi L. Diagnostic potential of fetal renal biopsy. Prenat Diagn 1994;14:415.
23. Gubler MC, Levy M. Prenatal diagnosis of nail-patella syndrorne by intrauterine kidney biopsy. Am J Med Genet 1993;47:122-4.
24. Elias S, Emerson DS, SimpsonJL, Shulrnan LP, Holbrook KA. Ultrasound-guided fetal skin sampling for prenatal diagnosis of genodermatoses. Obstet Gynecol 1994;83:337-41.
25. Bakharev VA, Aivazyan AA, Karetnikova NA, Mordovtsev VN, Yantousky Y. Fetal skin biopsy in prenatal diagnosis of sorne genodermatoses. Prenat Diagn 1990;10:1-12.
26. Buckshee Li, Parveen 5, Mittal 5, Verma K, Singh M. Percutaneous ultrasound-guided fetal skin biopsy: a new approach. Int J Gynaecol Obstet 1991 ;34:267-70.
27. Holbrook KA, Wapner R, Jackson L, Zaeri N. Diagnosis and prenatal diagnosis of epidermolysis bullosa herpetiformis (Dowling-Meara). In a mother, two affected children and an affected fetus. Prenat Diagn 1992;1 2:725-39.
28. Suzumori K, Kanzak 1. Prenatal diagnosis of Harlequirn ichthyosis by fetal skin biopsy; report of two cases. Prenat Diagn 1991 ;1 (1):451-7.
29. McGrath JA, McMillan JR, Dunnill MG, et al. Genetic bases of lethaljunctional epidermolysis bullosa in an affected fetus: implications for prenatal diagnosis in one family. Prenat Diagn 1995;15:647-54.
30. Shirnizu H, Onodera Y, Ikeda 5, Ogawa H, Suzumori K, Nishikawa T. Prenatal diagnosis of epidermolysis bullosa: first successful trial in Asia. Dermatology 1994;188:46-9.
31. Shimizu H, Ishko A, Kikushi A, Akiyarna M, Susumori K, Nishikawa 1. Prenatal diagnosis of tyrosinase negative oculocutaneous albinism by an electron microscopic dopa-reaction test of fetal skin. Prenat Diagn 1994; 14:442-50.
32. Akiyama M, Kim DK, Main DM, Otto CE, Holbrook KA. Characteristic morphologic abnormality of harlequin ichthyosis detected in amniotic fluid cells. J Invest Dermatol 1994; 102:210-3.
33. Rizzo WB. Sjögren-Larsson syndrome. Semin Dermatol 1993;12:210-8.
34. Akeo K, Shirai S, Okisaka S, et al. Histology of fetal ages with oculocutaneous albinism. Arch Ophthalmol 1996;1 (14):613-6.
35. Shimizu H, Niizeki H, Suzurnori K, et al. Prenatal diagnosis of oculocutaneous albinism by analysis of the fetal tyrosinase gene. J Invest Dermatol 1994;103:104-6.
36. Holbrook KA, Smith LI, Elias S. Prenatal diagnosis of genetic skin disease using fetal skin biopsy samples. Arch Dermatol 1993;129: 1437-54.
37. Normand J, Karasek MA. A method for the isolation and serial propagation of keratinocytes, endothelial cells and

fibroblasts from a single punch biopsy of human skin. Jn vitro Cell Dey Biol Anim 1995;31:447-55.

38. Evans MI, Krivchenia EL, Johnson MP, et al. In utero fetal muscle biopsy alters diagnosis and carrier risks in Duchenne and Becket muscular dystrophy. Fetal Diagn Ther 1995;10:71-5.
39. Fanin M, Pegoraro E, Angelini C. Absence of dystrophin and spectrin in regenerating muscle fibers from Becket dystrophy patients. J Neurol Sci 1994;123:88-94.
40. Lindahl M, Backman E, Henriksson KG, Gorospe JR, Hoffman EP. Phospholipase A2 activity in dystrophinopathies. Neuromusc Disord 1995;5: 193-9.
41. Benzie RJ, RayP, Thompson D, HunterAG, Ivey B, Salvador L. Prenatal exclusion of Duchenne muscular dystrophy in fetal muscle biopsy. Prenat Diagn 1994;14:235-8.
42. Evans MI, Hoffman EP, Cadrin C, Johnson MP, Quintero RA, Golbus MS. Fetal muscle biopsy: collaborative experience with varied indications. Obstet Gynecol 1994;84:913-7.
43. Evans MI, Quintero RA, King M, Kureshi F, Hoffman EP, Johnson MP. Endoscopically assisted, ultrasound-guided fetal muscle biopsy. Fetal Diagn Ther 1995;10:167-72.
44. Troyano JM, Clavijo MT, Clemente I, Marco OY, Rayward J, Mahtani VG. Kidney and urinary tract diseases: Ultrasound and biochemical markers. The Ultrasound Review of Obstetrics and Gynecology. 2002; 2(2): 92-109.
45. Bebatar A, Vaughan J, Nicolini U, Trotter S, Corrin B, Lincoln C. Prenatal pericariocentesis: its role in the management of intrapericardial teratoma. Obstet Gynecol 1992; 79 (5); (Pt2):859.

CHAPTER 9

Fetal Blood Sampling

Papantoniou Nikolas

INTRODUCTION

Fetal blood sampling was first performed by Valenti[1] in 1972 under endoscopic visualization during second trimester elective termination of pregnancies by cesarean section.

Two years later Kan[2] obtained fetal blood by direct placentocentesis in pregnancies with anterior placentas. At the same year 1974 Hobbins and Mahoney[3] reported the first transabdominal sampling of fetal blood using a 1.5 to 2.8 mm diameter fetoscope under ultrasonographic guidance.

Fetoscopy allowed fetal blood sampling without laparotomy, however the technique needed the use of local anesthesia and IV analgesia.

Pure fetal blood was obtained at 60 to 70% of the cases[4] with a fetal loss rate ranging between 3 and 5%[5,6] at the best hands. Additionally, chorio-amnionitis or premature rupture of membranes ranged between 18 and 30%.

In 1979, Rodeck and Campell[7] reported for the first time fetal blood sampling without any contamination from maternal blood by fetoscopy.

Finally, in 1983 Daffos et al[8] first reported the successful fetal blood sampling by the transabdominal route using a single needle under ultrasonographic guidance. The technique was named cordocentesis but similar terms exist such as a omphalocentesis, cordocentesis, or percutaneous umbilical blood sampling (PUBS). This technique combined the simplicity of amniocentesis with the effectiveness of fetoscopy and is a major breakthrough in prenatal diagnosis and fetal therapy.

INDICATIONS

During the decade of 1970 the commonest indications for fetal blood sampling was the diagnosis of hemoglobinopathies and red cell disorders, the diagnosis and management of Rh isoimmunization, as well as platelet disorders, intrauterine congenital infection, rapid karyotype and the diagnosis of immunodeficiency disorders (Table 9.1). Percutaneous umbilical blood sampling was widely adopted for prenatal diagnosis and therapy in the second half of the 80s and an exponential increase in number of procedures was observed for almost a decade.

Table 9.1: Prenatal diagnosis by fetal blood sampling

- Chromosomal
  - Karyotype
  - Mosaicism
  - Fragile X
- Fetal infections
  - Toxoplasmosis
  - Rubella
  - Varicella
  - Cytomegalovirus
  - Human parvovirus B19
- Isoimmunization
  - Rhesus disease
  - Other antigens
- Coagulopathies
  - Hemophilia A,B
  - von Willebrand's disease
  - Isolated factor deficiency
- Hemoglobinopathies and red cell disorders
  - Sickle cell anemia
  - α-thalassemia
  - β-thalassemia
  - Poikilocytosis
  - Spherocytosis
  - Diamond- Blackfan syndrome
  - Aase syndrome
  - Enzyme deficiencies, i.e. G6PD
- Immunodeficiencies
  - Severe combined immunodeficiency disorders
  - Chronic granulomatous disease
  - Chediak-Higashi syndrome
  - Wiskott-Aldrich syndrome
  - Ataxia telangiectasia
  - Homozygous C3 deficiency
  - Purine–nucleoside phosphorylase deficiency
- Platelet disorders
  - Alloimune thrombocytopenia
  - Autoimmune thrombocytopenia
- Other
  - Familial hypercholesterolemia
  - Hyperphenylalaninemia
  - Farber syndrome

Indications for fetal blood sampling have changed rapidly as new molecular biology techniques such as polymerase chain reaction (PCR) on chorionic villi or amniotic fluid cells can provide reliable diagnostic information for a variety of hereditary disorders, such as hemoglobinopathies, metabolic disorders and congenital infections with high sensitivity and specificity. Indications for erythroblastosis fetalis have also decreased significantly.

Nevertheless, at the beginning of the 21st century, there still exist some indications for fetal blood sampling which include

a. The presence of mosaicism at amniocentesis.
b. Rh isoimmunization.[9]
c. Hydrops of unknown origin.
d. Alloimune thrombocytopenia.
e. Fetal infections selected cases.
f. Prenatal diagnosis of hemoglobinopathies when DNA polymorphisms are not available for comparison.
g. Fetal blood grouping.
h. Thyroid disease, and finally.
i. Rapid karyotype in cases of delayed diagnosis of congenital malformations.

Cordocentesis has contributed significantly towards fetal therapy, with the use of intravascular intrauterine transfusions, or with drug administration digoxin, etc. The most common fetal pathologies that can be managed using cordocentesis are listed in Table 9.2.

Table 9.2: Common fetal pathology

i. Hemolytic disease
ii. Thrombocytopenia
iii. Agammaspherinemia
iv. Drug administration.

Prenatal Diagnosis of Hemoglobinopathies

Prenatal diagnosis is currently made with the use of molecular biology techniques.

If molecular techniques are not available, prenatal diagnosis of hemoglobinopathies can be performed on fetal blood obtained by cordocentesis by assessment of the rate of synthesis of different globin chain.[10]

In our department, Maternal Fetal Medicine Unit, Alexandra Hospital, University of Athens, we have performed more than 2000 cases of percutaneous fetal blood sampling for prenatal diagnosis of hemoglobinopathies, mainly beta-thalassemia. Since fetal loss rate is related to the indication of the procedure and the experience of the practitioner, and given the fact that in hemoglobinopathies fetuses are otherwise healthy, in our series fetal loss rate was low 1.6%.[39]

Beta-thalassemia can be caused by more than 60 different mutations. Four to six mutations account for over 90% of beta-thalassemia cases worldwide, so that most mutations can be detected by direct methods, such as PCR coupled with allele-specific oligonucleotide hybridization, restriction endonuclease digestion of amplified product, or both.[11-13] The accuracy of these tests is close to 100%.

The diagnosis of sickle cell anemia can be made reliably with the use of restriction endonucleases in cultured chorionic villi or amniotic cells.[14]

Alpha thalassemia is a condition with different presentation depending on the number of the four alpha-globin genes involved. The lack of one or two alpha-globin genes is generally asymptomatic. If three alpha-globin genes are missing hemoglobin H disease moderate or marked anemia is present since birth, though the condition is not lethal. If all four alpha-globin genes are deleted or inactive, fetal erythrocytes contain gamma-globin tetramers Hb Bart. The condition presents with nonimmune hydrops usually leading to fetal demise at 28 to 37 weeks. Prenatal diagnosis is indicated only in couples at risk for HB Bart's hydrops fetalis.

The accuracy of testing with the use of DNA techniques is greater than 99% since only three common deletions, in southeast Asia and eight common deletions throughout the world account for nearly all alpha-thalassemia mutations.[15]

Fetal Blood Sampling for Cytogenetic Diagnosis

Chorionic villous sampling and amniocentesis are the methods of choice for the prenatal diagnosis of chromosomal abnormalities.

The only remaining reasons for obtaining fetal blood for the diagnosis of chromosomal abnormalities are:

a. When karyotype results are necessary within a short time interval and the woman has presented in late pregnancy or when the time limit for legal termination is near, or delivery is imminent
b. When is a high risk of impeding fetal death, since determination of fetal karyotype may fail when performed at postmortem examination thus jeopardizing future genetic counseling and
c. When mosaicism or pseudomosaicism is detected at amniocentesis or chorionic villous sampling.

Fetal karyotype can also be obtained by transabdominal placental biopsy in the second and third trimesters of pregnancies, but fetal blood sampling is the method of choice, because the number of mitoses in trophoblastic tissue at this stage of gestation is lower than in those in blood cells.[16]

Another cytogenetic indication for fetal blood sampling is the presence of mosaicism at amniocentesis or CVS. Mosaicism has been reported in 2 to 3% of trophoblastic cell cultures,[17] but is confirmed by amniocentesis or fetal blood sampling only in 0.2 to 0.4% of the cases.[17] However, if mosaicism is not confirmed in fetal blood, patients should be informed that it is not possible to exclude that the mosaic cell line may be present in fetal tissues other than blood.

A supernumerary chromosome represents a heterogeneous group of disorders that can be inherited from one of the parents or arise *de novo*. Fetal blood sampling can be offered to the couple in order to rule out mosaicism for the marker chromosome in cases of *de novo* occurrences. Again, identification of mosaicism for marker chromosome in fetal blood is diagnostic but a negative result is not helpful.

Fetal Blood Sampling for Diagnosis of Congenital Infection

Indications for fetal blood sampling for the prenatal diagnosis of various congenital infections such as toxoplasmosis, rubella, cytomegalovirus, varicella, parvovirus and congenital syphilis,[18] have been significantly reduced due to extensive use of identification of specific DNA sequences of the infectious agents mentioned above with the use of PCR.

The general approach consists of obtaining fetal blood in order to isolate the infectious agent using standard microbiological techniques or PCR, or documenting a specific fetal immunoresponse, or serologic, hepatologic or hematologic studies indicative of fetal infection.

Fetal immunoresponse to the infectious is influenced by the maturity of fetal immune system, so that a consistent response may not be detected before 20 to 22 weeks. In addition the response can also be transient and therefore affected by the time interval between infection and blood sampling.

Moreover, fetal immunoresponse may be weak or undetectable and the formation of antigen-antibody complexes under condition of excess antigen may interfere with the immunologic assays used.

In conclusion, when fetal IgM is detected the diagnosis of fetal infection can be confirmed, while the absence of the specific antibody cannot exclude the diagnosis.

The fetal blood specimen is also examined for elevated WBC, elevated eosinophilic count, low platelet count and elevated liver enzymes, parameters which constitute nonspecific evidence of infection, but are important when fetal infection is strongly suspected and other techniques are inconclusive.

In our department, we have compared the sensitivity of amniotic fluid for mouse inoculation, amplification of *T. gondii* DNA by polymerase chain reaction PCR and fetal blood for detection of *T. gondii* specific IgM antibodies in ninety-three pregnant women with *T. gondii* seroconversion during pregnancy. The evidence of vertical transmission was 19.4%. The sensitivity for mouse inoculation was 61%, for PCR was 83.3%, while the combination for both tests allowed the prenatal diagnosis of 94.4%. In 13 cases where FBS was carried out had negative results. However, in two cases fetal infection was detected by amniotic fluid studies, which shows that a negative fetal IgM alone, cannot exclude the infection.

Similar sensitivities we have observed in 42 pregnancies with CMV primary infection. The sensitivity of amniotic fluid PCR 85.7% was superior to fetal IgM and in two cases fetal IgM studies were false-negative. This is generally due to timing or failure of the fetal immune system to sustain IgM response. Anemia, thrombocytopenia and elevated liver function tests were not observed in 13 cases where FBS was carried out, including the 2 false-negatives.

After the introduction of new molecular techniques over the last 15 years PCR, etc. amniocentesis after 20 to 22 weeks is the method of choice for the prenatal diagnosis of congenital infection, so that fetal blood sampling is limited only when amniocentesis fails to establish a diagnosis.

Intrauterine Assessment of IUGR Fetuses

In the presence of severely growth-restricted fetuses fetal blood sampling used to be the method of choice to identify possible causes such as aneuploidy or fetal infection or to assess the hematologic or acid-base status.[19]

Fetuses with severe growth restriction have signs of chronic hypoxia, as manifested by significantly increased levels of hemoglobin erythropoietin, and increased erythroblast count.[20] Since IUGR fetuses have a higher prevalence of hypoxia and academia as compared with normally grown fetuses, assessment of fetal oxygenation and acid-base balance in growth restricted fetuses has been proposed to optimize the timing of delivery. The acid-base status has been shown to correlate with noninvasive tests, such as Doppler velocimetry studies, nonstress test, and biophysical profile.[21, 22] The main indication for fetal blood sampling in IUGR fetuses today is for fetal karyotyping and simultaneous evaluation of pH and acid-base balance.

In our department we performed 73 blood samplings in 70 growth retarded fetuses. In three cases with abnormal karyotype the pregnancy was terminated. Six fetal losses 8.9% occurred in this group within two weeks of the procedure. In four fetuses metabolic acidosis was detected at the time of sampling, but because of the early onset of growth retardation a cesarean section was not taken into consideration. Three fetuses died *in utero* more than two weeks after the procedure, while four others died in the neonatal period. Two of the latter were found to have pulmonary hypoplasia, one intracranial hemorrhage and the other septicemia.

However, fetal blood sampling is an invasive procedure that cannot be performed for a longitudinal assessment of fetal wellbeing. Acid-base determination has not been shown to predict perinatal mortality in karyotypically normal, growth restricted fetuses without end-diastolic flow on Doppler velocimetry studies.[21]

Fetal wellbeing of the fetus is currently assessed by using biophysical profile and Doppler velocimetry therefore significantly decreasing the need of fetal blood sampling.

Hematologic Conditions Diagnosed by Fetal Blood Sampling

Hematologic indications for fetal blood sampling include assessment of fetal hematocrit in pregnant women with red cell isoimmunization and assessment of fetal platelet count in women with platelet alloimunization.

Rhesus Isoimmunization

The widespread use of Rh immune globulin has significantly reduced the incidence of hemolytic disease in 1/1000 liveborn infants as reported by the centers for Rh disease control.[23] Nevertheless, more than 400 other antigens are capable of producing hemolytic disease to the fetus. The inability to screen more than few Rh, Kell, Duffy, in the majority of pregnancies, has resulted in an incidence of hemolytic disease of 1 to 6.8/1000.

Efforts *in utero* treatment have been made since the era of Liley,[24] with intraperitoneal transfusions in the early 1960s and with poor results. They were successfully continued with intravascular transfusions via cordocentesis, a technique first shown by Daffos et al.[8]

Until the beginning of the new millennium all pregnancies complicated by alloimunization were followed with maternal indirect Coombs' titers, ultrasound markers, amniocentesis and fetal blood sampling. Several techniques for intravascular transfusion have been proposed, the most popular using the umbilical cord insertion site in the placenta. Fetal blood sampling for evaluation of fetal anemia carries a 1% fetal loss rate per procedure and according to some reports up to 2.7% up to 28 weeks of gestation.[25] Fortunately, only 10% of the estimated 1 to 6.8/1000 pregnancies affected by isoimmunization will require transfusion until the 34th week of gestation. Lately, noninvasive diagnosis of fetal anemia with the use of peak systolic velocity of the middle cerebral artery PSV-MCA[26] has been introduced in clinical practice and significantly reduced the need for fetal blood sampling in these pregnancies.[27] On the other hand, when Doppler studies are indicative of the presence of moderate or severe anemia, the only approach for evaluation and treatment remains through fetal blood sampling and intravascular transfusions (Figure 9.1). In our institution we have estimated the risk of fetal blood sampling in nonhydropic fetuses to be 1.3%, before the introduction of Doppler MCA-PSV in clinical practice. The overall perinatal survival rate in transfused fetuses was 83%.[28]

Prenatal Diagnosis of Coagulopathies

The majority of inherited coagulopathies can now be diagnosed by molecular genetic testing on amniocytes or chorionic villi.

Prenatal diagnosis of the lack of clotting factors can be performed by DNA polymorphisms analysis from chorionic villi sampling.[29] In cases where there is no information available for the family of the patient the only method is fetal blood sampling for direct measurement of the plasma levels of each clotting factor,[30] and other clotting studies.

Hemophilia A is inherited in an X-linked recessive pattern and its severity is related to the degree of reduction of factor VIIIC. Hemophilia B, or Christmas disease is also an X-linked recessive disorder due to deficiency in factor IX activity. In these cases low concentrations of the factor in combination with fetal sex will reveal the diagnosis.

von Willebrand disease is the most common inherited bleeding disorder and is characterized by a prolonged bleeding time associated with qualitative and quantitative abnormalities of vWF. More than 70% of von Willebrand cases are inherited as an autosomal dominant trait. Only homozygous cases of the disease warrant prenatal diagnosis due to severe hemorrhaging manifestations. Fetal blood sampling will reveal decreased levels of vWF, VIIIC and VIIIAg VIIIC: functional attribute of factor VIII, VIIIAg: antigenic expression of factor VIII as measured by immunoassays.

Platelet Disorders

Platelet disorders are either inherited or occur due to the passage of maternal antibodies through the placenta. The commonest platelet disorders that can be diagnosed by fetal blood sampling are listed in Table 9.3.

Table 9.3: Common platelet disorders

1. Wiskott Aldrich syndrome
2. May-Hegglin anomaly/TAR syndrome
3. Glanzmann's thrombasthenia
4. Alloimmune thrombocytopenia
5. Immune thrombocytopenic purpura

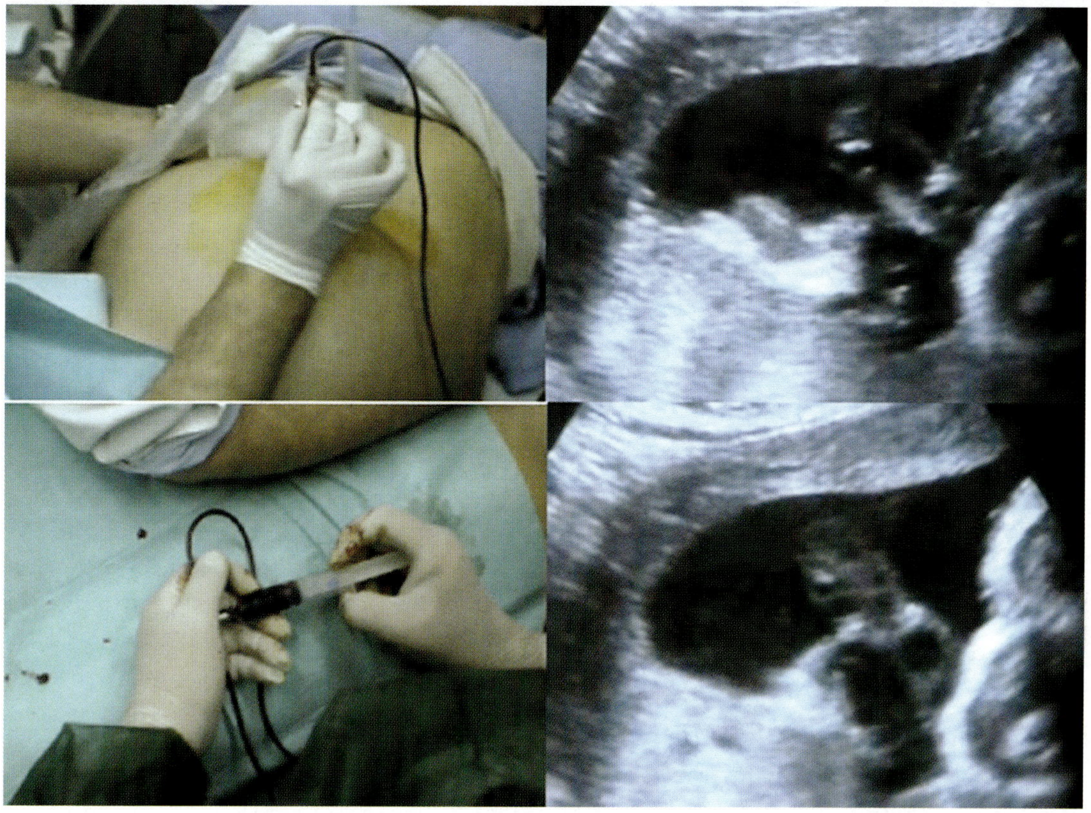

Figure 9.1: Fetal blood sampling and intravascular transfusion

Alloimmune thrombocytopenia occurs in about 1:5000 births, and in the majority of cases it involves the platelet-specific antigen PLA-1.The disease is the platelet equivalent of Rh isoimmunization. Severe fetal thrombocytopenia develops from transplacental passage of maternal antibodies and may lead to intracranial hemorrhage *in utero*. Fetal blood sampling is indicated in patients with previous pregnancies complicated by alloimmune thrombocytopenia to quantify the fetal platelet count and possibly begin antenatal therapy with maternal administration of intravenous gammaglobulin.

Idiopathic thrombocytopenic purpura ITP is much more common in obstetrics than alloimmune thrombocytopenia. In the setting of ITP maternal autoantibodies may cross the placenta and cause fetal thrombocytopenia, albeit much less frequently and of much less severity than with alloimmune thrombocytopenia. There is considerable debate as to whether the risks of fetal blood sampling are justified by the small risk of adverse fetal outcome from ITP. If fetal blood sampling confirms the presence of severe fetal thrombocytopenia in the setting of ITP at term, cesarean delivery may be performed.[31] No evidence exists, however, that such a management strategy improves perinatal outcome. Consequently, fetal blood sampling is being used less frequently in the contemporary management of ITP in pregnancy.

Since excessive bleeding after sampling in fetuses with coagulopathies has been reported.[32] Concentrated platelets for transfusion should be available at the time of fetal blood sampling in these cases.

Fetal Therapy

Access to fetal circulation offers the possibility of infusing biologic or pharmacologic agents for therapeutic purposes. This approach is necessary when the transplacental passage of the drug is poor, e.g., digoxin in hydropic fetuses with supraventricular tachycardia or when the drug must be administered as a bolus, e.g. adenosine in cases of persistent supraventricular tachycardia resistant to digoxin.

Another promising application is genetic therapy *in utero*, particularly of inherited disorders that can be treated with bone marrow transplantation, and extensive animal data are available to suggest that the earlier in pregnancy stem cells are transplanted, the lower the risk of rejection.[33]

TECHNIQUES OF FETAL BLOOD SAMPLING

Informed Consent

Fetal blood sampling is considered a surgical approach so that both the pregnant woman and the father of the baby to be born, must be completely informed about the technique and the risk to the fetus and mother.

Fetal losses depend on kinds of the procedure, i.e. cordocentesis, intrahepatic fetal blood sampling, cardiocentesis, and the existence of fetal pathology and ranges between 1 to 5%. However, information regarding Figure 9.2 of the tertiary center where the procedure takes place must also be given.

The couple must be informed about the limitations of the technique regarding obtaining blood, as well as the processing and analyzing the fetal blood.

Parents should always give their consent regarding the possible points of sampling umbilical cord, hepatic vein, fetal heart as well as the possibility of the need to abandon the procedure at any stage of the process if fetal life is considered in jeopardy.

Cordocentesis

An ultrasound examination is performed prior to the procedure in order to evaluate fetal viability, position and growth of the fetus, possible associated structural anomalies as well as the location of the placenta. The identification of the insertion site of the umbilical cord in the placenta or a fixed segment of cord is very important detail, since this information determines the target of the process. Color Doppler is very helpful in difficult cases to identify the branching of the vessels within the placental mass (Figures 9.2 and 9.3).

Prior to fetal viability the procedure of fetal blood sampling can be performed in an outpatient department. After viability, the procedure should be performed with an operating room available in order to proceed to cesarean section if it is required in case fetal distress develops during or after the procedure, as well as with adequate neonatal support available.

Cordocentesis is easiest when the placenta is anterior, because access to the target area of the cord with a posterior placenta is sometimes difficult due to the intervening fetus.

The abdomen is cleaned with an antiseptic solution and draped. The use of local anesthesia is a matter of choice.

A regular 22-gauge spinal needle, 9 cm long is used for cordocentesis. However, the length of the needle should take into account the thickness of maternal abdominal wall and the location of the target segment of the cord in the uterus. In such cases a15 cm length needle must be used. In cases of transfusion of packed red cells a 20-gauge needle is usually used. Nowadays, most of the experienced operators use a free-hand technique because of its flexibility in the adjustment of the needle path. A few centers still use the needle-within-needle technique.

The needle, under continuous ultrasonographic guidance enters the maternal abdominal wall and traverses slowly and steadily towards the targeted vessel.

In cases of a posterior placenta the needle goes through the amniotic cavity up until a few mm prior to the targeted vessel. Then advances slowly and steadily another 3 to 5 mm as to overcome the vessel wall resistance and insert the lumen. The proper insertion of the needle tip is confirmed sonographically as well as from the fact that blood is shown in the top of the used needle.

The volume of blood removed varies with the number of tests required and should take into account the gestational age. Usually up to 4 ml during the 2nd trimester and 6 ml during the 3rd trimester is considered as a safe quantity to be drawn.

Once the needle is in place the samples required are taken using different numbered syringes, and the transfer to the appropriate tubes should be done immediately after collection.

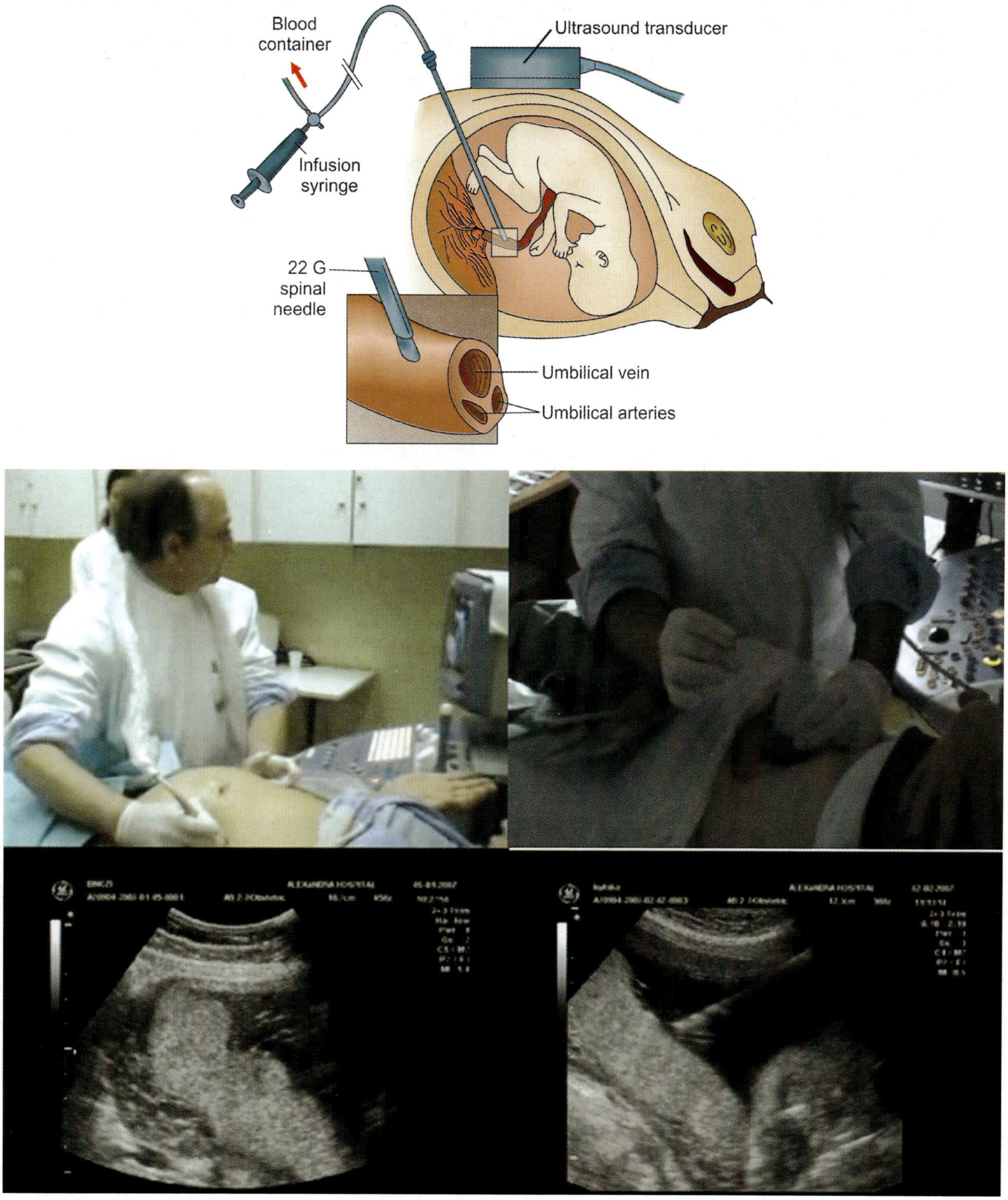

Figure 9.2: Technique of cordocentesis

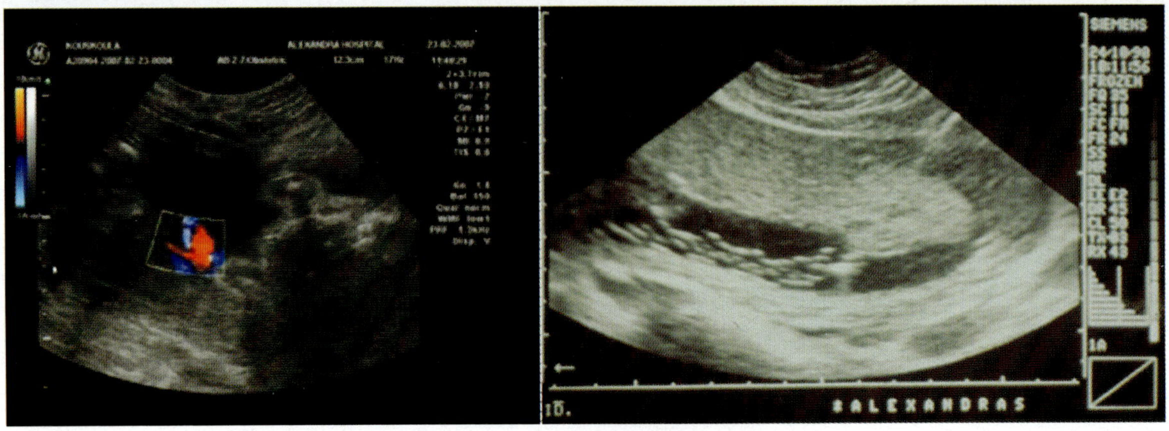

Figure 9.3: Color Doppler showing branching of vessels within fetal mass

Tubes containing citrate are for coagulation studies. Tubes with EDTA are for complete blood cell count and platelets, blood group typing requires serum and karyotype and molecular biology analysis require anticoagulation with sodium heparin. Finally, blood gas analysis can be performed directly on a sample in a heparin-primed syringe.

The puncture site is checked for bleeding for 10 minutes. All transdermal samplings tend to bleed thus requiring careful check until bleeding stops.

Fetal heart rate prior to the procedure must be within normal range, where in cases of viability post procedure checking time may reach up to 30 to 60 min. In cases of endometrial blood transfusion check must be done for the possibility of hematoma formation at the puncture site.

In cases of a Rh negative mother with a Rh positive or unknown Rh of the fetus, 300 mg of anti-D γ-globulin is administered.

The use of paralytic agents to decease fetal movements remains at the choice of the operator. In cases of procedures lasting more than 15 min. the preferred agents used are pancuronium (0.3 mg/kg of fetal weight), atracurium (0.4 mg/kg of fetal weight) and D tubocurarine (1.5-3.0 mg/kg of fetal weight) IV.

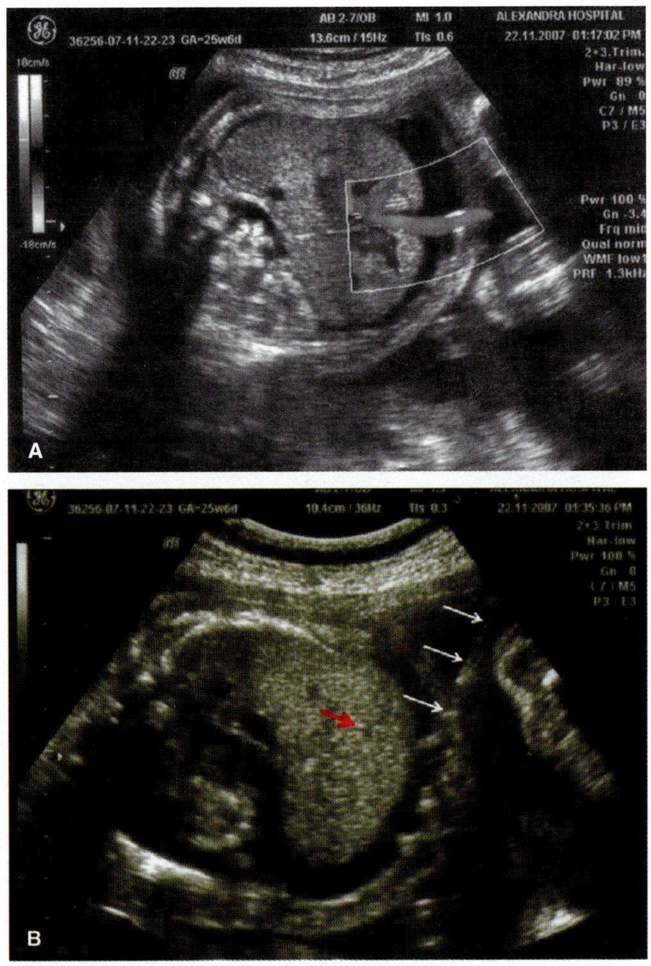

Figures 9.4A and B: Intrahepatic fetal blood sampling and intrauterine transfusion A. Visualization of intrabdominal course of the umbilical vein with color Doppler in fetus with ascites. B: Puncture of the vessel and intrauterine transfusion. White arrows show the needle course, and red arrow shows the hyperechogenic foci in fetal liver due to turbulence caused by the transfused RBCs

Intrahepatic Fetal Blood Sampling

This technique consists of the introduction of a 20-gauge needle into the fetal abdomen aiming for the intrahepatic portion of the umbilical vein or the left portal vein (Figures 9.4A and B).

Even though this procedure has some advantages compared to sampling of the umbilical cord such as avoidance of the of the umbilical arteries, certainty of the venous origin of the sample, and lack of need for immediate laboratory support to confirm the fetal origin of the sample it is considered to be second choice technique after cordocentesis because of its higher rate of fetal losses 6.2% in low risk patients.[34, 35]

Cardiocentesis

This method has limited indications due to the high risks of fetal loss involved 5.6%. Ideally the needle should enter the fetal heart, preferably the right ventricle though the anterior thoracic wall (Figures 9.5A and B).[36]

QUALITY CONTROL OF THE SPECIMEN'S ORIGIN

Most prenatal diagnostic tests require purity of the fetal blood sample, while for some of them this is essential. In cases of congenital infection, maternal blood contamination will give false-positive results. Amniotic fluid contamination will alter the results when coagulation factors are the target. Maternal cell in the sample may lead to mistakes in cases of cytogenetic analysis.

The most commonly used method to assess the purity of the sample is the estimation of the mean corpuscular volume of red blood cells since fetal red cells are larger that maternal. This difference decreases with advancing gestational age. Additional hematologic parameters can be used to distinguish between fetal and maternal blood.

Lymphocytes are the predominant white blood cells in the fetus whereas neutrophils are in the mother.

Kleihauer-Betke test may be used for second trimester samples, at which time it can accurately detect a maternal contamination of as little 0.5%,[37] but the utility of the test is limited during the late third trimester because fetal erythrocytes contain increasing amount of hemoglobin A.

Blood typing can confirm the fetal origin of a sample because the antigen I is present only in adult red cells. Determination of β-hCG, factors II, V, VII

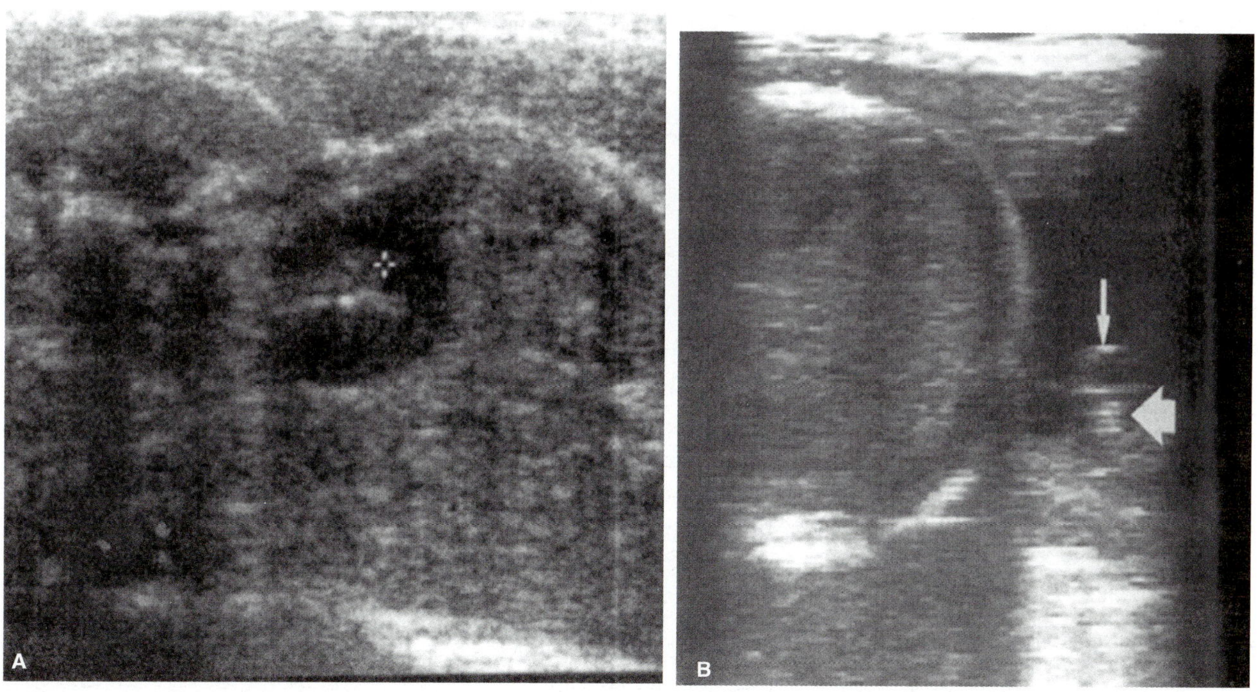

Figures 9.5 A and B: Intracardiac intrauterine transfusion. A: The needle is placed in the right ventricle (caliper) producing typical turbulence. B: Similar turbulence is produced in the umbilical arteries as the transfused RBCs enter into the fetal circulation [Sonography in Obstetrics and Gynecology. Eds: Fleisher A. et al. Appleton and Lange, 5th edition 1996, p 606]

and IX levels can be excellent markers for detection of maternal blood contamination in the specimen.

CONTRAINDICATIONS FOR FETAL BLOOD SAMPLING

No absolute contraindications exist but all contraindications are relative.

Obesity and decreased ability of ultrasound visualization are an indication to alter the site of target to free floating cord loops, hepatic vein or intracardiac aspiration. Oligohydramnios not necessarily represents a contraindication for fetal blood sampling since cord loops are usually packed and the site of cord insertion is probably visible, unless it is combined with fetal growth restriction.

Fetal bradycardia or uterine contractions prior to the procedure may be serious contraindications to be taken into account. Single uterine artery always manifests severe bradycardia post procedure.

Marginal cord insertion is a finding that must lead to another site of aspiration away from the cord insertion.

Finally, instable maternal condition, i.e pre-eclampsia, heart disease, etc. must be stabilized prior to any interventional procedure.

COMPLICATIONS FROM FETAL BLOOD SAMPLING

Failure to Obtain Fetal Blood

Failure to obtain an adequate fetal blood sample most likely dependents on the skill and experience of the operator, as well as on the gestational age that the procedure was performed. In one series of 1,320 fetal blood sampling performed between 16 and 24 weeks gestation, 97% of the procedures were completed successfully at the first attempt.[38]

If the fetal intrahepatic vein is the only target available for sampling, the failure rate to obtain fetal blood may be as high as 8.9%.[35]

Fetal Loss

Fetal blood sampling is associated with a higher risk of pregnancy loss than other invasive prenatal diagnostic techniques.[39]

However, it should be noted that fetuses selected for fetal blood sampling tend to have a higher background rate of adverse pregnancy outcome, mostly become such fetuses are more likely to have structural malformation, aneuploidy, infection or hematologic pathology. There are not studies available in which pregnancy loss rates have been compared between fetuses who had fetal blood sampling and an appropriately matched control group.

Various studies have reported fetal loss rates of 0.9 to 3.2%.[40,39]

In a review of 7,462 fetal blood sampling procedures the fetal loss rate within 14 days of the procedure was calculated at 1.1% per procedure.[41] However, this report may underestimate the real risk of the procedure since it is based on the operator's subjective impression as to whether a pregnancy loss was procedure related. In a more recent review of 1,320 procedures performed in a single center in Thailand the total fetal loss rate was 3.2% with a procedure related loss rate of 1% .[38]

Finally, Maxwell et at found that pregnancy loss rates vary greatly depending on the indication for the procedure, ranging from 1% to fetuses with structural malformation, and 25% for fetuses with nonimmune hydrops.[42]

Bleeding

Bleeding from the puncture site is the most common, usually benign complication of cordocentesis. It occurs in 41 to 53% of cases with a mean duration of 35 sec.[43]

At gestational ages <21 weeks has been associated with nearly a three-fold insease in the fetal loss rate.[44] Puncture of the umbilical artery is associated with a significantly longer duration of bleeding than venipancture.[44]

Cord Hematoma

In a pathologic study of 50 umbilical cords collected between 1 hour and 20 weeks after fetal blood sampling, hematomas were noted in 17% of the cases.[45] No relationship could be noted between transient fetal bradycardia or bleeding from the puncture site and the site of the hematoma. Hematoma is generally asymptomatic but it can be associated with prolonged bradycardia and rapid fetal deterioration.[45]

Bradycardia

A transient fetal bradycardia is a complication that occurs in 3 to 12% of the cases of fetal blood sampling[44] and it is usually a self limited event. In most cases bradycardias are thought to be the manifestation of a vasovagal response caused by local vasospasm in most cases. A significantly higher incidence of bradycardia has been noted among SGA than AGA fetuses 17.2 vs 4.1% respectively, $p = 0.001$ and among fetuses with absent diastolic flow to the umbilical artery as compared when diastolic flow is present 21.4 vs 5.3%.[44]

Fetomaternal Hemorrhage

Cordocentesis performed for therapeutic purposes is often associated with fetomaternal transfusion.

The mean estimated volume of hemorrhage is 2.4 ml 3.1% of the total fetoplacental blood volume,[44] and it is common when the procedure is performed with an anterior than a posterior placenta 65.6 vs 16.6%, $p<0.001$.[46]

No relation has been noted between degree of fetomaternal hemorrhage and number of attempts necessary, gestational age or type of procedure.

Preterm Delivery

In 7% of cases, cordocentesis is associated with an irregular pattern of uterine contraction.[47] The preterm delivery rate in a low-risk population was 5.0 to 5.7%.[47] Therefore, the procedure does not seem to increase the incidence of prematurity.

Chorioamnionitis

Chorioamnionitis seems to be a rare complication occurring in 1 in 600 procedures due to contamination from *Staphylococcus aureus*, or bowel microorganisms. However, prophylactic use of antibiotics has not be proven to be necessary.

SUMMARY

Percutaneous, ultrasound guided fetal blood sampling FBS since its introduction by Bang 1982[48] and Daffos 1983[8] has been universally practiced for various indications. Typical indications for FBS included prenatal diagnosis of genetic disorders, rapid karyotyping, diagnosis of fetal anemia and rhesus status and fetal infection. Advances in molecular biology PCR, ultrasound and Doppler, have reduced the number of indications through the years as already mentioned. The procedural risk of percutaneous umbilical blood sampling is also related to the indication and background fetal status.We have shown that it is directly related to the above, and it varies between 1 and 13%. The highest being in cases of abnormal fetal anatomy and growth restriction, 8.9 and 13.1% respectively.[39]

The preferable site of fetal blood sampling is always the insertion site of the cord to the placenta. Alternative sites are free loop of the cord, intrahepatic vein sampling and cardiocentesis. The relative simplicity of percutaneous fetal blood sampling has made cordocentesis available in a large number of centers and several thousands procedures are performed each year.

Percutaneous fetal blood sampling has a procedure related risk ranging between 0.2 and 2.7 % up to 28 weeks,[8,25,40,41] while intrahepatic vein sampling IHVS, and cardiocentesis carry a higher risk, 2.7 to 5.6% respectively and should be offered for prenatal diagnosis or therapy when other fetal blood sampling procedures are technically unfeasible.

In conclusion, percutaneous access to fetal circulation under continuous ultrasound guidance remains a valuable diagnostic and therapeutic technique which has altered clinical practice in perinatal medicine. Its application should be limited to the cases where other less invasive or noninvasive techniques are unable to establish diagnosis, or intravenous fetal therapy is mandatory.

REFERENCES

1. Valenti C: Antenatal detection of hemoglobinopathies. Am J Obstet Gynecol 1973; 115:851.

2. Kan YW, Valenti C, Camazza V, Guidotti R, Rieder RF. Fetal blood sampling in utero. Lancet 1974;1: 179.
3. Hobbins JC, Mahoney MJ. In utero diagnosis of hemoglobinopathies. N Engl J Med 1974; 290: 1065.
4. Kyle P, Harman CR. Invasive procedure in evolution. In Harman CR ed: Invasive Fetal Testing and Treatment. New York, Blackwell Scientific Publications, 1995; pp 341-400.
5. International Fetoscopy Group. The status of fetoscopy and fetal sampling. Prenat Diagn 1984;4:79.
6. Antsaklis A. Evaluation of diagnostic fetoscopy. J Foet Med 1982;2:41-4.
7. Rodeck CH, Campell S. Umbilical cord insertion as source of pure fetal blood for prenatal diagnosis. Lancet 1979;1: 1244.
8. Daffos F, Capella–Parlovsky M, Forestier F. A new procedure for fetal blood sampling in utero: preliminary results of fifty three cases. Am J Obstet Gynecol 1983;146:985.
9. Antsaklis AI, Papantoniou NE, Mesogitis SE, Koutra PT, Hassan S, Aravantinos DI. In utero diagnosis and treatment of severe rhesus isoimmunization by use of intravascular techniques 1991;11:171-4.
10. Alter BP. Prenatal diagnosis of haemoglobinopathies: Development of methods for study of fetal red cells and fibroblasts. Am J Pediatr Hematol 1985; 5:378.
11. Kazazian HH, Boehm C. Molecular basis and prenatal diagnosis of beta thalassemia. Blood 1988;72:1107.
12. Kazazian HH. Prenatal diagnosis of beta-thalassemia. Semin Perinatol 1991;15:15.
13. Lindeman R, Hu SP, Volpato F, et al. Polymerase chain reaction mutagenesis enabling rapid non radioactive detection of common beta-thalassemia mutations in Mediterraneans. Br J Haematol 1991;78:100.
14. Steinberg M. DNA diagnosis for the detection of sickle cell anemia. Am J Hematol 1993;43:110.
15. Lebo RV, Saiki RK, Swanson K, et al. Prenatal diagnosis of a-thalassemia by polymerase chain reaction and dual restriction enzyme analysis. Hum Genet 1990; 85: 293-9.
16. Pijpers L, Jahoda MJG, Reuss A, et al. Transabdominal chorionic villus biopsy in second and third trimesters of pregnancy to determine fetal karyotype. BMJ 1988; 297:822.
17. Hsu LYF, Perlis TE. United states survey on chromosome mosaicism and pseudomosaicism in prenatal diagnosis.Prenat Diagn 1984;4:97.
18. Rodis JF, Horvick TJ, Quinn DL, et al. Human parvovirus infection in pregnancy. Obstet Gynecol 1988;72:733.
19. Nicolaides KH, Soothill PW, Rodeck CH, et al. Ultrasound –guided sampling of umbilical cord and placental blood ta assess fetal well being. Lancet 1986;1:1065.
20. Cox WL,Daffos F, Forestier F et al. Physiology and management of intrauterine growth retardation: A biologic approach with fetal blood sampling. AJOG 1988;159:36.
21. Nicolini U, Nicolaidis P, Fisk NM, et al. Limited role of fetal blood sampling in prediction of outcome in intrauterine growth retardation. Lancet 1990;336:768.
22. Manning FA, Snijders R, Harman CR, et al. Fetal biophysical profile score. AJOG. 1993;169:755.
23. Chavez GF, Mulinare J, Edmonds LD. Epidemiology of Rh haemolytic disease of the newborn in the United States. J Am Med Assoc 1991;265: 3270-4.
24. Liley AW. Intrauterine transfusion of the foetus in haemolytic disease. Br Med J 1963;2:1107-9.
25. Moise KJ Jr. Management of rhesus alloimunnization in pregnancy. Obstet Gynecol 2002;100: 600-11.
26. Mari G. For the Collaborative Group for Doppler Assessment of the Blood Velocity in Anemic Fetuses. Non Invasive diagnosis by Doppler ultrasonography of fetal anemia due to maternal red cell alloimunization. N E J M 2000; 342:9-14.
27. Papantoniou N. Is there any role for cordocentesis and amniocentesis in assessment of Rhesus disease? Ultrasound Rev Obstet Gynecol 2004; 4: 239-44.
28. Antsaklis A, Papantoniou N, Mesogitis S, et al. In utero diagnosis and treatment of severe rhesus iso-immunisation by use of intravascular techniques. J Obstet Gynecol 1991; 11:171-4.
29. Tagliavacca L, Sacchi E, Mannucci PM. Carrier detection and feasibility of prenatal diagnosis of hemophilia B by multiplex polymerase chain reaction. Int Clin Lab Res 1993;23:169.
30. Daffos F, Forestier F, Kaplan C, et al. Prenatal diagnosis and management of bleeding disorders with fetal blood sampling. Am J Obstet Gynecol 1998;158:939.
31. Garmel SH, Craigo SD, Morin LM, Crowley JM, D' Alton ME. The role of percutaneous umbilical blood sampling in the management of immune thrombocytopenic purpura. Prenat Diagn 1995;15: 439-45.
32. Bussel J. Minutes of the Neonatal Subcommittee of Thrombosis and Haemostasis Working Party on Neonatal Alloimune Thrombocytopenia. Brussels, Belgium;1987.
33. Crombleholme TM, Langer JC, Harisson MR, et al. Transplantation of fetal cells. AJOG 1991;164:218.
34. Nicolini U, Santolaya J,Ojo OE et al. The fetal intrahepatic umbilical vein as an alternative to cord needling for prenatal diagnosis and therapy. Prenat Diagn 1988;8:665.
35. Nicolini U, Nicolaides P, Fisk NM, et al. Fetal blood sampling from the intrahepatic vein: Analysis of safety and clinical experience with 214 procedures. Obstet Gynecol 1990;76:447.
36. Antsaklis AI, Papantoniou NE, Mesogitis SE, Koutra PT, Vintzileos AM, Aravantinos DI. Cardiocentesis:an alternative method of fetal blood sampling for the prenatal diagnosis of haemoglobinopathies. Obstet Gynecol 1992;79:630.
37. Nikolaides KH, Clewell WH, Rodeck CH. Measurment of human fetoplacental blood volume in erythroblastosis fetalis. Am J Obstet Gynecol 1987;157:50.
38. Tongsong T, Wanapirak C, Kunavikatikul C, Sirirchotiyakul S, Piyarnongkol W, et al. Cordocentesis at 16-24 weeks of gestation: experience of 1320 cases. Prenat Diagn 2000;20:224-8.

39. Antsaklis AI, Daskalakis G, Papantoniou NE, Michalas S. Fetal blood sampling—Indication related losses. Prenat Diagn 1998;18:934-40.
40. Weiner CP, Okamura K. Diagnostic fetal blood sampling – technique related losses. Fetal Diagn Ther 1996;11:169-75.
41. Megerian G, Ludomirsky A. Role of cordocentesis in perinatal medicine. Curr Opin Obstet Gynecol 1994;6:30-5.
42. Maxwell DJ, Johnson P, Hurley P, Neales K, Allan L, et al. Fetal blood sampling and pregnancy loss in relation to indication. BJOG 1991;98:892-7.
43. Hogge WA, Thiagarajah S, Brenbridge AN, et al. Fetal evaluation by percutaneous blood sampling. Am J Obstet Gynecol 1988;158:132.
44. Weiner CP, Wenstrom KD, Sipes SL, et al. Risk factors for cordocentesis and fetal intravascular transfusion. Am J Obstet Gynecol. 1991;165:1020.
45. Jauniaux E, Donner C, Simon P, et al. Pathologic aspects of the umbilical cord after percutaneous blood sampling. Obstet Gynecol. 1989;73:215.
46. Nicolini U, Kochenour NK, Greco P, et al. Consequences of feto-maternal hemorrhage following intrauterine transfusion. BMJ 1988;297:1379.
47. Ghidini A, Sepulveda W, Lockwood CJ, et al. Complications of fetal blood sampling. AJOG 1993;168:1339.
48. Bang J, Bock JE, Trolle D. Ultrasound guided fetal intravenous transfusion for severe rhesus haemolytic disease. Br Med J 1982; 284: 373-4.

CHAPTER

10

Twin to Twin Transfusion Syndrome

Papantoniou Nikolas

INTRODUCTION

The incidence of multiple births has increased significantly during the past 20 years due to advances in assisted reproduction and changes in social attitudes of women resulting in advanced maternal age, both responsible for multifetal pregnancies. Today in the US, it is estimated that 1.5% of all pregnancies are multiple, but account for almost 10% of all perinatal morbidity and mortality.[1] All common complications of pregnancy like preterm birth, intrauterine growth restriction, etc. are found in increased frequency in multiple pregnancies. In addition, twin pregnancies present additional unique complications like TTTS, acardiac twins, conjoint twins and twin embolization with co-twin intrauterine death.

Twin to twin transfusion syndrome TTTS is a serious complication of monochorionic multiple pregnancies, with extremely high perinatal morbidity and mortality, and it occurs between 5.5 and 17.5% of all monochorionic pregnancies, affecting approximately 1:1600 pregnancies overall, if left untreated.[2] It affects two structurally normal fetuses that in the absence of the syndrome would have a good potential for infant survival as twins.

TTTS is perhaps the oldest syndrome recorded in medical history as some suggest that the twins of Isaac and Rebecca were affected by the syndrome. In 1882, Schatz showed the existence of anastomoses between the two fetal circulations.[3] In the same period it was also first stated that cerebral palsy was caused by intrapartum hypoxia, and not due to abnormal brain development. In a little more than a hundred years later, great advances have been achieved in the understanding of the pathophysiology of the syndrome. We now know that it is a complex cardiovascular disease resulting from unbalanced blood transfusion from the donor to the recipient due to one or more abnormal arteriovenous anastomoses (AVA) in the absence of adequate bidirectional superficial arterioarterial (AAA) and venovenous (VVA) anastomoses.

Several diagnostic approaches have been tried in the past decade, including placental pathology and Doppler studies. In clinical management, serial amnioreduction and laser ablation techniques, have been tried aiming to amelioration of the perinatal outcome. Nevertheless, perinatal mortality and long term morbidity are still unacceptably high, and for this reason clinical management of TTTS represents perhaps a major challenge in fetal medicine.

EMBRYOLOGY

Fertilization of two separate ova will result in dizygotic twin gestation which will result in dichorionic, diamniotic pregnancies with two separate placentas and two amniotic sacs. Dizygotic gestations account for two-thirds of twins. Monozygotic twins result from the fertilization of a single ovum. Division of the zygote fertilized ovum before day 4, when chorion differentiates, results in dichorionic, diamniotic gestation and accounts for 25% of monozygotic twins. Division between days 4 and 8, before amnion differentiation, results in monochorionic-diamniotic gestation and accounts for 75% of monozygotic twins. Beyond 8 days post fertilization, division of monozygotic twin gestation will result in monochorionic, monoamniotic gestation which occurs for 1% of monozygotic twinning. Division of embryonic disc, in more than 13 days will usually be incomplete and results in the formation of conjoint twins. Knowledge of chorionicity and amnionicity is critical in the assessment of multifetal pregnancy. With sonography it is possible to detect monochorionic-diamniotic gestations early in the first trimester and therefore identify the high risk group of twins for producing TTTS.

PLACENTAL ANATOMY

In 1882, Schatz first described the existence of TTTS. He observed that certain placental cotyledons could be perfused by an artery from one twin and a vein from the other twin. Injection of dye in placentas of monochorionic diamniotic twins, *ex vivo*, has shown that almost all placentas contain vascular anastomoses.[4] There are three general types of anastomoses, arterio-arterial AAA, venovenous VVA, and arteriovenous AVA. The first two types, AAA and VVA are superficial anastomoses and the blood flow can be bidirectional depending on alterations of hydrostatic pressures between the two fetal circulations. AVA are deep in the placental mass and are capable of unidirectional flow from one twin to another (Figures 10.1 and 10.2). In reality one artery from one twin enters the placental cotyledon from the chorionic plate and forms the classic villous capillary bed, while the corresponding vein drains blood to the co-twin. Deep AVA are present in almost all monochorionic pregnancies. AAA are found in most monochorionic pregnancies and VVA only in 25%.[5] It is estimated that an average of 3.1 anastomoses per placenta are found in the placentas of monochorionic twins and these anastomoses are responsible for net blood transfer from one twin to the other. On the other hand, monochorionic placentas have individually perfused cotyledons within which exchange of blood between the fetuses does not take place.

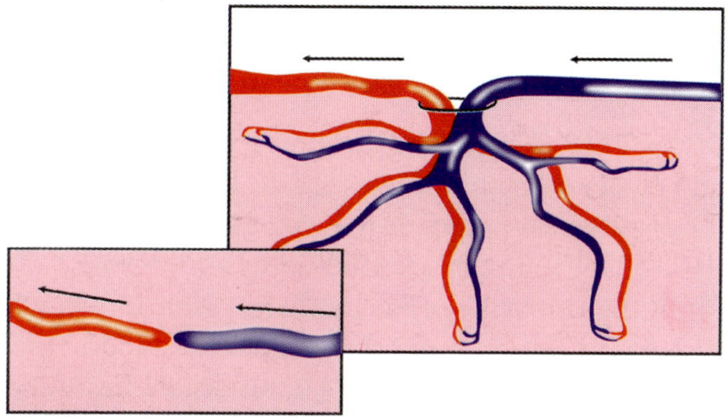

Figure 10.1: Schematic representation of deep arterio-venous anastomoses (AVA). [From Machin et.al USOBG 2000, page 215]

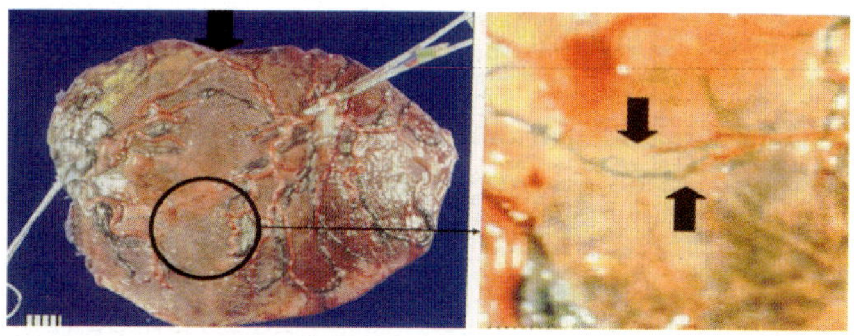

Figure 10.2: Arterio-arterial and arterio-venous anastomoses. On the left AAA is shown on the top of the placenta (black arrow), and AVA is circled and magnified on the right (black arrows). [Taylor et al. USOBG 2000, page 219]

TTTS results in only 15% of monochorionic-diamniotic pregnancies and occurs when the vascular architecture is such that forces blood flow from one twin to the other. The fetus who is providing the blood is the donor, and the one receiving is the recipient twin. From *ex vivo* placental studies, we now know that AVA are present in all TTTS placentas, while in other monochorionic-diamniotic pregnancies where the syndrome is not present their prevalence is 84%. In addition when one or more AVA are present and AAA are absent the prevalence of the syndrome is increased to almost 80%.[6] AAA play a significant protective role in monochorionic twin pregnancies, since their absence is associated with increased prevalence of the syndrome (61% versus 15%, or 8.6). AAA play a greater protective role compared to VVA due to their higher pressure differential due to their anatomic structure. Finally, computer modeling studies have confirmed that AAA are the anastomoses who offer greater protection from TTTS.[7]

PATHOPHYSIOLOGY

When TTTS is established, hypovolemia of the donor and hypervolemia of the recipient twin will lead to adaptive fetal responses. In the progress of the syndrome these adaptive responses will lead to fetal disease.

In the donor hypovolemia will result in growth restriction IUGR, redistribution of the blood flow and decreased perfusion of central organs resulting in multiorgan malfunction such as pneumonic hypoplasia, necrotizing enterocolitis and renal tubule dysgenesis and oligohydramnios. Apoptosis and ischemia contribute to renal tubular atrophy. Increased levels of renin are due to continuous hypoperfusion.[8] Hypovolemia will result in increased levels of angiotensin II which will further increase the donor's vasoconstriction and worsen the pathophysiologic consequences of growth restriction. Donor fetal adrenals will increase the production of aldosterone. In the recipient hypervolemia will result in high atrial natriuretic peptide ANP secretion, and suppression of antidiuretic hormone ADH which will lead to polyuria and polyhydramnios.[9] Hypervolemia elevates cardiac preload and produces consequent hypertension and cardiac dysfunction. Increased levels of endothelin are observed in the recipient. Cardiac disease will lead eventually to cardiac failure, detectable by ultrasound and Doppler studies. Cardiac hypertrophy in the recipient due to increased afterload may lead to functional right ventricular outflow obstruction. Recipient kidneys are enlarged and congested showing pathologic changes present in hypertensive disease. The renin-angiotensin-aldosterone system is also affected in the recipient through hemodynamic changes and possible transfer of renin, angiotensin and aldosterone from the donor through placental shunts.

SONOGRAPHIC FEATURES

Sonography plays a critical role in early diagnosis and clinical assessment of these pregnancies. During the first trimester sonographic assessment of chorionicity and amnionicity is most accurate. By the end of first trimester in diamniotic twins, the two amnios are opposed and form an intertwin membrane. In monochorionic twins the membrane is thin and composed of two layers of amnion, while in dichorionic twins, the intertwin membrane is thick composed of 4 layers, the two amnios and the two chorions. A cutoff of 2 mm is used to differentiate between mono- and dichorionic gestations.

In cases of dichorionic placentas, adjacent and fused along their borders sonographically is impossible to differentiate between monochorionic-diamniotic gestation with one placenta and dichorionic-diamniotic gestation. "twin peak sign" or "lambda sign". Figures 10.3A and B refer to the appearance of intertwine membrane at its insertion from the placenta. In dichorionic gestations, a triangular projection of trophoblastic tissue, extending from the placental surface is observed which in combination with the membrane thickness establish an early diagnosis of dichorionic twins. In monochorionic gestations, the intertwin membrane is thin (< 2 mm) and there is no projection of the placenta due to the single continuous chorion. The appearance of the intertwine membrane in monochorionic-diamniotic gestations is described as "T" sign.

Increased nuchal translucency (NT) at 10 to 14 weeks has a 3.5 likelihood ratio for developing TTTS. Nevertheless, in a reported series from UK only 28% of cases were predicted[10] (Figure 10.4). Sonographic features of TTTS are obvious from 15 to 25 weeks onward. Folding of the intertwin membranes is found in ¼ of monochorionic-diamniotic pregnancies and almost half of them 43% will present with the syndrome[10] (Figure 10.5).

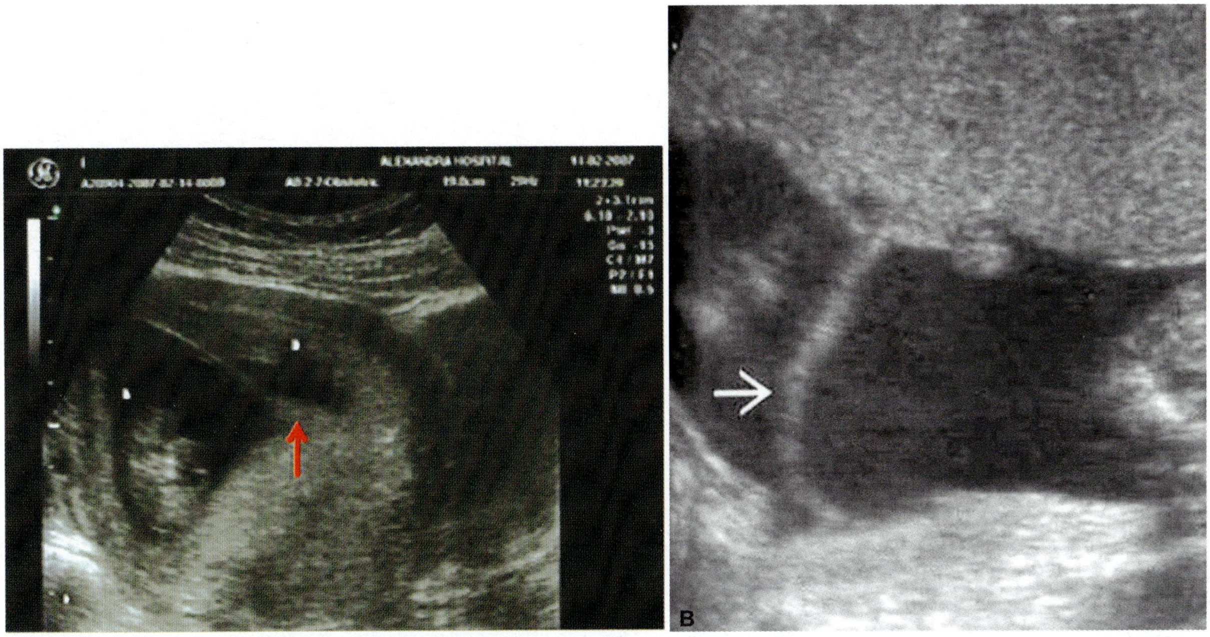

Figure 10.3: Twin pregnancies – (A) Dichorionic with twin peak sign or lamda-sign (red arrow). (B) Monochorionic with "T" sign (white arrow). [Diagnostic Imaging Obstetrics Eds: Woodward et al. Amirsys, 2005, chp13,p5]

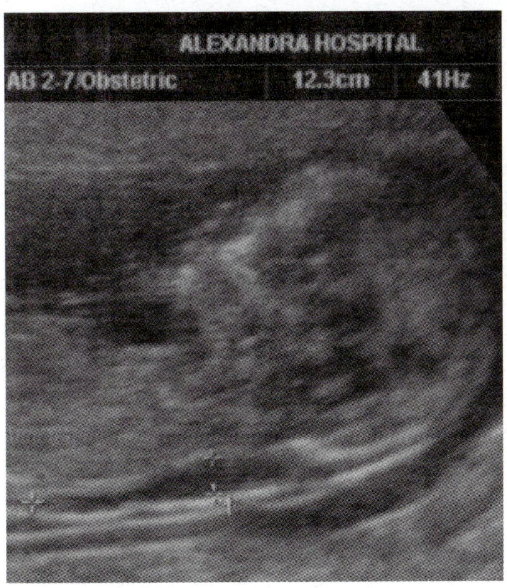

Figure 10.4: NT

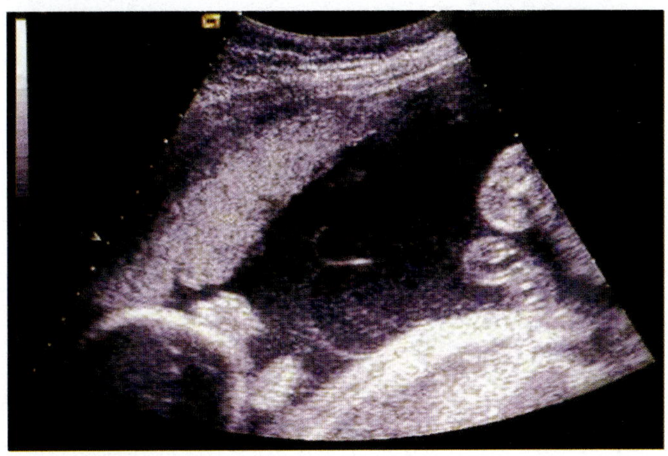

Figure 10.5: Intertwin membrane folding. Due to discordant amniotic fluid in 2nd trimester monochorionic twin pregnancy. [High Risk Pregnancy, Management Options. Eds: D. James et al. Philadelphia, Elsevier Saunders 3rd edition, 2006. p 544]

The sonographic diagnosis of TTTS is made by noting the presence of significant growth discordance (>20%) accompanied by polyhydramnios in one fetus and oligohydramnios in the other, in a monochorionic-diamniotic twin pregnancy. Sonographic features of TTTS are listed in Table 10.1. Polyhydramnios is defined when a maximum vertical pocket (MVP) is greater than 8 cm and oligohydramnios when a (MVP) is less than 2 cm.

Table 10.1: Sonographic features of TTTS

	Donor	*Recipient*
Size*	Small	Large
Mobility	Normal/reduced	Reduced
Amniotic fluid	Reduced	Increased
Umbilical cord	Normal/Small	Enlarged
Bladder	Small/non visible	Large
Abnormal Doppler studies	+ / –	+ / –

*Growth discordance >20%

In TTTS there are also evident signs of intrauterine growth restriction in the donor, concerning fetal biometry (< 3rd centile) and abnormal Doppler studies (AEDF/REDF) in the umbilical artery. Circulatory redistribution will be evident from Doppler studies of MCA and ductus venosus (absent or reversed A wave) (Figure 10.6). A nonvisible or small urinary bladder is an important sonographic criterion of worsening of fetal condition.

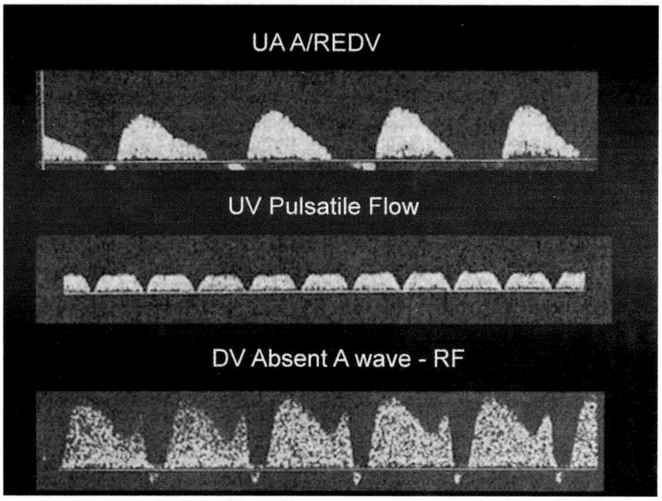

Figure 10.6: TTTS: Critical abnormal Doppler studies

Sonographic features of the recipient due to hypervolemia include polyhydramnios, visceromegaly, abnormal Doppler flow of ductus venosus (absent or reversed A wave), pulsatile flow in the umbilical vein and marked tricuspid regurgitation. Worsening of cardiovascular disease will lead to total hydrops for the recipient (Figures 10.7A and B).

Single amniotic fluid discordance but not meeting the above mentioned criteria can be present in monochorionic twins without TTTS manifestations. Isolated polyhydramnios (MVP > 10 cm) can be of various, (i.e. congenital malformations) unknown aetiology. In TTTS cases it is an important sonographic feature which warrants therapy. Isolated oligohydramnios can occur in several cases without the presence of the syndrome, i.e. renal agenesis, intrauterine growth restriction of one fetus, premature undiagnosed rupture of the membranes of the one fetus, and does not need initiation of therapy for TTTS.

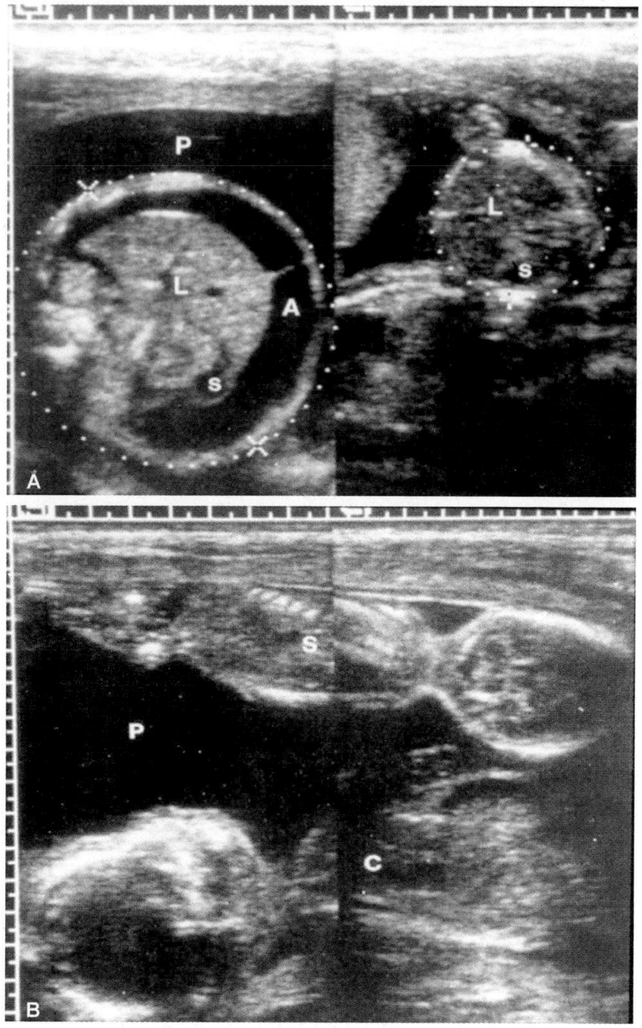

Figure 10.7: TTTS. A: Hydrops of the recipient-hydramnios and growth retardation of donor, B: Significant growth discordance. Donor presents with severe oligohydramnios-"stuck" twin and significant growth retardation. Recipient presents with hydramnios and visceromegaly. [Diagnostic Ultrasound of Fetal Anomalies. Eds: Nymberg D, Philadelphia, Mosby 2004; pages 600, 608].

In 35% of cases of this twin oligohydramnios - polyhydramnios sequence (TOPS) one fetus the recipient will appear with marked polyhydramnios and the other, the donor, will be immobilized or stuck in a sac with very little or no amniotic fluid. In some cases the amniotic fluid of the donor is nonexistent and the intertwine membranes are not separated from the donor and therefore cannot be recognized.

Monozygotic twins have the same genes and theoretically should have identical parameters if measured at the same time. Difference in fetal-estimated weight with growth discordance more than

20% is no longer a valid criterion for diagnosis of the syndrome, since it is reported in 23% of monozygotic twins without TTTS.[11] Nevertheless, increased morbidity and mortality is reported in these cases. The causes of discordance are diverse. Aneuploidy and inequality of placentation (one twin supported by inadequate placenta) are two significant factors for growth discordance. TTTS with its unbalanced vascular shunting leads to growth discordance but other significant sonographic features are also present and confirm the diagnosis. The differential diagnosis of TOPS by ultrasound is listed in Table 10.2.

Table 10.2: Sonographic differential diagnosis of TOPS in growth discordant MC diamniotic twins

1. TTTS
2. Inequality of placentation
3. Isolated polyhydramnios in growth discordant twins
4. Isolated oligohydramnios due to IUD, IUGR, PROM, renal disease or agenesis
TOPS: Twin oligohydramnios-polyhydramnios sequence
IUGR: Intrauterine growth restriction
PROM: Premature rupture of membranes
IUD: Intrauterine death

Arteriovenous anastomoses are identified *in vivo*, with colored Doppler,[12] showing a unidirectional arteriovenous flow from twin to the other, with typical Doppler waves (Figures 10.8A and B). Arterioarterial anastomoses (AAA) play a significant protective role in TTTS and are detectable after 18 weeks with spectral and color Doppler, with reported high sensitivities and specificities (85% and 97%). A typical "speckled pattern" due to bidirectional flow is shown on color Doppler (Figure 10.9). The absence of AAA implies a high risk for development of TTTS (OR86). Nevertheless, in 30% of TTTS placentas AAA are present but higher perinatal survival is reported in these cases.[13]

STAGING AND PROGNOSIS

Presentation of TTTS is not homogeneous. Based on observational data, the disease follows an individualized time course for the development of renal failure, abnormal Doppler studies, heart failure, hydrops, and finally, intrauterine fetal death. Quintero proposed a staging system which categorizes disease severity and is based on worsening clinical features identified with sonography[14](Table 10.3).

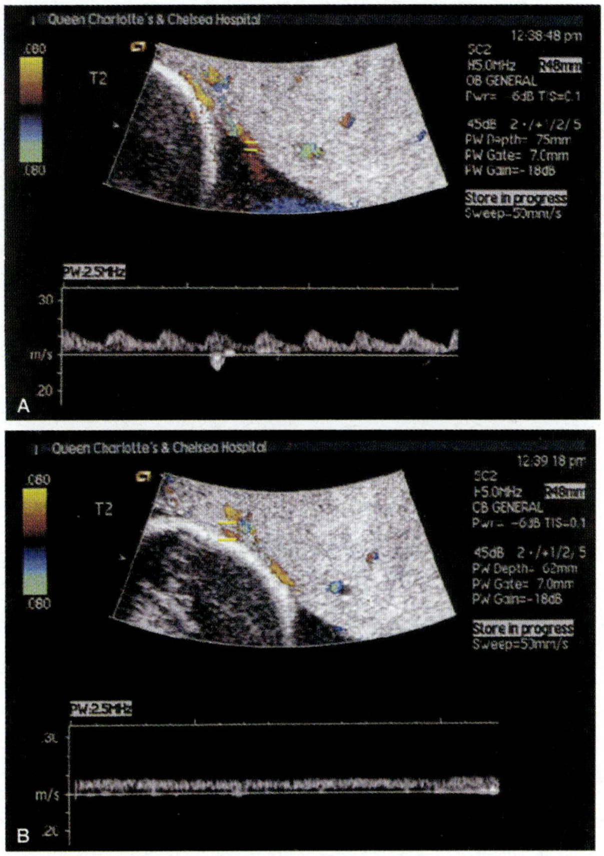

Figure 10.8: Arterio-venous anastomoses (AVA). A: arterial Doppler waveform from fetus A, continuing with venous waveform towards fetus B (same color–direction of flow) [Taylor et. al. USOBG 2000, page 219]

Table 10.3: Staging of TTTS (Quintero 2003)

Stage I	The bladder of the donor is still visible.
Stage II	The bladder of the donor is not visualized in more than 60 min. The fetus is considered in renal failure.
Stage III	Critically abnormal Doppler studies (AEDF/REDF) in the donor umbilical artery or reverse flow in ductus venosus or pulsatile flow in the umbilical vein of the recipient.
Stage IV	Hydrops in the recipient.
Stage V	Fetal demise in one or both twins.

Quintero staging of TTTS has been proven useful in clinical practice for various purposes. It is helpful

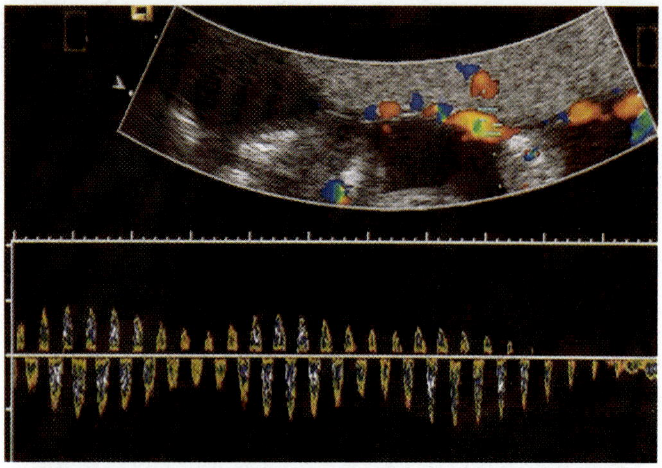

Figure 10.9: Arterio-arterial anastomosis (AAA): characteristic speckled pattern due to bidirectional flow on color Doppler. [Tony Tan et al. Obstet Gynecol 2004 103;1176]

in standardizing criteria for treatment and evaluating the results of several therapeutic approaches, by recognizing the stage of disease of first treatment, expectant management and worst ever stage.

In a recent stage dependent report of 52 consecutive cases, stage III was present in 63% at presentation, 45% of these cases progressed to a more advanced stage and 18% fell into a lesser stage. An interesting observation in this series was that 20% of stage II progressed to an advanced stage; while in 60% fetal condition was improved regressing to stage I. There was no significant influence of the stage at presentation on survival. When the worst ever stage was considered as prognostic factor, survival was well correlated. Survival was better when in the course of the disease the fetus fell into a lesser stage.[15]

A modified staging system has been proposed and incorporates the presence of protective AAA. The stage is characterized by an "a" if AAA are identified and "b" if they are absent. In an analysis of 96 pregnancies complicated by TTTS the presence of an AAA showed a stage depended survival improvement for stages I to III. Of notice was that in this report survival was better for stage III a than for IIb. The authors believe that this modification improves prognosis and significantly helps clinical decision for treatment.[16]

TREATMENT

Treatment of TTTS remains perhaps the most challenging and controversial aspect in perinatal medicine. It is challenging because it affects two otherwise healthy fetuses, which in the absence of treatment have unacceptably high perinatal mortality (>80%) and morbidity. Treatment remains controversial because there are a variety of therapeutic approaches, mainly interventional, and on the other hand, investigators have not adhered to standard diagnostic sonographic criteria. Lately, Quintero's staging system has contributed significantly in the objective evaluation of the different therapeutic approaches.

Expectant management or medical treatments with digoxin, or indomethacin, have place only in cases of stage I at presentation, diagnosed after 24 weeks and with MVP less than 10 cm. Digoxin has been administered aiming to improve the cardiac function of the recipient with questionable results.[17] Others have given indomethacin to control polyhydramnios in the recipient but in our opinion it is wrong because of its effects on the already compromised renal function of the donor.[18]

Interventional therapeutic alternatives include serial aggressive amnioreduction (AR) aiming to removal of large volumes of amniotic fluid, septostomy disruption of the dividing membranes, laser ablation of anastomotic vessels, and umbilical cord occlusion.

Serial Amnioreduction

Polyhydramnios and PROM may lead to prematurity which is responsible for increased mortality and morbidity. The most obvious and simple therapeutic approach which has been widely practiced until now, is serial aggressive AR. There is not standard technique for AR concerning the type of needles and the use of suction and local anesthesia and maternal sedation. An 18-gauge Echotip needle and local anesthesia and maternal sedation has been used by Quintero's group. In our department of MFM in the University of Athens, we use 18-gauge needles, under local anesthetic without maternal sedation. Extension tubing is attached to the needle and the amniotic fluid evacuates freely into a urine collection plastic bag. Serial AR is recommended when maximum vertical pocket (MVP) is estimated 10 cm or more, or amniotic fluid index (AFI) is greater than 40 cm. Large quantities of amniotic fluid >3 lit may be drained in each procedure, until reaching a MVP of 5 to 6 cm. Ten centimeters of amniotic fluid index (AFI) correspond to 1 liter of amniotic fluid. The procedure must be repeated when polyhydramnios recurs. Procedure-related risks include PROM, placental abruption and chorioamnionitis.

The results of the International Amnioreduction Registry, which is a retrospective study of 223 sets of twins, between 26 centers, showed an overall 78% survival at birth, and 60% after the neonatal period.[19] Both fetuses survived the neonatal period in 48% and at least one in 70.8%. Serious neurological morbidity PVL was 12% in this series.

The Australian and New Zealand TTTS Registry, with 112 sets of twins reported an overall 62% survival rate. One twin survival was 72.3%, and long-term neurological sequele due to PVL was 10.8%, while intact neurologic survival was 21%.[20]

In another report from England *of* cases with severe TTTS treated with serial AR, there was 60% survival. When survival of both twins was considered, it was 20% and single perinatal survival was 50%.

In conclusion from retrospective trials, AR has been shown to improve fetal survival significantly with a 66% success rate when at least one twin survived, and an average risk of cerebral palsy of 15%.[21] Nevertheless, survival rates of 18 to 83% have been reported in the literature, and neurologic complications ranging between 5 and 58%.[22] It is important to emphasize at this point that although AR controls polyhydramnios, it is not an etiologic therapy of TTTS.

Amniotic Septostomy

The creation of an artificial opening between the two gestational sacs is referred as amniotic septostomy. The goal of the iatrogenic disruption of the dividing membranes is to allow amniotic fluid from the recipient to enter the cavity of the donor and thus equilibrate pressures between the two cavities. The mechanism of improvement after septostomy remains unclear, suggesting that the donor may correct the oligohydramnios by oral rehydration. Another theory suggests that improvement of the donor status is due to a decrease of pressure on the umbilical vessels of the donor, improvement of blood flow and diminishing of the shunting effect. On the other hand, it has not been shown that a difference of amniotic fluid pressure exists between the two cavities, after disruption, while other reports have shown that pressures are equal despite the large differences of amniotic fluid volumes between them.[23] There are very few reports of amelioration after septostomy, and immediate improvement and high survival rates.[24] There are also reports of cord entanglement and fetal demise.[25]

In general this technique has been of limited use and some think it should be abandoned since it has not a solid theoretical etiological background for fetal therapy, and might actually harm the pregnancy by diminishing the ability to perform laser therapy or serial AR.

Laser Therapy

Laser therapy is the only etiological treatment for TTTS, since it aims to the cessation of the anastomotic vessels AVA responsible for intertwin transfusion. Typically, a modern fine embryoscope is introduced into the uterus, transabdominally, in a preselected area by ultrasound in the recipient's sac. Photocoagulation of anastomotic vessels under direct vision follows with the use of Nd: Yag Laser applied through a 400 to 600 μm optic fiber introducing it from the side channel of the fetoscope (Figures 10.10A to C).

Nonselective Fetoscopic Laser Ablation

Nonselective fetoscopic laser ablation was first introduced in the mid 90s through laparotomy incision and entrance of the fetoscope in a predetermined area

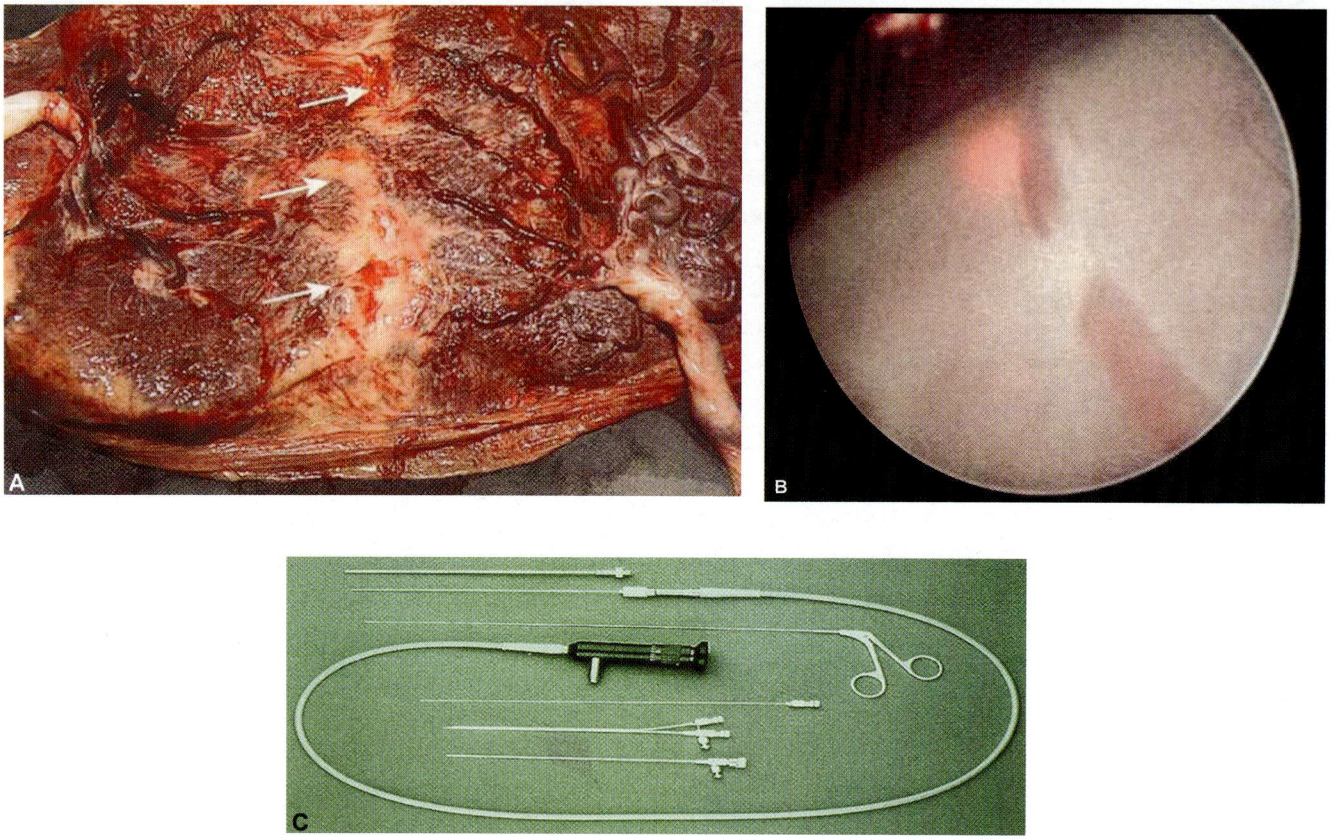

Figures 10.10A to C: Fetoscopic laser ablation: A. Placenta with obvious scars from previous laser ablation. B. Fetoscopic picture during laser ablation. C. Fetoscope: High risk pregnancy, management options. (Eds: D. James et al. Philadelphia, Elsevier Saunders 3rd edition, 2006)

by ultrasound.[26] All surface placental vessels approaching or crossing the intertwin membrane were ablated. This initial technique was characterized as non selective laser ablation. The initial overall survival was between 55 and 69% and at least one survivor 73 to 82%.[26-28] These survival rates did not differ significantly from those of serial AR and although in one series with 132 patients, laser ablation was followed by AR.[27] The most likely explanation of this lack of improvement is that the intertwin membrane has in reality very small relationship with responsible anastomotic vessels. The membranous equator usually lies close to the donor cord insertion and is also transversed by normal vessels, AAA and AVA which play a protective role against presentation of TTTS. Besides, destruction of the vessels of normal cotyledons leads to devitilization and worsening of fetal condition. The donor is usually more affected by the non selective laser technique. Complications like high procedure related fetal loss rate[27] full thickness placental necrosis,[29] PROM, prematurity and chorioamnionitis have been reported initially. Rare fetal and maternal complications have been reported including aplasia cutis, amniotic bands, limb necrosis, maternal pulmonary edema, and adult respiratory distress syndrome (ARDS) but is not possible to establish a direct causal relationship between them and the procedure.

Selective Laser Photocoagulation of Communicating Vessels

Selective laser photocoagulation of communicating vessels (SLPCV) was introduced in clinical practice in the end of 90s.[30] This technique aimed to the ablation of only the responsible AVA anastomoses involved in the twin to twin transfusion syndrome. All arteries near the intertwine membrane were followed endoscopically to their terminal end in the placenta. The returning vein from the insertion point of the artery studied, should normally return to the same twin. If the vein drained blood to the other twin, the presence of a deep AVA was confirmed and the responsible vessels were ablated. AAA and VVA are easily identified endoscopically by the lack of a terminal end in the placental surface and therefore reserved.[31,32] It is important to mention that endoscopic identification of all vessels responsible has not been validitated with classical placental *ex vivo* injection of dye studies. From *ex vivo* studies, it has been shown that even under optimal endoscopic conditions, only two-thirds of AVA were identified. Targeted sonography with the use of spectral and color Doppler can identify arterio-venous anastomoses. Sonoendoscopic delineation of these AVA prior to selective fetoscopic laser ablation is theoretically the best treatment modality, because it facilitates this highly selective procedure and shortens the procedure time. Nevertheless, the reported sensitivity of the technique is 55% and with at least one survivor 70%.

Laser Ablation of the Placental Equator

Laser ablation of the placental equator has been proposed as an alternative to selective and non-selective procedures. In this technique the vessels crossing the placental vascular equator are identified and coagulated. In this manner the pathologic arteriovenous anastomoses (AVA) are destroyed, while the normal anastomoses (AAA-VVA) close to the donor are left intact. A significant advantage of this technique is the shorter operating time compared to selective ablation.[33]

Laser Versus AR

Undoubtedly, one of the most controversial topics in TTTS is the choice of treatment, between laser and serial AR. The controversies exist mainly due to lack of standard sonographic inclusion criteria for the syndrome, different gestational ages at inclusion between studies and staging at presentation.

Selective laser photocoagulation of the communicating vessels has higher survival rates as expected compared to non selective laser ablation. Quintero et al from the US reported survival of 83% of at least one fetus after selective procedure, compared with 61% in non selective and 67% after serial AR managed by the same group.[32] Hecher et al from Europe reported similar results in 200 pregnancies with severe TTTS with overall survival of 68% in selective, 61% in nonselective and 51% in the AR group. Survival of at least one fetus was 81%, 79% and 60% respectively for these three groups.[31,34]

AR when used alone as treatment modality has also improved survival. The results of the International AR Registry have shown an overall perinatal survival of 78% and at least one fetus in 70.8%. The interval between last AR and delivery was 17.5 days (0-138) and 60% of twins survived the neonatal period.[19]

The Australian New Zealand Twin-Twin Transfusion Registry reported a 62 % overall perinatal survival and 72.3% one twin survival.[20] Another reported issue besides survival in selecting between AR and laser is the rare serious neurological sequelae. In a stage based treatment with 173 pairs of twins, there was significantly lower incidence of neurologic sequelae in the laser vs the AR group, 4.2% vs 24.4% respectively.[35] Similar results have been shown from another study from Europe, by Hecher's group, who reported a 6% vs 18% incidence in neurologic sequelae in laser and AR respectively.[31] The same group has published the results of a follow up study of these survivors of TTTS for 14 to 33 months. They reported a 22% incidence of neurologic sequelae in the SLPCV group and 11% of these infants suffered from cerebral palsy.[36] The incidence between donors and recipients was similar. In cases of single intrauterine death the incidence of neurologic sequelae was significantly higher reaching 27% vs 8% in cases of double twin survival. In the prospective randomized European trial,[22] there was also a 6% vs 14% difference in favor of the laser group. In general neurologic complications after laser treatment were lower and ranged between 5 and 11%.

All the above mentioned studies comparing AR and laser therapy were retrospective and thus could be biased.

The need of a prospective randomized trial with staging of patients at presentations was obvious and a multicenter trial from Europe was carried out.[22] It included 144 sets of twins, 70 allocated in the AR group and 72 in the laser group. They assessed perinatal survival of at least one twin as prespecified primary outcome, survival of at least one twin at 6 months of age, and survival without neurological complications at 6 months of age. The overall perinatal survival was 57% for laser and 41% from the AR group. One twin survival was 76% vs 56% in favor of the laser group, which was statistically significant (p =0.009). The incidence of neurologic sequelae (PVL) was also lower in the laser group 6% vs 14% as already mentioned. At six months of age 52% of the infants from the laser group were free of neurologic complications, compared with 31% of the AR group. These improved outcomes in the laser group might be explained by the prolongation of pregnancy by 4 weeks. The impressive results of this prospective randomized study lead to the conclusion that SLPCV should be the treatment of choice in TTTS before 26 weeks. Nevertheless there are some aspects of concern regarding the results.

The assessment of perinatal survival of at least one twin is a prior acknowledgment that almost half of the babies will be lost even with laser treatment. The percentage of patients with stage I disease was 8% and stage IV was 1%, which does not really address the issue of TTTS since there is a broad spectrum of the disease and in some cases the disease falls into greater or lesser severity. Furthermore 9% of the AR group changed to laser treatment and there was a significant difference in percentages of pregnancy terminations in this study, 16% in the AR group vs 0% in the laser group, parameters which may have altered survival and neurological morbidity rates. It is of notice, that although the trial was prospective and generally patients in these trials have better results, the survival rate in the AR group was surprisingly low 41%, compared with other retrospective trials 66%.[21] Another important issue was that anterior placentas which are more difficult to manage with laser were less common compared to the AR group. Finally the improved neurological outcome in the laser group may be due to prolongation of the gestation by 4 weeks in the laser group, which is in favor of this therapeutic approach.

In conclusion, the very optimistic results in favor of laser treatment as a sole therapeutic modality by the recent European trial should be treated with caution. Furthermore, a stage based analysis of TTTS including the presence of AAA showed that laser treatment had better results for stages III and IV and AR in stages I and II.[19] We also know that 20% of stage II patients may ameliorate to stage I after the first AR.

CONCLUSION

Twin to twin transfusion syndrome if left untreated results in unaccepted rates of perinatal survival (10%). Since the problem is anatomical and the fetuses are otherwise healthy, TTTS is a major therapeutic challenge in perinatal medicine.

Several interventional therapeutic approaches have been tried but the main controversy remains between selective laser photocoagulation of communicating vessels (SLPCV) and AR. There are several retrospective studies comparing the two techniques with comparable results in survival ranging between 57 to 64% for the laser group, and 41 to 78% for AR. Neonatal and infant morbidity is reduced with laser treatment, a fact that may be explained by the prolongation of gestation reported in some studies.

The choice of the therapeutic modality remains controversial. To our opinion it should be individualized according to stage of disease, taking into account the presence of AAA. For stages I and II AR may be suffice and about 20% of cases of stage II disease may improve to stage I after initial treatment with AR. If the syndrome shows signs of deterioration or at presentation the disease is already at stage III, then laser treatment with consequent AR may be the sole option. We should always keep in mind that the availability of SLPCV in clinical practice is limited and training and expertise is not easily acquired. Finally, even with laser coagulation therapy, only one third of affected pregnancies with TTTS will result in two healthy infants, and more importantly the couple has a two out of three chance of delivering a dead or brain damaged baby. Although great progress has been achieved in the management of the disease, perinatal mortality and morbidity in the form of severe neurological handicap (CP), remain high. The major therapeutic challenge of TTTS treatment exists and perhaps with careful staging at presentation and individualization of treatment and acquirement of more expertise in laser techniques, results may improve even more.

REFERENCES

1. Fisk NM, Taylor MJO. The fetus with twin- twin transfusion syndrome. In Harrison M, Evans M, Adzick S, Holzgreve W (Eds): The Unborn Patient: The Art and Science of Fetal Therapy. Philadelpia Company; 2000.
2. Quintero R. Twin-twin transfusion syndrome. Clinics in Perinatology 2003; 591-600.
3. Cincotta RB, Fisk NM. Current thoughts on TTTS. Clinical Obstetrics and Gynecology 1998;140(2):290-302.
4. Bajoria R, Wigglesworth J, Fisk NM. Angioarchitecture of monochorionic placentas in relation to twin-twin transfusion syndrome. AJOG 1995; 172:856-63.
5. Machin G, Still K, Lalani T. Correlations of placental vascular anatomy and clinical outcomes in 69 monochorionic twin pregnancies. AJ Med Genet 1996; 61:229-36.
6. Denbow ML, Cox P, Taylor M, et al. Placental Angio-architecture in monochorionic twin pregnancies: relationship to fetal growth, fetofetal transfusion syndrome, and pregnancy outcome. AJOG 2000; 182: 417-26.
7. Umur A, van Gemert MJ, Nikkels PG et al. Monochorionic twins and twin-twin transfusion syndrome: the protective role of arterio-arterial anastomoses. Placenta 2002;23: 201-9.
8. De Paepe ME, Stopa E, Huang C, et al. Renal tubular apoptosis in twin-twin transfusion syndrome. Pediatr Dev Pathol 1992; 2:25-32.
9. Bajoria R, Ward S, Sooranna SR. Atrial natriuretic peptide mediated polyouria: pathogenesis of polyhydramnios in the recipient twin-twin transfusion syndrome. Placenta 2001;22:716-24.
10. Sebire NJ, Souka A, Skentou H, et al. Early prediction of severe twin to twin transfusion syndrome. Hum Reprod 2000;l5:2008-10.
11. Taylor, et al. USOBG 2000, V16, 3:218-22.
12. Sonntag J, Waltz S, Schollmeyer T, et al. Morbidity and mortality of discordant twins up to 34 weeks of gestational age. Eur J Pediatr 1996; 155:224.
13. Taylor MJ, Denbow ML, Tanawattanacharoen S, et al. Doppler detection of arterio-arterial anastomoses in monochorionic twins feasibility and clinical application. Hum Reprod 2000; 15:1632-6.
14. Quintero R, Morales W, Allen M, Bornick P, Johnson P, et al. Staging of twin-twin transfusion syndrome. J Perinatol 1999;19:550-5.
15. Taylor MJ, Govender L, Jolly *Js/L,* et al. Validation of the Quintero staging system for twin-twin transfusion syndrome. Obstet Gynecol 2002; 100:1256-65.
16. Tan TYT, Taylor MJ, Wee LW, et al. Doppler for artery - artery anastomoses predicts stage independent survival in twin-twin transfusion. Obstet Gynecol 2004.
17. De Lia J, Emery M, Sheafor S, et al. Twin transfusion syndrome: successful in utero treatment with digoxin. Int J Gynecol Obstet 1985;23:197-201.
18. Jones J, Sbarra A, Dilillo L, et al. Indomethacin in severe twin to twin transfusion syndrome. Am J Perinatol 1993;10:24-6.
19. Mari G, Roberts A, Detti L, et al. Perinatal morbidity and mortality rates in severe twin-twin transfusion syndrome: results of the International Amnioreduction Registry. Am J Obstet Gynecol 2001;185:708-15.
20. Dickinson JE, Evans SF. Obstetric and perinatal outcomes from the Australian and New Zealand twin -twin transfusion syndrome registry. AJOG 2000;182:706-12.
21. Quintero R. Twin-twin transfusion syndrome. Clinics in Perinatology 2003;30:591-600.
22. Senat MV, Deprest J, Boulvain M, et al. Endoscopic laser surgery versus serial amnioreduction for severe twin to twin transfusion syndrome. N E J M 2004; 351:136-44.
23. Quintero *R,* Quintero L, Morales W, et al. Amniotic fluid pressures in severe twin twin transfusion syndrome. Prenat Neonat Med 1998;3:607-10.
24. Berry D, Montgomery L. Amniotic septostomy for the treatment of the stuck twin sequence. AJOG 1997;176:S19.
25. Gilbert WM, Davis SE, Kaplan C, et al. Morbidity associated with prenatal disruption of the dividing membrane in twin gestations. Obstet Gynecol 1991; 78:623.
26. De Lia JE, Kuhlmann RS, Harstad TW, et al. Fetoscopic laser ablation of placental vessels in severe previable twin-twin transfusion syndrome. AJOG, 1995; 172:1202-8.
27. Ville Y, Hecher K, Gagnon A, et al. Endoscopic laser coagulation in the management of severe twin-twin transfusion syndrome. BJOG 1998;105:446-53.

28. Ville Y, Hyett J, Hecher K, Nicolaides K. Preliminary experience with endoscopic laser surgery for severe twin-twin transfusion syndrome. NEJM 1995;332:224-7.
29. De Lia JE, Cruikshank DP, Keye WR Jr. Fetoscopic neodymium: YAG laser occlusion of placental vessels in severe twin-twin transfusion syndrome. Obstet Gynecol 1990; 75:1046-53.
30. Quintero R, Morales W, Mendoza G, et al. Selective photocoagulation of placental vessels in twin-twin transfusion syndrome: evolution of a surgical technique. Obstet Gynecol Surv 1998;53: s 97-103.
31. Hecher K, Plath H, Bregenzer T, et al. Endoscopic laser surgery versus serial amniocenteses in the treatment of severe twin-twin transfusion syndrome. AJOG 1999; 180:717-24.
32. Quintero R, Comas C, Bornick PW, et al. Selective versus non selective laser photocoagulation of placental vessels in twin-twin transfusion syndrome.Ultrasound Obstet Gynecol 2000;16: 230-6.
33. B. Thilaganathan, D.J. Gloeb, S. Sairam, A. Tekay. Sono-endoscopic delineation of the placental vascular equator prior to selective fetoscopic laser ablation in TTTS. Ultrasound Obstet Gynecol 2000;16: 226-9.
34. Hecher K, Diehl W, Zikulnig L, et al. Endoscopic laser coagulation of placental anastomoses in 200 pregnancies with severe mid-trimester twin-twin transfusion syndrome. Eur J Obstet Reprod Biol 2000;92:135-9.
35. Quintero R, Dickinson JE, MoralesWJ, et al. Stage-based treatment of twin-twin transfusion syndrome. AJOG 2003;188:1333-40.
36. Banek CS, Hecher K, Hackeloer BJ, et al. Long-term neurodevelopmental outcome after intrauterine laser treatment for severe twin-twin transfusion syndrome. AJOG 2003;188:876-80.

CHAPTER

11

Fetal Pleural Effusion

Castagno Romina, Carreras Moratonas Elena, Toran Nuria, Higueras M Teresa, Sánchez Durán M Angeles

INTRODUCTION

Unlike trace pericardial fluid, which can be seen in normal fetuses, any fluid in the pleural space is abnormal.[1, 2] The incidence of fetal pleural effusion is unknown, but has been estimated to occur in 1 in 15,000 pregnancies in tertiary care centers.[2,3, 28] The actual incidence of primary fetal hydrothorax may be even higher if one considers that in many cases the condition may remain undiagnosed, it may resolve spontaneously, the fetus may be aborted, or death may occur soon after birth in outlying hospitals before transfer to a tertiary care center.[2]

Fetal hydrothorax, either unilateral or bilateral, is a pleural effusion that may be primary, due to chylous leak, or secondary, in which the effusions are part of a generalized fluid retention associated with immune or non-immune hydrops.[2,4] The management of pleural effusion in the fetus is complicated by the difficulty in distinguishing primary from secondary hydrothorax. Chylothorax is the most common cause of pleural effusion in the newborn. Secondary fetal hydrothorax is far more common in the fetus than in the neonate. Irrespective of the underlying cause, fetal pleural effusions may be potentially responsible of fetal and neonatal death.[3,4] This complication occurs as a consequence of pulmonary hypoplasia due to chronic intrathoracic compression, to hydrops developed from mediastinal shift, cardiac compression, and vena caval obstruction, which diminishes venous return to the heart, resulting in a low-cardiac output state[5] and to the prematurity as a consequence of an excess of amniotic fluid secondary to the esophagic compression. Infants affected by pleural effusions usually present in the neonatal period with severe, and often fatal, respiratory insufficiency. This is either a direct result of pulmonary compression caused by the effusions, or due to pulmonary hypoplasia secondary to chronic intrathoracic compression.[3, 28] The overall mortality of neonates with pleural effusion is 25%, with a range from 15% in infants with isolated hydrothorax to 95% in those with gross pleural effusions.[6,7, 28] More recently, Longaker et al reported that the mortality rate in cases of antenatally diagnosed chylothorax was 53%.[2]

Sometimes, it exists an associated maternal morbidity, as in the mirror syndrome characterized by a generalized edema, due to the hydropic placenta that produces vasoactive substances.[8, 28]

NATURAL HISTORY

Fetal pleural effusion may occur as a primary abnormality, in which case one conclude that it is a primary condition after excluding other structural abnormalities, chromosomal abnormalities, other causes of hydrops or after evidencing resolution of hydrops after placing a shunt; or as a secondary manifestation of another condition that causes hydrops fetalis.[3,9,10]

Primary pleural effusions are generally chylous in origin, which occurs as a consequence of an accumulation of lymphatic fluid due to atresia, agenesia or fistulas of the lymphatic duct. Aspirated fluid of a chylous effusion in the feeding infant or adult is characteristically "milky" in appearance because of the presence of chylomicrons in the lymph fluid. Aspirates of fetal chylothoraces yield fluid, which is clear and "straw" colored because the lymph fluid does not contain chylomicrons as a consequence of the "fasting" state of the fetus. Cellular analysis of chylous effusion in the fetus typically shows a large number of lymphocytes, and some suggest that > 80% lymphocytes in the fluid is pathognomonic for a chylous effusion.[27] Others found the cell count in the aspirated fluid to be less consistent.[10]

Congenital pulmonary lymphangiectasia is another rare cause of primary fetal pleural effusion. This is a congenital pulmonary disease, characterized by a subpleural, interlobar, perivascular or peribronchial lymphatic dilatation. Both incidence and etiology remain understood. Some sporadic and even some infrequent familial cases are reported. Recent advances in neonatal intensive care have modified the ominous prognosis of affected newborns. Those who survive present chronic pulmonary complications[11,12] (Figures 11.1 and 11.2).

Pleural effusion is thought to be one of the earliest signs of hydrops fetalis.[12,13] The causes of pleural effusions with hydrops include those of immune hydrops fetalis and non-immune hydrops fetalis: cardiac and vascular diseases 50%,[14] chromosomal abnormality more frequently trisomy 21 and Turner's syndrome 7 to 10%,[3] anemia and hematological diseases, pulmonary or digestive abnormalities, hepatic or metabolic diseases, infections

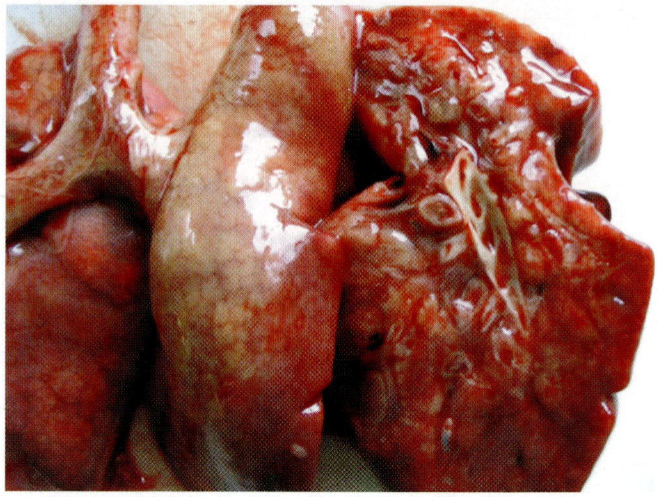

Figure 11.1: Pleural effusion secondary to pulmonary lymphangiectasia. Macroscopic appearance of pulmonary edema and subpleural lymphatic ectasia that gives a fine reticular aspect to the visceral pleural surface

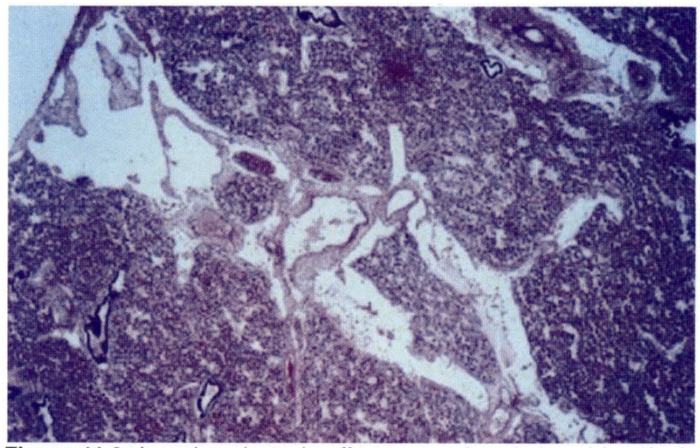

Figure 11.2: Lymphangiectasia affects not only subpleural lymphatic vessels but those located in the interlobar spaces and those adjacent to the vascular vessels

including TORCH, parvovirus B19, skeletal dysplasia and placental or funicular abnormalities. Other major congenital abnormalities are found in 25 to 40% of fetuses with non-immune hydrops fetalis: congenital diaphragmatic hernia, extralobar sequestration, congenital adenomatoid pulmonary disease, thyroid teratoma or congenital fetal goiter.[28] And perinatal mortality is > 90% in hydropic fetuses with pleural effusion if another structural abnormality is identified. This underscores the necessity for a complete anatomic survey in any hydropic fetus with hydrothorax. The risk of chromosomal abnormality is also increased in association with non-immune hydrops fetalis or isolated fetal pleural effusion (6 to 10%). While the underlying cause of a secondary fetal pleural effusion may be evident from detailed sonographic examination and karyotype analysis, in many instances the etiology remains obscure even after a postmortem examination[3] (Figures 11.3 to 11.16).

The prognosis associated with a fetal hydrothorax is determined by many features that are observed with sonography, by this way the cause can sometimes be established and also generalized hydrops may be excluded. The assessment should begin with confirmation of the presumed primary and isolated nature of the hydrothorax by ruling out all secondary hydrothorax etiologies and any associated malformation. The maternal assessment serves as a starting point and should include a review of past obstetrical and medical history, along with a current pregnancy evaluation. Maternal serologies should be verified for all known congenital infections toxoplasmosis, rubeola, CMV, parvovirus B19, adenovirus, syphilis, herpes. Other laboratory tests may be performed (complete blood cell count, blood type and antibody screen). In cases in which hemoglobinopathy is suspected a hemoglobin electrophoresis is performed and if there is a concern about maternal fetal transfusion, Kleihauer-Betke test is recommended. Fetal karyotype must always be confirmed, as most authors agree that there is a 6 to 10% associated chromosomal anomalies. A detailed ultrasound examination is recommended because major congenital abnormalities are commonly found in association with hydrops (41% in one series)[1] and also any subtle sign that may suggest a genetic syndrome must be individualized.[13,14, 28]

A detailed echocardiographic examination is also performed to identify any structural or rythmogenic abnormality that can explain fetal pleural effusion. A careful sonographic inspection should be made to detect subtle signs of hydrops, hydramnios and placental or umbilical cord's associated anomalies.

SONOGRAPHIC FINDINGS

Although the earliest gestational age at which prenatal diagnosis has been made sonographically, is 17 weeks, the vast majority of cases are not diagnosed until third trimester.[2]

Sonographically, pleural effusions appear as anechogenic fluid collections in the fetal chest and

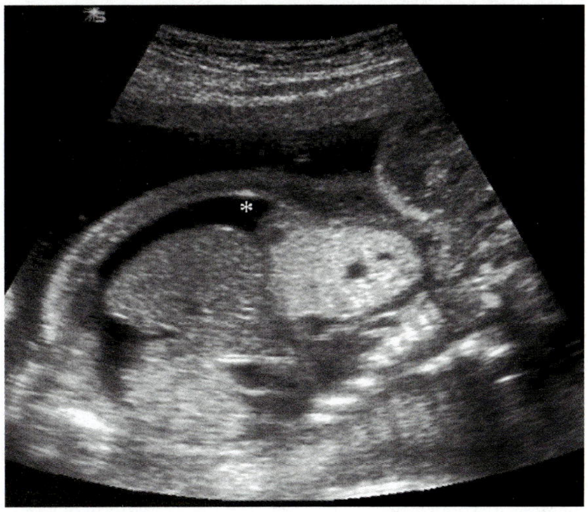

Figure 11.3: MAQ. Oblique section of the fetal thorax. The pulmonary mass is responsible for the mediastinal shift that develops hydrops fetalis. It constitutes a poor prognostic sign. Ascites*

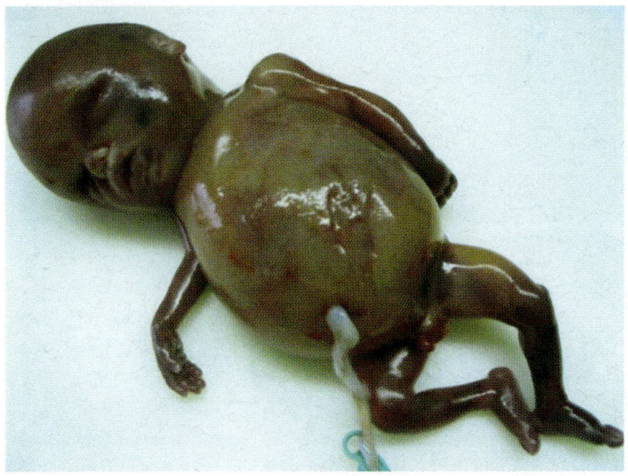

Figure 11.4: A 20 weeks male fetus with an hydropic aspect, distended abdomen

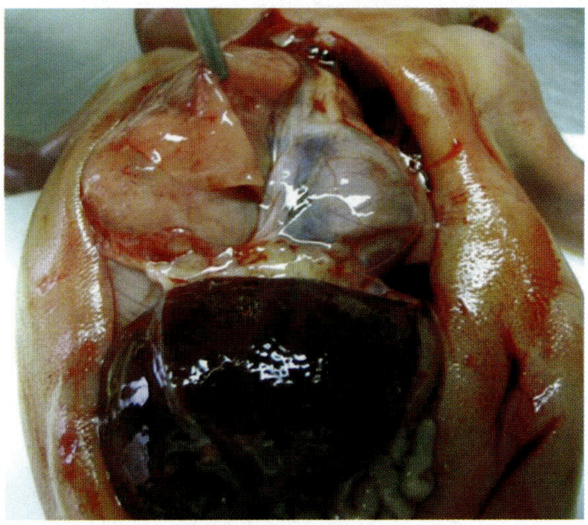

Figure 11.5: After the incision at postmortem autopsy a mass that shifts the mediastinum and collapses fetal heart and left lung with a central right hepatic lobule is exposed

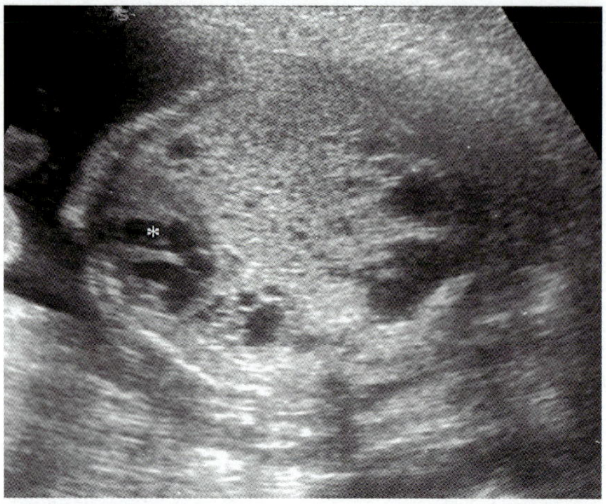

Figure 11.6: MAQ II. Hyperrefringent mass with median size cysts occupying all the right lung and collapsing the contralateral one. Evident cardiac shift (*)

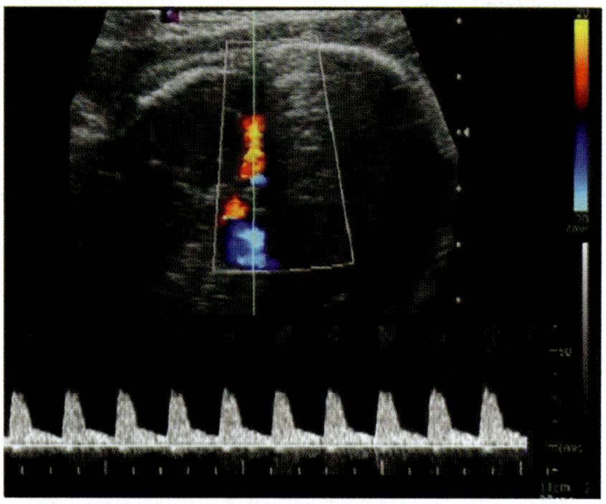

Figure 11.7: Hydrops. During diagnostic evaluation a meticulous US must be performed in order to detect fetal or placental malformations and to exclude fetal anemia by Doppler study of the peak systolic velocity of the middle cerebral artery

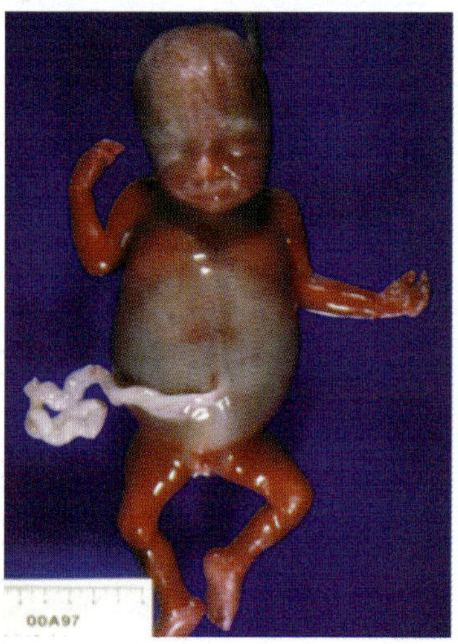

Figure 11.8: Hydrops fetalis of infectious etiology. Distended abdomen as a consequence of an important congestive hepatomegaly

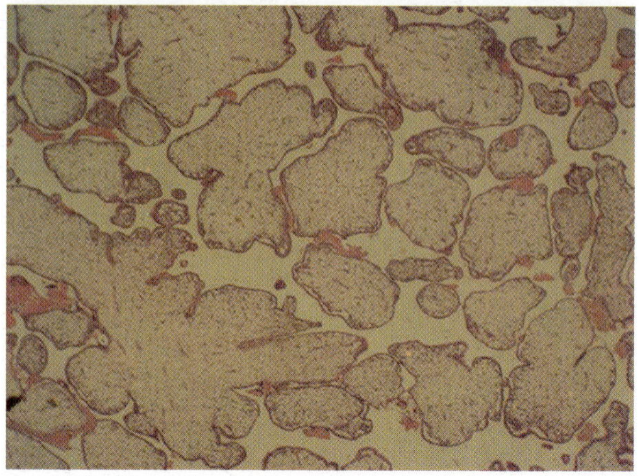

Figure 11.9: Placental microscopic aspect of a parvovirus B19 congenital infection. Generalized edema of chorionic villous

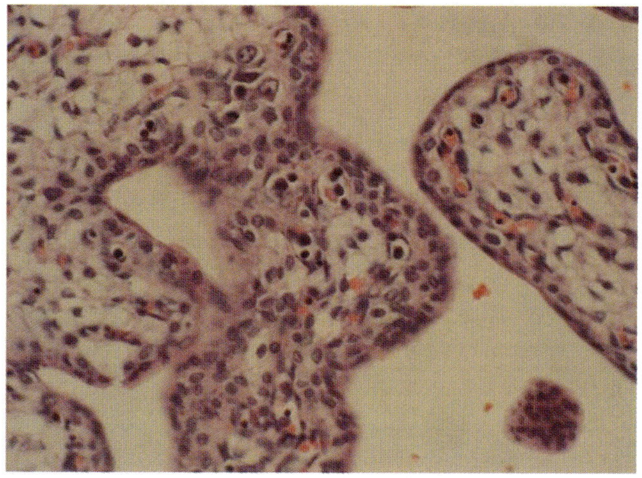

Figure 11.10: Placental microscopic aspect of a parvovirus B19 congenital infection. Microscopic aspect of a chorionic villous showing numerous erythroblasts circulating in fetal capilliaries

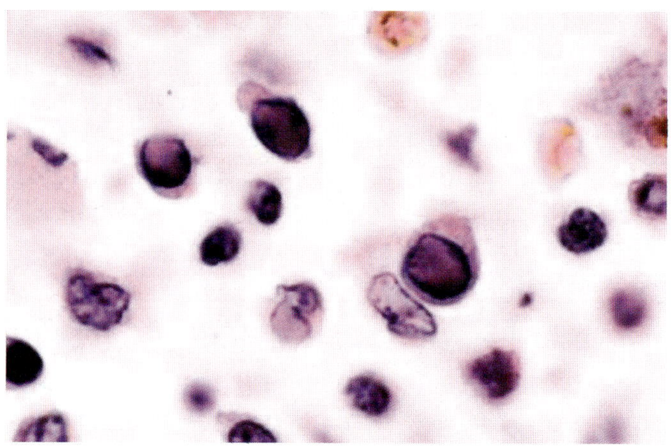

Figure 11.11: Placental microscopic aspect of a parvovirus B19 congenital infection. Intrahemopoietic inclusions typically found in parvovirus infection

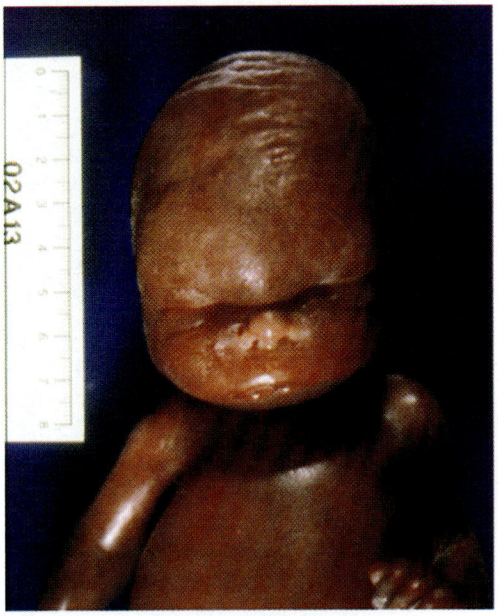

Infectious hydrops fetalis

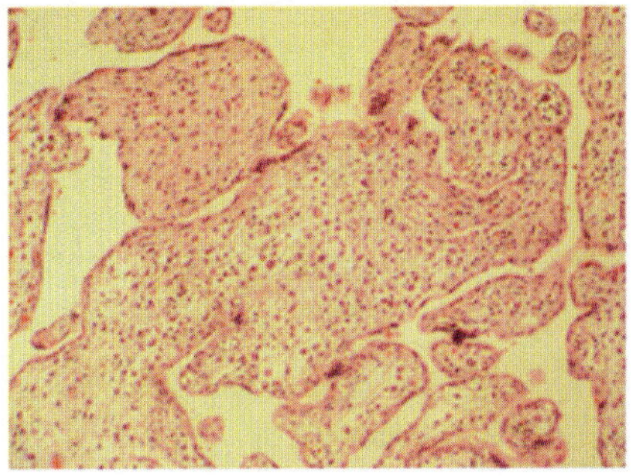

Chorionic villous edema

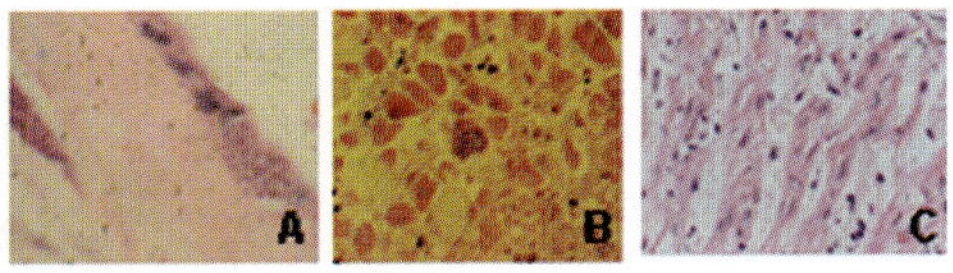

Toxoplasma cysts in funicular surface (A), adrenals (B) and myocardiac tissue (C)

Figure 11.12: Congenital toxoplasmosis infection

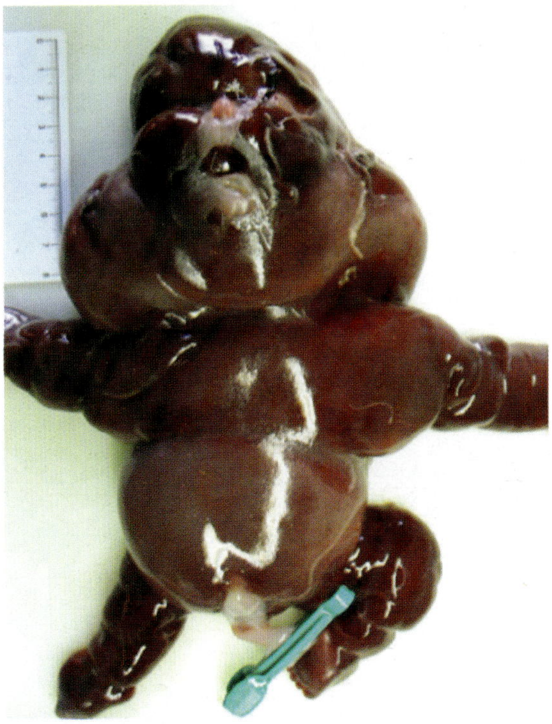

Figure 11.13: Metabolic cause of hydrops fetalis

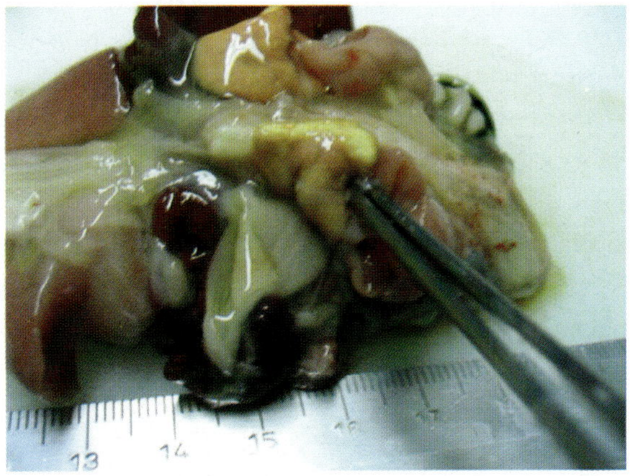

Figure 11.14: Metabolic hydrops fetalis. Wolman's disease. Transverse section of fetal adrenal gland showing an increased size and yellow aspect as a consequence of lipidic storage

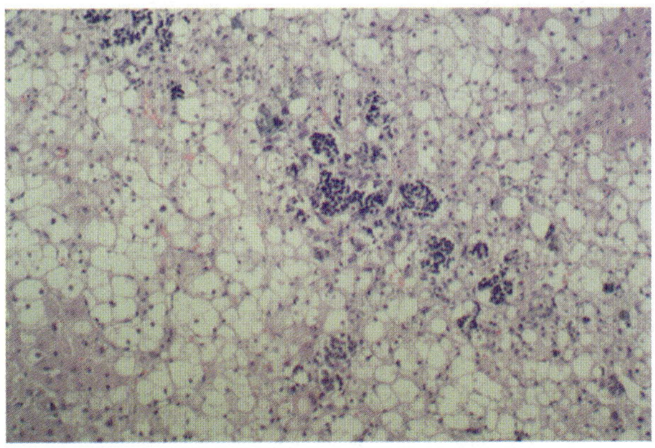

Figure 11.15: Wolman's disease: Adrenal gland's histological section that shows an adipous degeneration of the cortex surrounding medullary neuroblasts and granular calcifications (*)

diaphragmatic contour. When unilateral and large, the hydrothorax can demonstrate considerable mass effect on the diaphragm, fattening or inverting it and displacing the heart and mediastinal structures into contralateral hemithorax. The latter are usually

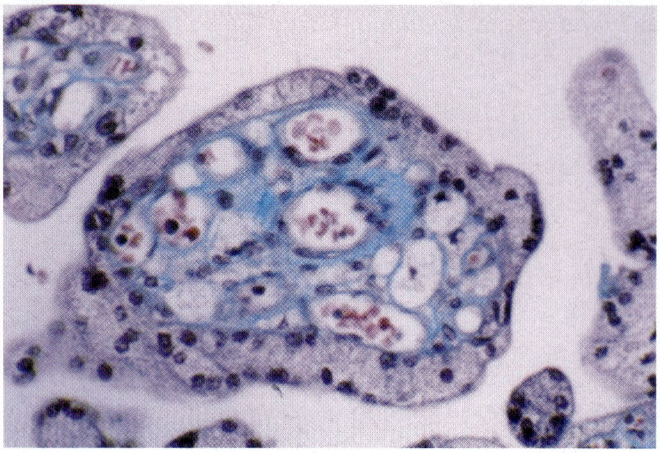

Figure 11.16: Mucolipidosis: vacuolization of syncytiotrophoblast cells

primary fetal pleural effusions. Secondary hydrothoraces tend to be more symmetric in size with little mediastinal shift. The presence of septations or solid components within the intrathoracic fluid collection suggests alternative diagnoses.[2, 14, 15] Fetal hydrothorax has been reported in association with congenital diaphragmatic hernia, congenital cystic adenomatoid malformation of the lung and bronchopulmonary sequestration, but it can usually be differentiated from simple hydrothorax by its more echogenic appearance.[2]

Fetal pleural effusion may be the first sign of non-immune hydrops, and a careful sonographic inspection should be made to detect signs of hydrops fetalis. Congenital heart disease is observed in up to 50% of cases of antenatally diagnosed hydrothoraces.[28] Large pleural effusions with shift of the mediastinum and cardiac compression may limit delineation of cardiac anatomy on fetal echocardiography. Evacuation of these effusions by fetal thoracocentesis will shift the heart to the midline and may facilitate an imaging of the heart (Figures 11.17 to 11.25).

In up to 70% of cases hydramnios is associated with fetal hydrothorax,[2,3,10] as a consequence of interference with fetal swallowing due to mediastinal shift.

The prognosis associated with a fetal hydrothorax is influenced by many features that can be observed by sonography. One of the most important contributions of sonography is determining whether

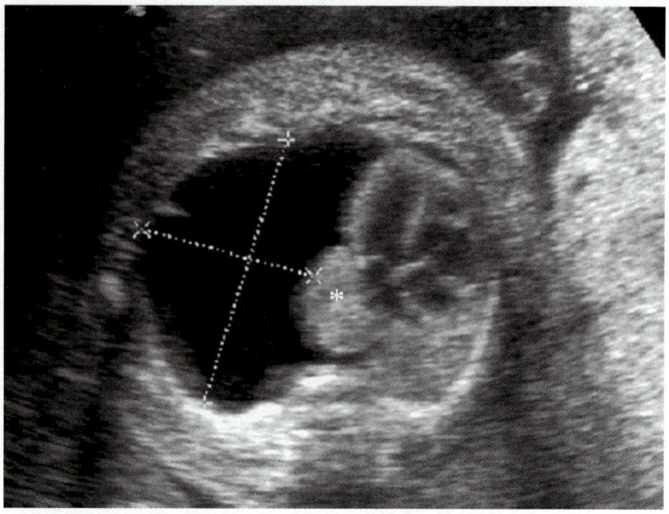

Figure 11.17: Severe left pleural effusion as shown. Transverse section of the fetal thorax showing right shift of the heart. Left lung compressed by the effusion (*)

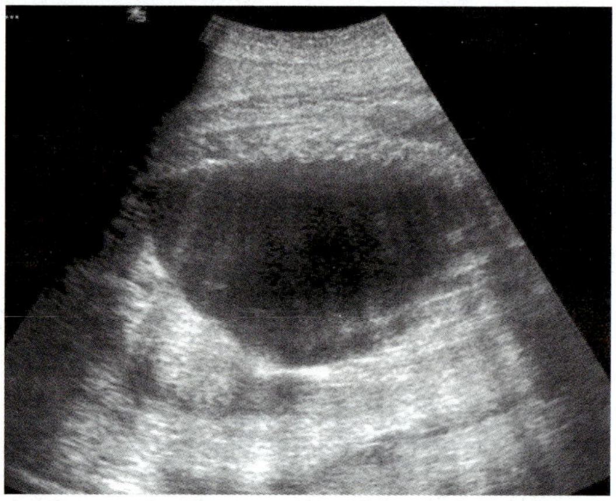

Figure 11.18: Severe pleural effusion in a term fetus. Longitudinal section of the thorax. Antenatal thoracocentesis is performed in order to facilitate newborn reanimation

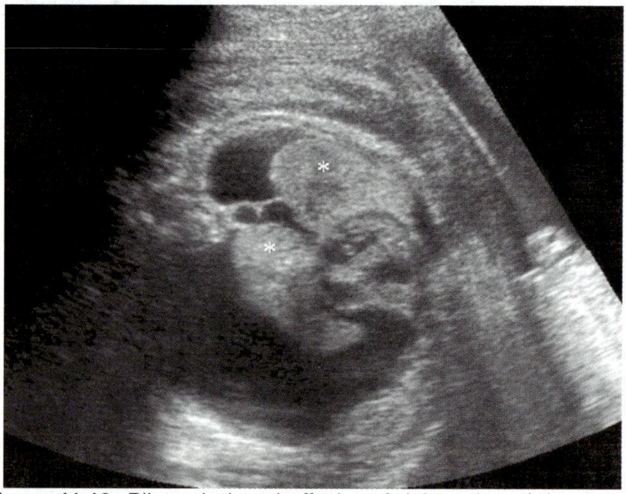

Figure 11.19: Bilateral pleural effusion. Axial section of the thorax. Both lungs appear collapsed (*) at both sides of the heart

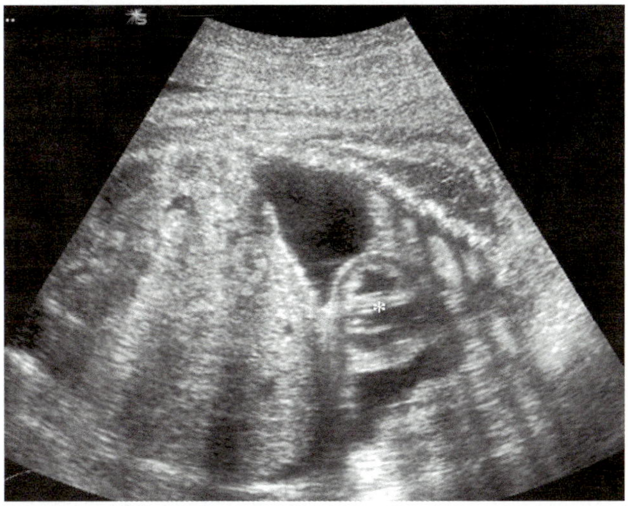

Figure 11.20: Bilateral severe pleural effusion. Coronal section of the trunk. Heart (*) No signs of ascites

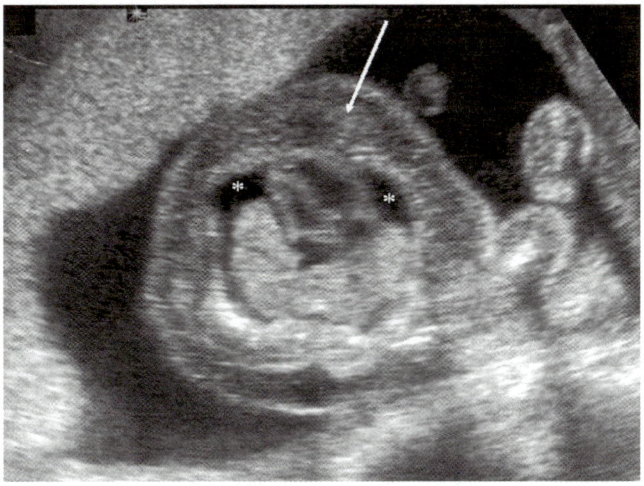

Figure 11.21: Hydrops. Axial section of fetal thorax showing bilateral hydrothorax (*) and evident subcutaneous edema white arrow

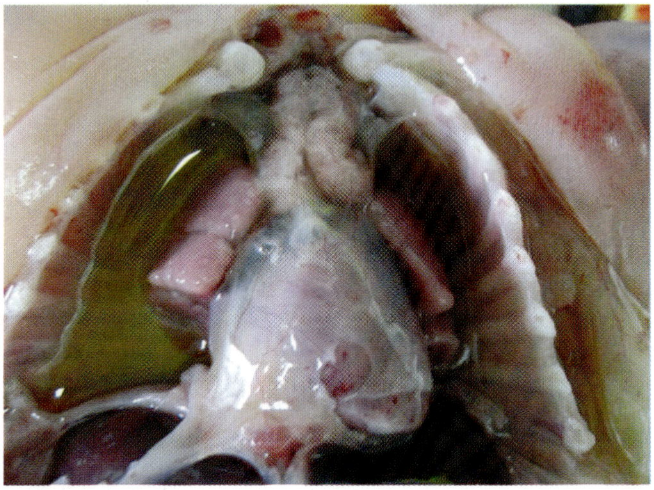

Figure 11.22: Atelectasia and pulmonary hypoplasia secondary to bilateral pleural effusion

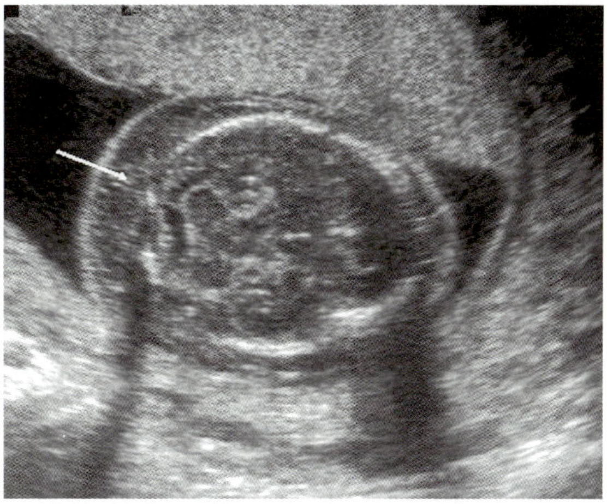

Figure 11.23: Hydrops. Transversal section of fetal vault showing evident subcutaneous edema (white arrow)

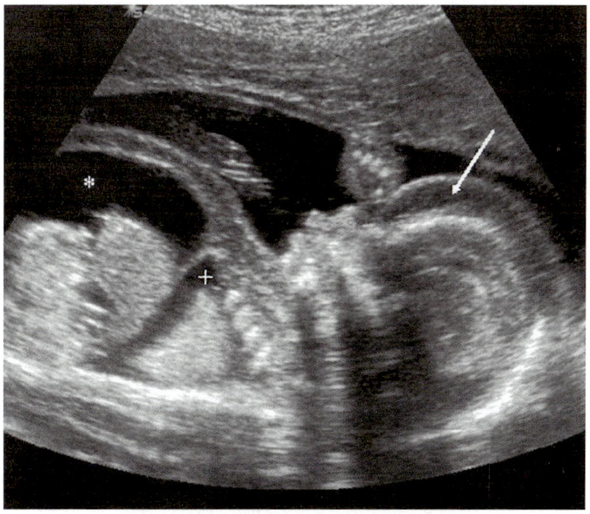

Figure 11.24: Hydrops. Severe ascites(*), pleural effusion(+) subcutaneous edema (white arrow)

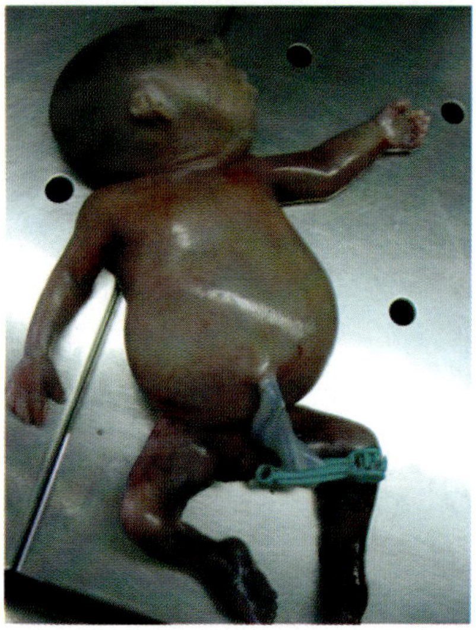

Figure 11.25: 22 weeks of gestation fetus with generalized hydropic aspect. Subcutaneous edema and abdominal distention secondary to ascites

the hydrothorax is a primary or secondary abnormality.

Sonographic features suggestive of primary fetal pleural effusion include the following:

- The hydrothorax is unilateral, or bilateral, very asymmetric.
- The unilateral hydrothorax occurs as an isolated finding no other abnormalities.
- There is considerable mediastinal shift implying mass effect from the hydrothorax. If there are other serous effusions (i.e. ascites), the pleural fluid is disproportionately large compared with other effusions.

These observations are oriented to aid the examiner in recognizing a primary hydrothorax because hydrops caused by a chylothorax is one of the most treatable causes of non-immune hydrops fetalis.[16, 17]

PROGNOSIS

Overall, the clinical course of fetal pleural effusions is unpredictable.[13] This fact difficult both management and parental counseling.

The natural history of fetal pleural effusion is significantly different from chylothorax in the newborn and carries a much poorer prognosis. The mortality rate for chylothorax in the newborn is at most 15%, but the mortality rate for prenatally diagnosed fetal pleural effusion is 53%.[2] The reported mortality rate in cases of secondary hydrothorax with associated hydrops may be as high as 95%.

The major concern in a fetus with a large primary hydrothorax is the potential development of hydrops and pulmonary hypoplasia.

Spontaneous resolution or regression has been reported to occur in 9 to 22% of primary fetal hydrothoraces, even in cases of large,[1, 7, 9, 15] and has been associated with nearly 100% of survival.[15] Unfortunately, it is not possible to predict accurately which effusions will resolve or progress based on finding of a single ultrasound examination. One can nevertheless try to define the characteristics of fetal pleural effusion cases which spontaneously resolve: diagnosis is generally made early in second trimester 67%, they are more often unilateral 65%, they are not associated with hydramnios 69%, there is not hydrops 90%. If regression is possible, worsening is, however more frequently reported in the literature.[13] Spontaneous resolution of fetal hydrothorax has occurred in approximately 5 to 10% of cases.[2,3,10] Because of the possibility of spontaneous resolution, a period of observation and follow-up is warranted in all cases. In some cases the fetal pleural effusion remains stable a satisfactory postnatal treatment may be undertaken.[2,16]

To better define prognostic features, several investigators reported outcomes of fetuses with antenatal diagnosed hydrothoraces. Aubard et al summarized the information reported in 35 untreated fetuses. Overall mortality was 39% in this series, similar to 35 to 50% mortality reported by other authors.[1, 2] Adverse prognostic indicators included bilaterality, presence of hydrops, absence of spontaneous resolution and premature delivery.[13]

Of all the poor prognostic indicators, hydrops is probably the most important. The development of hydrops in a fetus with primary fetal hydrothorax is a poor prognostic sign, with a mortality rate of 52%.[2] It is thought that hydrops develops from mediastinal shift, cardiac compression, and vena caval obstruction, which diminishes venous return to the heart, resulting in low cardiac-output state.[5]

The mortality rate associated with primary fetal pleural effusion is still significantly better than the 95 to 98% mortality rate observed in secondary fetal pleural effusion.[1, 2] In the report of Longaker et al of 32 fetuses with hydrothorax, the absence of hydrops was associated with 100% survival. The best outcomes are reported with unilateral effusions and no more anomalies.

In cases of fetal hydrothorax diagnosed prior to 33 weeks, the survival rate was only 43%, versus 80% if it was diagnosed before that gestational age. Similarly, a gestational age of less than 35 weeks at delivery had a survival rate of only 30%, versus 79% if delivered after 35 weeks.[2]

Hydramnios has no independent prognostic significance, except that it results in uterine over distention, predisposing to preterm labor and delivery.[17, 29]

Even in the absence of hydrops, large pleural effusions can cause pulmonary hypoplasia due to compression. It is likely that time of onset, size, and duration of the pleural effusion probably influence the development of pulmonary hypoplasia. The most common cause of neonatal death in a fetus diagnosed with hydrothorax is respiratory insufficiency due to pulmonary hypoplasia.[17, 29]

MANAGEMENT OF PREGNANCY

Fetal pleural effusion is frequently associated with extrathoracic anomalies. The risk of an abnormal karyotype in fetal hydrothoraces is small, but significant up to 7% in most series. Prenatal karyotyping is recommended, especially if fetal intervention is considered. The incidence of Down's syndrome in fetal pleural effusion is 4.9%.[1] Because the incidence of associated congenital heart disease may be as high as 5% most authors agree in recommending to perform a meticulous fetal echocardiography. As previously mentioned sometimes it is not until the effusion's evacuation that a congenital heart disease is detected.

The fetus with a pleural effusion is at significant risk for the development of hydramnios and preterm delivery. Most authors recommend a careful follow-up, with ultrasound examination every 1 to 2 weeks for early detection of signs consistent with tension hydrothorax, such as mediastinal shift, diaphragmatic eversion, development of hydrops, and hydramnios.

The fetus affected by a hydrothorax is also at significant risk for pulmonary hypoplasia and respiratory distress following delivery. It seems convenient that fetuses with large pleural effusion be delivered in a tertiary care center. Prenatal consultations with a pediatric surgeon, neonatologist, geneticist, and pediatric cardiologist may be indicated.

The presence of hydrothorax does not influence the mode of delivery. Cesarean delivery should be reserved for obstetrical indications (Flow chart 11.1).

Fetal Intervention

The goals of antenatal therapy, as described by Weber and Philipson[1] are:

- Prevention of lung compression, allowing normal development
- Prevention or reversal of hydropic changes and hydramnios, avoiding fetal death and preterm delivery
- Improved postnatal respiratory function.

The primary goal of any intervention is to avoid progression of an otherwise frequently fatal disease. Then it is crucial to select fetuses that could be candidates for intrauterine therapy.

There are several options in the management of fetuses with isolated hydrothorax; the options depend on gestational age, severity of effusion, evidence of progression, and the presence or absence of hydrops, hydramnios or mediastinal shift. The outcome of fetal pleural effusion is significantly worsened by prematurity less than 32 weeks of gestation, the presence of hydrops and lack of prenatal therapy.[1] Therefore, occurrence of fetal pleural effusion at less than 32 weeks of gestation should be treated prenatally for the majority of authors.

When the hydrothorax is small, isolated, and well tolerated, frequent surveillance may be most prudent because of the possibility of spontaneous resolution. If the fetal pleural effusion is very large or increases over time with signs of fetal decompensation, i.e. hydrops, a fetal intervention may be needed.

Prenatal therapy for pleural effusion can include a single thoracocentesis, serial thoracocentesis or catheter placement to drain fetal fluid into the amniotic fluid. Thoracocentesis is considered the initial procedure of choice because it can provide cytologic and biochemical diagnostic information as well as a relief of intrathoracic compression.

Thoracocentesis

Thoracocentesis was proposed for the first time as a treatment of fetal hydrothorax by Petres et al in 1982.

It is a diagnostic maneuver to obtain pleural fluid for cell count, differential, and culture and to establish whether the effusion is chylous. Additionally, the diagnosis of an underlying cardiac abnormality or other intrathoracic lesion may become apparent only after effective decompression and return of the mediastinum to its normal position. It may be useful in the prenatal diagnosis of pulmonary hypoplasia

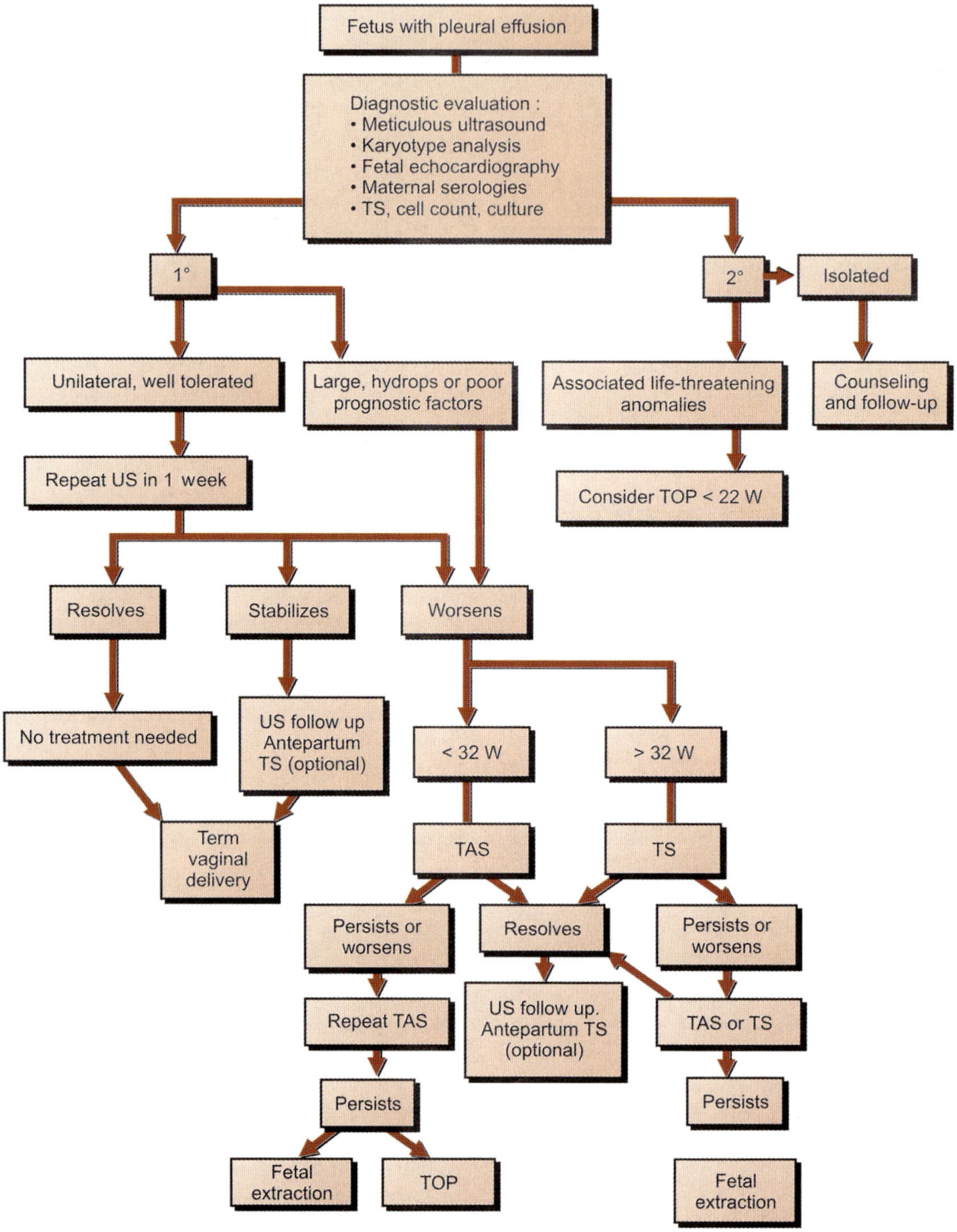

Flow chart 11.1: Algorithm for the management of pleural effusions. TS= thoracocentesis, TAS= thoracoamniotic shunting, TOP= termination of pregnancy

because in such cases the lungs often fail to expand after the procedure.

It may also be done in the immediate prepartum period to help improve the neonatal respiratory status.

Clinical outcomes after fetal thoracocentesis alone are variable. There are several reports of thoracocentesis for fetal pleural effusion, performed with either complete resolution or a good outcome despite reaccumulation.[16,18,19, 30] In their summary, Aubard et al reported that 16 of 29 (55%) fetuses treated by thoracocentesis had good outcomes. Others have had disappointing results with repeated thoracocentesis for fetal hydrothorax because of rapid accumulation of the effusion and neonatal death from respiratory insufficiency.[1-3] Thoracocentesis cannot adequately decompress the fetal chest to allow pulmonary expansion and prevent pulmonary hypoplasia.[2]

Thoracocentesis may be extremely useful before delivery or for temporary stabilization of the fetus, but this treatment alone is often not effective earlier in gestation owing to the rapid accumulation of fluid in most 76% of cases.[13]

However, if the effusion reaccumulates, thoracoamniotic shunting is felt to be less traumatic than repeated aspiration.[34]

Pleuroamniotic Shunting

When the pleural fluid reaccumulates rapidly after the initial tap, and if the condition worsens with the development of fetal hydrops, a thoracoamniotic shunt should be considered for permanent *in utero* drainage. This may be especially useful in fetus < 32 weeks of gestational age because of the higher risk of preterm delivery.

Use of this technique to drain primary fetal hydrothoraces was first proposed by Seeds and Bowes in 1986.[31] Presently, the most commonly used technique for pleuroamniotic shunting is that described by Rodeck et al.[32] This technique has been successfully used in the treatment of isolated hydro- or chylothorax and more rarely in cases of pleural effusion secondary to congenital lung abnormalities such as pulmonary sequestration or cystic adenomatoid malformation.[33]

To accomplish thoracoamniotic shunting, a metal trocar with cannula is introduced through the maternal abdominal wall and uterus into the fetal thorax as close as possible to the midaxillary line of the fetus. Once the trocar has been introduced into the thorax, a double pig-tail catheter is passed through the trocar, and the "internal" loop is deployed into the thorax with an introducer rod. As the trocar and introducer are removed, the "external" end of the catheter is left in the amniotic space. Situated in this way, the catheter creates a permanent communication between the pleural space and the amniotic cavity.

The mechanism by which shunting benefits the fetus is by allowing the pleural fluid to decompress to the pressure of the amniotic fluid. This allows the lungs to expand, potentially reducing the risks of pulmonary hypoplasia, and also reduces pressure on the venous system, increasing venous return to the heart and improving coexisting heart failure. However there are no randomized trials of its use, nor are there data from animal models confirming these mechanisms of action in cases of fetal pleural effusion.[34]

This has been accomplished in many fetuses; two larger series were reported by Nicolaides and Azar (n=35) and Mussat et al (n=18). Aubard et al summarized 80 reports of thoracoamniotic shunting in fetuses with bilateral or unilateral pleural effusions. This series suggests that shunting has the most dramatic effect on survival among fetuses already showing signs of hydrops.[13] In the series of Aubard et al, only 10% of hydropic fetuses survived after thoracocentesis alone, whereas 67% of hydropic fetuses survived after thoracoamniotic shunting. Other series reported similar survival rate ranging between 50 and 75% after in uterus pleuroamniotic shunting.[3, 32] Shunt failures were reported in 26% of cases.[13, 20, 21, 25]

The risks of thoracocentesis and shunt placement to mother and fetus have been minimal and far outweighed by the potential benefits. Few complications have been reported for either fetal thoracocentesis and thoracoamniotic shunts. In the series of Smith et al of 23 cases of shunting, one ended in a fatal fetal hemorrhage at the time of shunt insertion at 23 weeks and one in a neonatal death following the procedure-related abruption at 30 weeks of gestation.[34] Migration of the catheter has been a consistent problem. It has been found in the intra-amniotic cavity, maternal peritoneal cavity, neonatal subcutaneous tissue and the neonatal intrathoracic cavity.[21] Drainage of amniotic fluid into the fetal pleural cavity has been reported.[32] Acute maternal compromise has occurred due to amniotic fluid leakage into the maternal peritoneal cavity.[35] It should be recognized that these procedures have the potential for infection, bleeding, premature rupture of membranes, preterm labor and injury to the fetus.[2] Procedure risks may be increased by maternal obesity, hydramnios or fetal position. After delivery, delay in clamping of the catheter can result in temporary neonatal compromise.

The prognosis after shunting is determined by the underlying cause of the effusion. There is no evidence that fetuses that had a successful intervention suffer later from any chronic respiratory disease. Thompson et al described a series of 17 survivors after a successful intervention, all of them had a normal pulmonary development and an adequate functional capacity[24, 25] (Figures 11.18 to 11.28).

CONCLUSION

Published studies emphasize on the fact of the vast heterogeneity of fetal hydrothorax etiology. A careful sonographic evaluation is then mandatory.

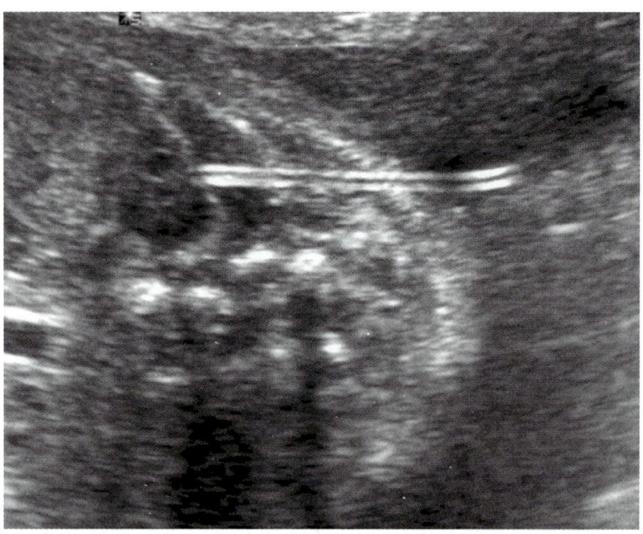

Figure 11.26: MAQ II. Placement of a catheter in one of the cysts connecting with the amniotic cavity

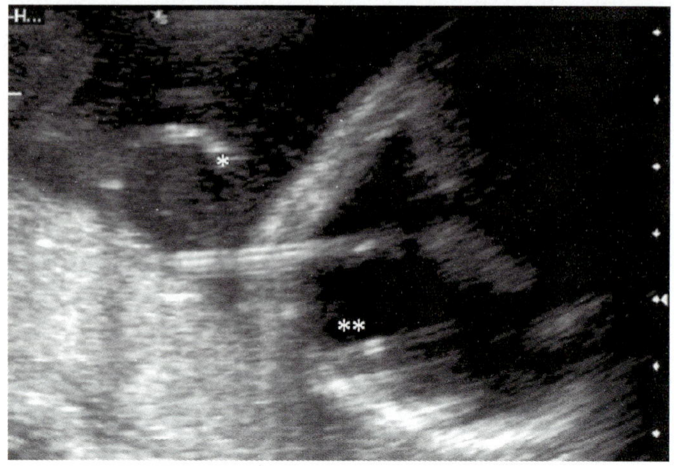

Figure 11.27: Left pleural effusion. Pleuroamniotic shunting (pig tail). One of the ends is within the amniotic cavity (*) the other (**) in the pleural cavity. It allows to drain the effusion, decompress the lung and prevent pulmonary hypoplasia

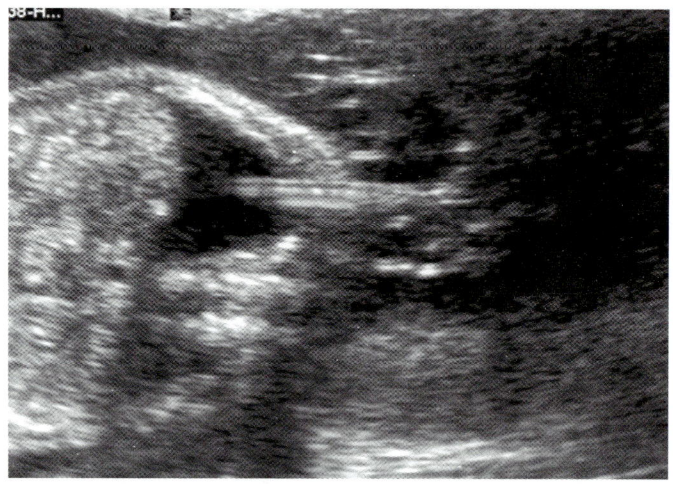

Figure 11.28: Thoracoamniotic shunt

The clinical course of primary fetal hydrothorax is highly variable, ranging from complete resolution with good outcome to progression to hydrops fetalis and perinatal death.

The more accurate targeting of therapeutic approaches to particular cases may allow us to significantly ameliorate the somber overall prognosis of this condition, and make infant survival without sequelae more feasible.

This condition is rare in prenatal medicine but it does nevertheless warrant special attention.

REFERENCES

1. Weber AM, Philipson EH. Fetal pleural effusion: a review and meta-analysis for prognostic indicators. Obstetrics and Gynecology 1992; 79: 281-6.
2. Longaker MT, Laberge JM, Dansereau J, Langer JC. Primary fetal hydrothorax: natural history and management. Journal of Pediatric Surgery 1989; 24: 573-6.
3. Nicolaides KH, Azar GB. Thoraco-amniotic shunting. Fetal Diagnosis Therapy 1990; 5: 153-64.
4. Estroff JA, Parad RB, Frigoletto Jr FD, Benacerraf BR. The natural history of isolated fetal hydrothorax. Ultrasound in Obstetrics and Gynecology 1992; 2: 162-5.
5. Bessone LN, Ferguson TB. Chylothorax. Ann Thorac Surg 1971; 12: 527-50.
6. Beischer ND, Fortune DW. Non- immunologic hydrops fetalis and congenital anomaly. Obstetrics and Gynecology 1971; 38: 89-95.
7. Klam S, Bigras JL, Hudon L. Predicting outcome in primary fetal hydrothorax. Fetal Diagnosis and Therapy 2005; 20: 366-70.
8. Brochot C, Collinet P, Pronost N. Mirror syndrome due to parvovirus B19 hydrops complicated by severe maternal pulmonary effusion. Prenatal diagnosis 2006; 262: 179-80.
9. Mussat P, Dommergues M, Parat S, Mandelbrot L. Congenital chylothorax with hydrops: postnatal care and outcome following antenatal diagnosis. Acta Paediatrica 1995; 84: 749-55.
10. Eddleman KA, Levine AB, Chitkara U, Berkowitz RL. Reliability of pleural fluid lymphocyte counts in the antenatal diagnosis of congenital chylothorax. Obstetrics and Gynecology 1991; 78: 530-2.
11. Stevenson DA, Pysher TJ, Ward RM. Familial congenital non- immnune hydrops, chylothorax and pulmonary lymphangiectasia. American Journal of Medical Genetics 2006; 140A 4: 368-72.
12. Bellini C, Boccardo F, Campisi C. Pulmonary lymphangiectasia. Lymphology 2005; 38 3: 111-21.
13. Aubard Y, Derouineau I, Aubard V, Chalifour V. Primary fetal hydrothorax: A literature review and proposed antenatal clinical strategy. Fetal Diagnosis and Therapy 1998; 13: 325-33.
14. Skoll MA, Sharland GK, Allan LD. Is the ultrasound definition of fluid collections in non- inmune hydrops fetalis helpfull in defining the underlying cause or predicting outcome? Ultrasound in Obstetrics and Gynecology 1991; 1: 309-12.
15. Aguirre OA, Finley BE, Ridgway LE, Bennett TL. Resolution of unilateral fetal hydrothorax with associated non-immune hydrops after intrauterine thoracocentesis. Ultrasound in Obstetrics and Gynecology 1995; 5: 346-8.
16. Cardwell MS: Aspiration of fetal pleural effusions or ascites may improve neonatal resuscitation. South Medical Journal 1996; 89:177-8.
17. Defoort P, Thiey M. Antenatal diagnosis of congenital chylothorax by gray- scale sonography. J Clin Ultrasound 1978; 6: 47.
18. Petres RE, Reawing TO. Congenital bilateral chylothorax: antepartum diagnosis and successful intrauterine surgical management. JAMA 1982; 248:1360-1.
19. Picone O, Benachi A, Mandelbrot L, Ruano R, Dumez Y. Thoracoamniotic shunting for fetal pleural effusions with hydrops. American Journal of Obstetrics and Gynecology 2004; 191: 2047-50.
20. Sase M, Miwa I, Hasegawa K, Sumie M. Successful treatment of primary fetal hydrothorax with double basket catheter. American Journal of Perinatology 2002; 19: 405-11.
21. Wittman B, Martin KA, Wilson RD, Pecock D. Complications of long-term drainage of fetal pleural effusion: case report and review of the literature. American Journal of Perinatology 1997; 14: 443-7.
22. Thompson PJ, Greenough A, Nicolaides KH. Respiratory function in infancy following pleuro-amniotic shunting: fetal diagnosis therapy 1993; 8:79-83.
23. Lien JM, Colmorgan GHC, Gehret JF. Spontaneous resolution of fetal pleural effusion diagnosed during the second trimester. Journal of Clinical Ultrasound 1990; 18: 54-6.
24. Smoleniec J, James D. Predictive value of pleural effusions in fetal hydrops. Fetal diagnosis and Therapy 1993; 10: 95-100.
25. Nakayama h, Kukita H. Long-term outcome of 51 liveborn neonates with non-immune hydrops fetalis. Acta Paediatrica 1999; 88:24-8.
26. Defoort P, Thiey M. Antenatal diagnosis of congenital chylothorax by gray-scale sonography. J Clin Ultrasound 1978; 6:47.
27. Lange IR, Manning FA. Antenatal diagnosis of congenital pleural effusions. Am J Obstet Gynecol 1981;140:839-40.
28. Gratacós E. Terapia Fetal: indicaciones y técnicas actuales. Ediciones Mayo, 2002;147-54.
29. Carroll B. Pulmonary hypoplasia and pleural effussions associated with fetal death *in utero*: Ultrasonic findings. AJR 1977; 129:749.
30. Benacerraf BR, Frigoletto FD. Midtrimester fetal thoracocentesis. J Clin Ultrasound 1985; 13: 302-4.
31. Seeds JW, Bowes WA. Results of treatment of severe fetal hydrothorax with bilateral pleuroamniotic catheters. Obstet Gynecol 1986; 68: 577-80.
32. Rodeck CH, Fisk NM. Long-term in utero drainage of fetal hydrothorax. N Engl J Med 1988; 319: 1135-9.
33. Becher R, Arabin B. Successful treatment of primary fetal hydrothorax by long term drainage from week 23. Case report and review of the literature. Fetal Diagn Ther 1993; 8: 331-7.
34. Smith RP, Illanes S, Soothill PW. Outcome of fetal pleural effusions treated by thoracoamniotic shunting. Ultrasound Obstet Gynecol 2005; 26: 63-6.
35. Ronderos-Dumit D, Nicolini U. Uterine- peritoneal amniotic fluid leakage: an unusual complication of intrauterine shunting. Obstet Gynecol 1991; 78: 913-5.

CHAPTER 12

Invasive Procedure and Therapy in Fetal Hydrocephalus

Iniesta S, Salazar FJ, Bajo JM

INTRODUCTION

Hydrocephalus is defined as ventriculomegaly and macrocephaly associated with an increased intracranial pressure. It results from an abnormal increase in the volume of the cerebral ventricles compared with that of brain substance.

It is one of the most common congenital abnormalities and it is found in 1 to 3 of every 1000 born children, being the incidence of isolated hydrocephalus lower, in a range between 0.39 and 0.87 per 1000 births.[1]

The most common cause of congenital hydrocephalus is the obstruction of cerebrospinal fluid flow,[2,3] specially at the cerebral aqueduct congenital defects in the developing of the cerebrospinal fluid circulation pathways, with the resulting increase in intracraneal pressure. But there are many other causes of hydrocephalus, such as the increase in cerebrospinal fluid production or a relative decrease in the amount of brain substance.

Hydrocephalus may be associated with a variety of chromosomal abnormalities,[4,5] including triploidy, trisomy 13, trisomy 18, trisomy 21, mosaicisms and certain balanced translocations,[6-9] specially the congenital stenosis of the aqueduct of Sylvius, that has been inherited in some cases as an X-linked recesive trait,[10,11] and can be also associated with intrauterine infections,[12-17] but many cases of diagnosed hydrocephalus cannot be assigned to any of the causes described before.[18]

The etiology of the hydrocephalus has been described for some authors as a major determinant of the outcome in the children with early postnatal surgical treatment of fetal hydrocephalus.[19]

DIAGNOSIS

Many techniques can be used for the diagnosis of ventriculomegaly.

The prenatal diagnosis of hydrocephalus is usually made by the demonstration of a dilated ventricular system in an ultrasound examination, by measuring the atrium of the lateral ventricles (Figures 12.1 and 12.2).

The width of the lateral ventricle remains nearly the same during the second an third trimesters,[20,21] so it is a good measure to use for the diagnosis, and some authors have even described the possibility of exclusion of fetal ventriculomegaly with a single

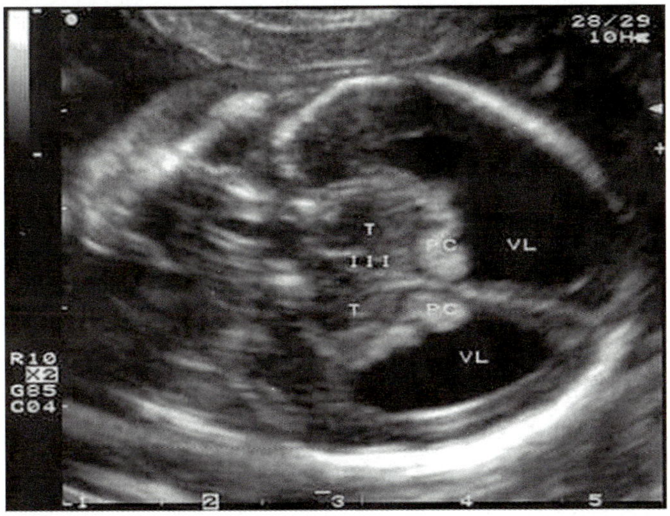

Figure 12.1: Bilateral fetal hydrocephalus diagnosed by a dilatation of the atrium diameter, demonstrated by a single ultrasound exploration. T: thalamus; III: third ventricle; PC: choroid plexus; VL: lateral ventricles

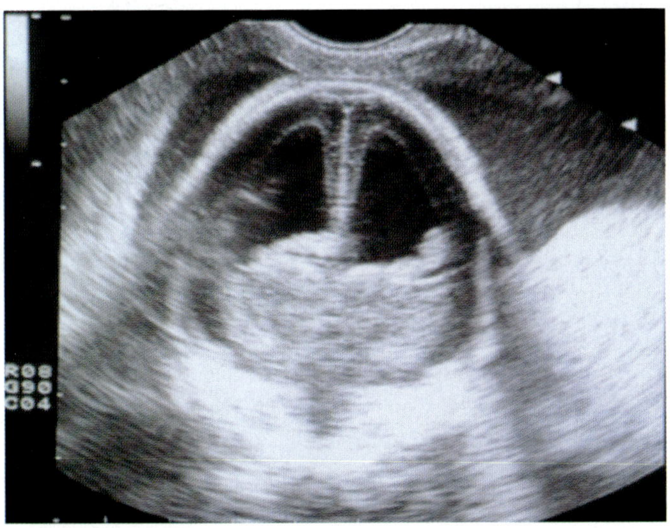

Figure 12.2: Fetal hydrocephalus diagnosed at 20 weeks of gestation. Dilatation of both lateral ventricles

measurement of the width of the lateral ventricular atrium.[22]

Other morphologic criteria, such as the lateral ventricle to hemispheric width ratio, the asymmetric appearance of the choroid plexus or the size and configuration of the horns, have been described by some authors as useful in the diagnosis of hydrocephalus at earlier stages of the pregnancy.[20,23,24]

Although ultrasound remains the gold standard in fetal imaging, *in utero* magnetic resonance imaging of the fetal nervous system has been described for some authors as an useful complementary imaging procedure in the late stages of pregnancy, especially in pregnant women in whose fetuses ultrasound examination had shown hydrocephalus and neural tube defects.[25-27]

ASSOCIATED ANOMALIES

In nearly 50% of the cases, hydrocephalus is associated to other anomalies, both intracranial and extracranial ones, that have to be excluded prior to have an accurate diagnosis and classification of this condition.

Hydrocephalus is described as *isolated* when the fetus is free of other anomalies and is not the direct result of the ventricular enlargement or increased intracranial pressure.

Most of the anomalies that can be associated with hydrocephalus are described in Table 12.1. The most common one is the meningomyelocele.

Table 12.1: Most common associated anomalies with fetal hydrocephalus

▪ Intracranial anomalies	Microcephaly Encephalocele Arachnoid cyst Agenesis of corpus callosum Arteriovenous malformations
▪ Extracranial anomalies	Myelomeningocele Scoliosis Spinal dysraphism Vertebral body anomalies
▪ Renal system abnormalities	Hydronephrosis Dysplastic kydneys Uni/bilateral renal agenesis
▪ Cardiac abnormalities	Ventricular septal defects Fallot's tetralogy Hypoplastic left heart syndrome
▪ Gastrointestinal malformations	Omphalocele Gastroschisis Tracheoesophagial fistula Malrotation of the bowel
▪ Chromosomal abnormalities	Trisomies 21, 13 and 18 Balanced translocations Mosaicisms

When a hydrocephalus is diagnosticated, an adequate exploration must include a systematic evaluation of the central nervous system (posterior fossa, third and fourth ventricles, subarachnoid space), a careful examination of the fetal spine and a careful examination of other systems, as we describe in Table 12.1. It is also recommended a chromosomal study (amniocentesis) because of the high risk of aneuploid anomalies (3-27%),[28-30] especially when other abnormalities are present.

PROGNOSIS

The mortality for hydrocephalus is nearly 67%, but this high percentage decreases to 37% for fetuses without anomalies outside the cental nervous system.

The incidence of early neonatal death and poor neurologic outcome and life expectancy are directly related to the etiology[31] and to the presence and severity of the associated anomalies.[32]

It has not been demonstrated the correlation between the thickness of the cortical mantle and the neurological prognosis,[6] as some authors suggested at the beginning.

Newborns with isolated, moderate ventriculomegaly, but without other abnormalities have the best prognosis, with a good neurological outcome.[33-35] It is also described a significantly poor postnatal functional outcome in those fetal hydrocephalus diagnosed in the early gestation.[19]

MANAGEMENT

Once the diagnosis of fetal hydrocephalus is done, it is very important to distinguish between the isolated hydrocephalus and the hydrocephalus associated with other anomalies, especially with those of the central nervous system. As we have described before, the neurological outcome will depend on this factor, being dismal in the last case.

So before taking any treatment decision, we do have to do an accurate diagnosis, by performing a detail ultrasound examination, to exclude another associated anomalies, an amniocentesis for the determination of fetal karyotype, as well as virus cultures.

Obstetric management would vary from vaginal delivery, with or without the need of a cephalocentesis, or cesarean section. The place of shunting procedures has no place at the moment, although some studies are trying to introduce them again during the last few years, after the failure of the first trial of fetal neurosurgery in the 1980s.

In all cases, therapeutic options need to be discussed in detail with the parents.

Cephalocentesis consists in removing fluid from the fetal ventricular system to assure the overlapping of the cranial sutures by introducing transabdominally or transvaginally a needle (14- to 18-gauge) under ultrasound guidance.[36] This technique would be indicated in those cases of fetal hydrocephalus with macrocephaly and severe associated anomalies that assure a dismal prognosis,[6,36] this technique followed by a vaginal delivery may be the most appropiate form of manegement in these cases of poor outcome.[6]

Only about 37% of fetus wih hydrocephalus diagnosticated have some degree of macrocephaly,[32] so it is not recommended to perform a cesarean section in all the cases. Cesarean delivery would be indicated in those cases of fetal hydrocephalus with macrocephaly, without associated malformations, in those cases of fetal hydrocephalus associated to meningomyelocele, or for obsterics indications.[6]

If there is not any of the previous conditions, a vaginal delivery would be the most appropriate (no macrocephalic fetuses, with a vertex presentation).[6]

In Utero Shunting Procedures

The use of this kind of techniques has been discussed during the last years, after its failure during the 1980s, and at the present time it has no indications, until more studies assess its therapeutic benefit.

It seems rational to try to prevent the progressive damage by using a ventricular shunting drainage, but the efficacy and safety of these decompression techniques have not been yet demonstrated.[37]

The placement of shunts in compressive pathologies have been used for almost twenty years, and at the begining, its use in experimental models fetal rhesus monkeys in the case of hydocephalus, had encouraging results.[38] But the experience in human gestations did not find the same results.[39-40]

It has been described a non-slight mortality, nearly 10%, in one large series, but with a very low rate of normal developement on the liveborn infants.[41]

For some authors the reason of this "failure" of shunting procedures was the incorrect diagnosis of the pathologies unknowing the etiology of hydrocephalus,[42] its application is not well selected cases,[42] and the use of not advanced surgical techniques.[43] With the recent improvements in fetal imaging, such as magnetic resonance imaging, and the advances in fetal surgical techniques, and the important role of neurosurgery procedures at the present time, it is possible that, in some years, we could offer the possibility to properly selected fetuses with hydrocephalus to be benefited from an *in utero* intervention.[42]

During the last few years, many studies are emerging to try to reproduce the physiopathology of hydrocephalus, and to try to find the preoperative predictors of success in the shunting procedures.[44-46]

For some authors, there is only a small group of fetuses with hydrocephalus diagnosticated that might benefit from prenatal shunt placement; the prerequisites are not still well defined, but would be fetuses with a gestational age between 24 and 32 weeks, with a progresive hydrocephalus of non-infectious origin and with normal caryotype.[47,48]

At this moment, the value of this shunt procedure in the management of fetal hydrcocephalus has to be disscussed, and further clinical investigation is necesary to assess its usefulness, potential benefits and potential harms.

REFERENCES

1. Vintzileos A, Ingardia CH, Nochimson D. Congenital hydrocephalus: a review and protocol for perinatal management. Obstet Gynecol 1983:62:539.
2. Drugan A, Krause B, Canady A, et al. The natural history of prenatally-diagnosed ventriculomegaly. JAMA 1989; 261:1785-8.
3. Chervenak FA, Berkowitz RL, Romero R, et al. The diagnosis of fetal hydocephalus. Am J Obstet Gynecol 1983;147:703-16.
4. Jouet M. The role of genetics in understanding hydrocephalus and spina bifida. An update. Eur J Pediatr Surg 1996;6:35-6.
5. Zlotogora J, Sagi M, Cohen T. Familiar hydrocephalus of prenatal onset. Am J Med Genet 1994;49:202-4.
6. Chervenak FA, Berkowitz RL, Tortora M, Hobbins JC. The manegement of fetal hydrocephalus. Am J Obstet Gynecol 1985;151:933-42.
7. Hungstschlager M, Mittermayer C, Prusa AR, et al. Prenatal diagnosis of a de novo inversion of chromosome 2 p21q11. Arch Gynecol Obstet 2003: 268:230-2.
8. Morava E, Bartsch O, Czaco M, et al. Small inherited terminal duplication of 7q with hydrocephalus, cleft palate, joint contractures, and severe hypotonia. Clin Dysmorphol 2003;12:123-7.
9. Urban M, Bommer C, Tennstedt C, et al. Ring chromosome 6 in three fetuses: case reports, literature review, and implications for prenatal diagnosis. Am J Med Genet 2002;108:97-104.
10. Hamada H, Watanabe H, Sugimoto M, et al. Autosomal recessive hydrocephalus due to congenital stenosis of the aqueduct of Sylvius. Prenatal Diagn 1999;19:1067-9.
11. Koh S, Boles RG. Cerebral aqueductal stenosis as a presentation of deletion 6q25-qter. Clin Genet 1998;53:317-8.
12. Hoppen T, Eis Hubinger Am, Schild RL, et al. Intrauterine herpes simplex virus infection. Klin Pediatr 2001;213:63-8.
13. Seidman DS, Nass D, Mendelson E, et al. Prenatal ultrasonographic diagnosis of fetal hydrocephalus due to infection with parainfluenza virus type 3. Ultrasound Obstet Gynecol 1996;7:52-4.
14. Katz VL, McCoy MC, Kuller JA, Hansen WF. An association between fetal parvovirus B19 infection and fetal anomalies: a report of two cases. Am J Perinatol 1996;13:43-5.
15. Guiffre R, Pastore FS, De Santis S. Connatal fetal hydrocephalus: an acquired pathology? Childs Nerv Syst 1995;11:97-101.
16. Kawehara H, Tahyama J, Ingaki M, Ohno K. Congenital hydrocephalus due to intrauterine HTVL-I infection. Lancet 1990;336:1442.
17. Senat MV, Bernard JP, Delezoide A, et al. Prenatal diagnosis of hydrocephalus—stenosis of the aqueduct of Sylvius by ultrasound in the first trimester of pregnancy. Report of two cases. Prenatal Diagn 2001;21:1129-32.
18. Relkin N, Marmarou A, Klinge P, et al. Diagnosing idiopathic normal-pressure hydrocephalus. Neurosurgery 2005;57:4-16.
19. Mori K, Shimada J, Kurisaka M, et al. Classification of hydrocephalus and outcome of treatment. Brain Dev 1995;17:338-48.
20. Benaceraff B, Birnholz J. The diagnosis of fetal hydrocephalus prior to 22 weeks. J Clin Ultrasound 1987;15:531.
21. Pilu G, Reece A, Goldstein I, et al. Sonographic evaluation of the normal developmental anatomy of the fetal cerebral ventricles: II. The atria. Obstet Gynecol 1989;73:250.
22. Cardoza J, Goldstein R, Filly R. Exclusion of fetal ventriculomegaly with a single measurement: the width of the lateral atrium. Radiology 1988;169:711.

23. Chinn DH, Callen PW, Filly RA. The lateral cerebral ventricle in early second trimester. Radiology 1983;148:529-31.
24. Chervenak FA, Berkowitz RL, Tortora M, et al. Diagnosis of ventriculomegaly before fetal viability. Obstet Gynecol 1984;64:652.
25. Turgut F, Turgut M, Onur E, Baskaya V. In utero MR imaging and management of foetal hydrocephalus and NTDs in the third trimester. J Neuosurg Sci 2001;45:189-92.
26. Teksam M, Ozyer U, McKinney A, et al. Fetal MRI of a severe Dandy-Walker malformation with an enlarged posterior fossa cyst causing severe hydrocephalus. Fetal Diagn Ther 2005;20:524-7.
27. Williamson RA, Weiner CP, Yuh WTC, Abu-Yousef MM. Magnetic resonance imaging of anomalous fetuses. Obstet Gynecol 1989;73:952.
28. Goldstein RB, LaPidus AS, Filly RA, Cardoza J. Mild lateral cerebral ventricular dilatation in utero: clinical significance and prognosis. Radiology 1990;1761:237-42.
29. Twining P, Jaspan T, Zuccollo J. The outcome of fetal ventriculomegaly. Br J Radiol 1994;67793:26-31.
30. Gupta JK, Bryce FC, Lilford RJ. Management of apparently isolated fetal ventriculomegaly. Obstet Gynecol Survey 1994;4910:716-21.
31. Futagi Y, Suzuki Y, Toribe Y, Morimoto K. Neurodevelopmental outcome in children with fetal hydrocephalus. Pediatr Neurol 2002;27:111-6.
32. Nyberg D, Mack L, Hirsh J, et al. Fetal hydrocephalus: sonographic detection and clinical significance of associated anomalies. Radiology 1987,163:187.
33. Beke A, Csabay L, Rigo J Jr, et al. Folow-up studies of newborn-babies with congenital ventriculomegaly. J Perinatal Med 1999;276:495-505.
34. Pilu G, Falco P, Gabrielli S, et al. The clinical significance of fetal isolated cerebral borederline ventriculomegaly: report of 31 cases and review of the literature. Ultrasound Obstet Gynecol 2000;15:265-7.
35. Lipitz S, Yagel S, Malinger G, et al. Outcome of fetuses with isolated borderline unilateral ventriculomegaly diagosed at mid-gestation. Ultrasound Obstet Gynecol 1998;12:23-6.
36. Chasen ST, Chervenak FA, McCullough LB. The role of cephalocentesis in modern obstetrics. Am J Obstet Gynecol 2001;185:734-6.
37. Glick PL, Harrison MR, Halks-Miller M, et al. Correction of congenital hydrocephalus in utero II: efficacy of in utero shunting. Journal of Pediatric Surgery 1984;19:870-81.
38. Michejda M, hodgen GD: In utero diagnosis and treatment of non-human primate fetal skeletal anomalies. I. Hydrocephalus. JAMA 246:1093, 1981.
39. Clewell WH, Johnson ML, Meier PR, et al. A surgical approach to the treatment of fetal hydrocephalus. N Engl J Med 1982;306:1320.
40. Holzgreve W, Evans MI. Nonvascular needle and shunt placements for fetal therapy. West J Med 1993;159:333-40.
41. Manning FA, Harrison MR, Rodeck C, et al. Catheter shunts for fetal hydronephrosis and hydrocephalus. N Engl J Med 1986;315:336.
42. von Koch CS, Gupta N, Sutton LN, Sun PP. In utero surgery for hydrocephalus. Childs Nerv Syst 2003:197-8:574-86.
43. Oi S. Diagnosis, outcome, and management of fetal abnormalities: fetal hydrocephalus. Childs Nerv Syst 2003;193:508-16.
44. Babapour B, Oi S, Boozari B, et al. Fetal hydrocephalus, intrauterine diagnosis and therapy considerations: an experimentall rat model. Childs Nerv Syst 2005;21:365-71.
45. De Keersmaecker B, Vloeberghs M, Ville Y. Fetal hydrocephalus and intrauterine cerebral ventriculoscopy: an animal model. Fetal Diagn Ther 2005;20:445-9.
46. Penn RD, Lee MC, Linninger AA, et al. Pressure gradients in the brain in an experimental model of hydrocephalus. J Neurosurg. 2005;102:1069-75.
47. Cavalheiro S, Moron AF, Zymberg ST, Dastoli P. Fetal hydocephalus-prenatal treatment. Childs Nev Syst 2003;197-8:561-73.
48. Davis GH. Fetal hydrocephalus. Clin Perinatol 2003;303:531-9.

CHAPTER 13

Amniocentesis

M Theodora, S Mesogitis, AJ Antsaklis

HISTORY

Amniocentesis is the oldest invasive procedure for prenatal diagnosis. It was first used toward the end of the 19th century for evacuative paracentesis in a pregnancy that involves hydramnion.[1] At the beginning of the 1950s it was used to determine the amniotic composition in cases of rhesus isoimmunization.[2] However, for diagnostic reasons amniocentesis was used in the '50s, as a method for sex determination by the identification of Barr bodies in the noncultured amniocytes.[3] About ten years later the karyotype of the embryo was determined through an amniotic fluid cell culture.[4] Since then, amniocentesis has been established as a basic invasive method for the prenatal diagnosis of various problems found in the fetus, such as karyotype examination, examination for metabolic or enzymatic diseases, examination of the hemolytic disease gravity, examination of pneumonic maturity, examination for endometrial infections, the infusion of various drugs into the amniotic cavity, determining the composition of the amniotic fluid, and finally, for evacuation of hydramnion.

INDICATIONS

Amniocentesis is used for both prenatal diagnosis and fetal therapy.

Chromosome and DNA Analysis

Examination of the number and structure of fetal chromosomes (fetal karyotyping) is the main indication for amniocentesis and it is offered to the women in cases when the risk for fetal aneuploidies is high such as advanced maternal age (traditionally ≥ 35 years), previous fetal aneuploidy, parental balanced translocation, positive screening test in the first or second trimester, identification of aneuploidy markers in genetic sonogram, etc. Another indication is an ambiguous result from a previous test such as mosaic karyotype obtained by the CVS. Fetal karyotype is examined either in cultured cells or with PCR technology. The result of the latter technique however should always be confirmed with culture.

Fluorescent labeled *in situ* hybridization (FISH) allows for DNA study, with direct probing and therefore the diagnosis of fetuses with gene diseases such as hemophilia, β-thalassemia, cystic fibrosis, etc.

Fetal Infection

Diagnosis of fetal infection from toxoplasmosis, CMV, etc, in cases of maternal seroconversion is possible by examination of amniotic fluid with PCR based technologies.

Lung Maturity

Fetal lung maturity can be assessed indirectly using both qualitative and quantitative characteristics of amniotic fluid. Pulmonary maturity can be assessed by the measurement of lecithin-sphingomyelin ratio or the concentration of phosphatidyl glycerol in amniotic fluid. Similarly, the detection of lamellar bodies and the study of other characteristics of the amniotic fluid test may give information about lung maturity. However, the improvement in neonatal care and the accurate confirmation of gestational age with ultrasound early in pregnancy have diminished the need for examination of amniotic fluid and thus amniocentesis in order to confirm lung maturity.

Chorioamnionitis

Premature rupture of the membranes (RPOM) and preterm labor has been associated with amniotic fluid bacterial colonization by various series.[5] Thus amniocentesis and Gram's stain, microscopy and culture of the amniotic fluid have been advocated in cases of premature rapture of membranes or premature labor. Researchers who advocate for amniocentesis state that early diagnosis and management is possible and may result in better perinatal outcome. However, spontaneous labor within 24 hours after rapture is very common and thus there are no data that can support amniocentesis as a clinical standard in cases of PROM.

Biochemistry

Amniotic fluid collection and estimation of enzymes' level were used in order to diagnose metabolic diseases and other conditions such as cystic fibrosis or congenital adrenal hyperplasia before DNA techniques were applied. Nowadays, this practice has been replaced by the most accurate detection of gene mutation responsible for the disease in fetal cells collected by amniocentesis or chorionic villus sampling.

Another indication of amniocentesis that has been abandoned is the evaluation of fetal hemolytic anemia in cases of rhesus alloimunization. Amniocentesis and amniotic fluid spectrophotometry are not preformed since middle cerebral artery (MCA) Doppler velocimetry is being used as a routine test for evaluation of hemolysis and fetal anemia.

Obstetric Cholestasis

Amniocentesis is used in obstetric cholostastis in order to diagnose meconium-stained amniotic fluid which is common complication of this pregnancy-related disorder and related to intrauterine fetal demise. However, improvements both in understanding the pathophysiology of the disease and in means of management of these cases have led to decreased need for amniocentesis with this indication.

Fetal Therapy

Amniocentesis is used for uterine decompression in case of hydramnios and twin to twin transfusion syndrome in monochorionic twin. Amnioinfusion has been also used in cases of severe oligohydramnios but research is needed in order to define both the indications and the outcome of such an intervention. Finally, thyroxine has been injected into amniotic fluid to treat goitrous hypothyroidism of the fetus.

TECHNIQUE

Amniocentesis for prenatal diagnosis of genetic diseases of the fetus is traditionally carried out between 15 and 18 weeks of gestation when the fundus of the uterus is easily accessible. Additionally, in this gestation age, the volume of amniotic fluid is 150 to 200 ml, which permits the removal of 15 to 20 ml of amniotic fluid which is adequate for this test without creating problems whatsoever. In addition, at this gestation stage, the relationship between the viable and non-viable cells of the amniotic fluid is the best possible one in order to have results. For all the above reasons, amniocentesis should be carried out at this time.[6] Early amniocentesis (between 11 and 14 weeks) has been associated with increases risk of fetal malformations mainly clubfeet and has been abandoned.

In any case, before amniocentesis is preformed, a detailed ultrasound examination must be done in order to determine the number of fetuses, gestation age, cardiac function, possible abnormal formation, amniotic fluid quantity, position of the placenta, existence of fibromas in the uterus, existence of tumor adnexas, and finally, possible cervical inadequacy. When this ultrasound examination has been completed, the entry site of the needle into the amniotic cavity is determined.[7, 8] Preferred pockets are located away from the fetal face. Sites that must also be determined and avoided as much as possible during amniocentesis is the umbilical cord and—depending on its position—the placenta. However, none of these is absolutely necessary to obtain amniotic fluid safely. The skin around the entry site of the needle is carefully cleaned with an antiseptic solution. A disposable 22 G spinal needle (Figure 13.1) is carefully guided into the amniotic cavity while under continuous ultrasound monitoring and when it finally enters the corresponding area, the inner needle is removed and a syringe is attached to the needle hub. If freely flowing fluid is not obtained, the needle is then repositioned. Failure to aspirate amniotic fluid is most commonly due to membrane testing. When this occurs, the needle appears inside the amniotic cavity, but the needle tip has not actually penetrated the amniotic sac. This usually occurs when an early amniocentesis is carried out, when the amnion and the chorion have not yet fused. In this case, it is recommended that the inner needle is replaced and the needle's entry point to the amniotic cavity is carefully changed so as to avoid injuring the fetus or the umbilical cord. Another reason for failing to take a sample of amniotic fluid is when the fetal membranes plug up the opening of the needle, due to the negative pressure that is exerted here. If this occurs, we then slightly change the needle site without exerting negative pressure. The first 1 to 2 cc of amniotic fluid that is aspirated is discarded because in theory it may contain some of the mother's cells and thus give us inaccurate prenatal results. An amount of approximately 20 cc amniotic fluid is considered to be enough for the results we require, when amniocentesis is carried out between the 15th and 20th weeks of gestation. An ultrasound examination is performed after the amniocentesis has been completed to document fetal cardiac activity and to look for evidence of bleeding into the amniotic cavity. The pregnant woman is then advised to rest and avoid intercourse for several days and informed as to possible complications that may occur, such as persistent uterine cramping, fever, bleeding or leakage of the amniotic fluid, and for which she must report timely.

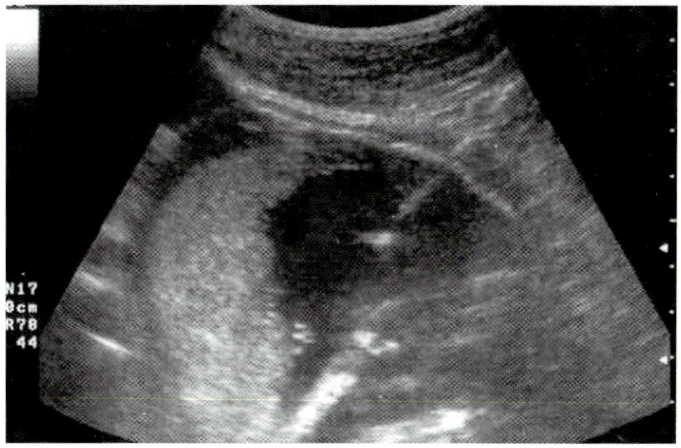

Figure 13.1: Amniocentesis in singleton. Note that the whole length and the tip of the needle can be identified then the procedure is done under ultrasound guidance

COMPLICATIONS

Amniocentesis is an interventional procedure and since fetomaternal unit is injured, a number of complications are related to it. Maternal complications are rare and include perforation of the intra-abdominal viscera with subsequent intra-abdominal infection, bleeding, blood group sensitization and uterine contractions.[9] On the other hand fetal complications are more of a concern and include fetal loss, needle puncture injuries, placental abruption, preterm labor, injury due to withdrawal of amniotic fluid (e.g. amniotic bands) and rupture of the membranes. Amniocentesis may also cause intra-amniotic infections through the introduction of micro-organisms into the amniotic cavity via the needle that is used to perform it and this may therefore lead to the abortion or death of the fetus. In order to eliminate the possibility of an infectious condition, rules of aseptic procedures which apply in all surgical procedures case must be applied here, such as the aseptic cleaning of the skin and using aseptic gloves and needles. However, endometrial infections are not always related to amniocentesis, but may pre-exist before the prenatal intervention.[10, 11]

Fetal Loss

Fetal loss is the major risk of second trimester genetic amniocentesis. When amniocentesis was first introduced in the clinical practice the risk of miscarriage related to the procedure was not clear mainly because there was lack of ultrasound guidance and lack of determination of fetal viability before the procedure. Since fetal miscarriage does not occur only when amniocentesis is performed it is essential to take into consideration the background loss rate which is associated with the gestation age, parity and any other underlying risk factors such as pathological conditions of the mother (e.g. uncontrolled diabetes mellitus, severe hypertension induced by lupus, etc) and the fetus (e.g. structural anomalies, chromosomal abnormalities, etc) as well. Gestational age at the procedure is an important determinant of the observed fetal loss rate, since the earlier the pregnancy the greater is the preprocedure risk of miscarriage.

The safety of amniocentesis has been evaluated by several series from single centres and a number of multicentric studies. The difficulties in evaluating of procedure related loss risk have been shown by the controversial results of these studies.

In 1976 the National Institute of Child Health and Human Development (NICHD) conducted a case-control/cohort study to evaluate the safety and accuracy of second trimester amniocentesis for prenatal diagnosis and reported that the study group who underwent amniocentesis had a 3.5% total loss rate while the controls had 3.2%.[9] The study group also concluded that the loss risk was unrelated to previous miscarriage, volume of aspirated fluid or number of attempts. In the same year, the Canadian Collaborative Study reported a loss rate 3.2% but there were no controls.[12] In this study, an increased risk of loss was reported in cases of failed attempts and large bore needles (>19). The third collaborative case control study was conducted by the British Working Party on Amniocentesis in 1978[13] and the writers reported a loss rate of 1.5% related to amniocentesis. They reported a 2.4% fetal loss rate <28 weeks in study group and I.2% in controls. This study however was strongly criticized mainly on the selection of control individuals who we recruited in the study later in gestation and on the replacement of some of the matched controls who had aborted.

The only randomized trial for the estimation of miscarriage risk related to amniocentesis was done in Denmark in 1986.[14] This study randomized 4,606 low-risk women aged 24 to 35 years to have or not to have an amniocentesis, which was carried out using a 20-gauge needle under realtime ultrasound guidance. Most procedures were performed at between 16 and 18 weeks of gestation. The amniocentesis group had a loss rate which exceeded the control group by 1% (1.7% and 0.7% respectively), a figure which has often been quoted in counseling. More than half of the procedures were performed by one operator and the rest by four less experienced operators. The placenta was avoided whenever possible but was perforated in 15% of cases and the study indicated that perforation of the placental was associated with a relative risk of 2.6% for miscarriage.

Since then a lot of studies reported amniocentesis related fetal loss rate between 0.2 and 0.9%.

In 2001, JW Seeds preformed a systematic review of 29 controlled and uncontrolled studies with a total of 68,119 amniocenteses[15] and he concluded that amniocentesis with concurrent ultrasound guidance in controlled studies appears to be associated with a procedure-related rate of excess pregnancy loss of 0.6% (95% CI, 0.31, 0.90) (Table 13.1). The use of concurrent ultrasound guidance appears to reduce the number of punctures and the incidence of bloody fluid and eliminates the direct fetal needle trauma. Finally, the review did not substantiate an increased

Table 13.1: Fetal loss rate in review*

Ultrasound use	*Preamniocentesis scan*	*Concurrent ultrasound guidance*	*P value*
All studies			
Losses (n/N)			
Amniocentesis	714/33975 (2.1%)	478/34144 (1.40%)	<0.0001
Control subjects	88/6457 (1.4%)	130/12097 (1.08%)	NS
Difference (%)	0.74	0.33	
P value	<0.0001	<0.0007	
95% CI for difference	0.37, 1.1	0.09, 0.56	
Only controlled studies			
Losses (n/N)			
Amniocentesis	170/8607 (2.0%)	191/11372 (1.68%)	NS
Control subjects	88/6457 (1.4%)	130/12097 (1.08%)	NS
P value	0.0042	<0.0001	
Odds ratio	1.46	1.57	
Difference (%)	0.6	0.6	
95% CI for difference	0.19, 1.03	0.31, 0.9	

*From John W. Seeds. Diagnostic mid trimester amniocentesis: How safe? Am J Obstet & Gynec 2004;191: 608-16

rate of pregnancy loss if placental puncture is required.

In 2006, another trial was published in order to quantify the contemporary procedure-related loss rate after midtrimester amniocentesis using a database generated from patients who were recruited to the First and Second Trimester Evaluation of Risk for Aneuploidy (FASTER) trial.[16] A total of 35,003 unselected patients from the general population with viable singleton pregnancies were enrolled in this trial and 3,096 of them underwent midtrimester amniocentesis. The total spontaneous fetal loss rate less than 24 weeks of gestation in the study group was 1.0% and was not statistically different from the background 0.94% rate seen in the control group (P_.74, 95% confidence interval –0.26%, 0.49%). The researched stated that the odds of pregnancy loss were actually lower in patients who underwent amniocentesis because of advanced maternal age or screen positive results compared with those who did not and they concluded that this is likely due to the fact that spontaneous pregnancy loss is so strongly associated with aneuploidy, and patients who have an amniocentesis would presumably terminate aneuploid fetuses in most cases before a spontaneous loss could occur. They stated that it is not surprising that patients in these categories who elected not to undergo amniocentesis, had a higher rate of spontaneous loss because they were carrying a higher proportion of aneuploid fetuses.

Recently, F Mujezinovic and Z Alfirevic compiled a systematic review of complications related to genetic amniocentesis and chorionic villus sampling (CVS) to provide benchmark data for counseling and performance assessment of individual operators.[17] Twenty-nine articles of amniocentesis were included and pooled pregnancy loss within 14 days was 0.6% (95% confidence interval [CI] 0.5– 0.7), rising to 0.9% (95% CI 0.6 –1.3) for pregnancy loss before 24 weeks and 1.9% (95% CI 1.4 –2.5) for total pregnancy loss (Table 13.2). However, the writers noted that since most of the reviewed studies do not take into account the background risk, and therefore, do not address the issue of added, procedure-related risk, these figures may be useful only for counseling purposes in a broad sense. The writers identified five studies which have included control groups in order to quantify the background risk. Overall, these studies reported higher pregnancy losses compared with uncontrolled case series and the pooled results showed a relative increase of 25% for total pregnancy loss after amniocentesis and 46% for pregnancy losses

Table 13.2: Pregnancy loss after amniocentesis

Type of pregnancy loss	*Combined total (n/N)*	*Combined proportion (%)*	*95% CI*
Less than 20 weeks of pregnancy	22/2.133	1.1	0.7-1.5
More than 20 weeks of pregnancy	17/1,775	0.9	0.5–1.4
Less than 24 weeks of pregnancy	122/14,057	0.9	0.6-1.3
More than 24 weeks of pregnancy	57/4,195	1.0	0.5–1.8
Less than 28 weeks of pregnancy	283/14,915	1.7	1.3–2.2
More than 28 weeks of pregnancy	134/14,596	0.9	0.7.7–1.2
Less than 14 days after AC	102/17,047	0.6	0.5–0.7
Less than 30 days after AC 85/10,727 0.8 0.4–1.2	85/10,727	0.8	0.4–1.2
Less than 60 days after AC	66/9,406	0.7	0.5–0.9
Total pregnancy loss	627/49,413	1.9	1.4–2.5
Multiple insertions	226/12,142	2.0	0.9–3.6
Bloody or discolored tap	468/10,908	4.1	1.1–8.7

CI, confidence interval; AC, amniocentesis.

F Mujezinovic, Z Alfirevic. Procedure-related complications of amniocentesis and chorionic villous sampling: a systematic review. Obstet Gynecol 2007;110:687-94

before 24 or 28 weeks' gestation. However, the results for the later were quite heterogeneous, resulting in very wide, statistically no significant confidence intervals. The absolute risk difference between cases and controls was quite similar, showing that second trimester pregnancy loss and total fetal loss after an amniocentesis increase by approximately 0.6%. The reviewers noted that although the risks of pregnancy loss are relatively low, lack of adequate controls tends to underestimate the true added risk of prenatal invasive procedures.

Midtrimester amniocentesis does not appear to further increase the already increased risk for second-trimester spontaneous abortion in pregnant women with myomas in uterus.[18]

Preterm Delivery

The association of second trimester and amniocentesis and delivery before 37 weeks was evaluated by a case control study in 2003 by the EUROPOP Group.[19] Three thousand and ninety-one preterm births and 5,298 controls randomly selected from singleton births born at term during 1994 to 1997 were analyzed. An increased risk of preterm delivery was found in women having second trimester genetic amniocentesis after taking account of other risk factors and confounding variables (odds ratios (OR) ¼ 1:59, 95% confidence intervals (95%CI): 1.31–1.92). The association was statistically significant and similar for spontaneous preterm delivery and induced preterm delivery. Since the data are limited, further research on the etiologic role of this prenatal diagnostic technique is needed.

Fetal Trauma

The risk of direct fetal needle injury often is presumed to be reduced with the use of simultaneous ultrasound guidance, but several case reports document or attribute cases of fetal injury to the amniocentesis needle, despite the use of simultaneous guidance for the procedure.[15] Although several case reports document or attribute cases of fetal injury to the amniocentesis needle, despite the use of simultaneous guidance for the procedure,[20-22] the attribution has been generally by association only and not on the basis of direct evidence.[21,23-31]

Alloimmunization

Feto-maternal hemorrhage occurs in approximately 50% of all women[32] and during amniocentesis in one out of six women.[33] The attributed risk is 1% greater than the background risk of 1.5%.[34] As for preventing the rhesus sensitization of the mother and when the husband is rhesus positive, every rhesus negative mother must be given 300 μg anti-D IgG immediately after amniocentesis, provided of course the indirect Coombs' is negative.[35,36]

Other means to minimize the risk is the use of small gauge needles and to avoid transplacental approach.[36]

Respiratory Distress

A significant although small increase of neonatal respiratory distress was noted in some studies but not to others.[9,37] This complication has been attributed to chronic oligohydramnios which might follow amniocentesis.

Orthopedic Abnormalities

The British collaboration study[13] implied that amniocentesis is associated with talipes equinovarus, congenital dislocation and subluxation of the hip. This trend was not confirmed by other studies. This complication has been attributed to chronic oligohydramnios which might follow amniocentesis.

Transmission of Viral Diseases

Before antiretroviral therapy use mother-to-child HIV infection considered as an relative contraindication for amniocentesis and invasive prenatal procedures. Since maternal antiretroviral therapy has been used, amniotic fluid virus load is usually undetectable even if the virus was detectable in maternal blood samples. This finding raises the possibility to perform amniocentesis, when it is indicated, to provide the mother with an adequate antiretroviral treatment.[38]

Leakage of Amniotic Fluid and Vaginal Bleeding

Uterine contractions and vaginal spotting are quite common (2 to 3%) after amniocentesis however they are almost always transient and self limited. Leakage of amniotic fluid occurs in 1% of women who underwent second trimester amniocentesis. It is usually small amount and the outcome is normal in 90% of the patients who experienced fluid leakage.[39]

SPECIAL CIRCUMSTANCES

Discolored Amniotic Fluid

The presence of blood in the amniotic fluid occurs in a very small number of cases. It is usually derived from the mother and under no circumstances does it affect the development or multiplication of the cells. However, the presence of blood in the amniotic fluid is related to the increased possibility that the outcome of the pregnancy will not be good. Thus the percentage of fetal losses in these cases reaches 33% of all cases.[40-42] If at the same time, the bloody or discolored amniotic fluid is accompanied by increased levels of α-fetal protein (AFP), then in almost all instances the prenatal results will not be good.

Amniocentesis in the Presence of Bleeding

The fetal loss following amniocentesis in women who have had bleeding before the procedure is probably increased. Antsaklis et al found an excess loss rata of 0.6% in women who had experienced bleeding before amniocentesis.[43]

History of bleeding is not a contraindication for the procedure but patients should be counseled about the risks.

Amniocentesis in Multiple Gestations

Amniocentesis has been recognized as a relatively safe procedure for prenatal diagnosis in singletons. Amniocentesis can be safely preformed on twins or higher multiple gestations as long as the sacs have been defined through ultrasound examination. The amniocentesis technique in multiple gestations is different to that used in a single gestation and therefore should be referred to experienced centres. The number of fetuses, their positions, the number of gestation sacs and placentas, the gender, the age and the degree of development of each fetus and finally the fetal anatomy, are all important and necessary elements of the ultrasound examination that precedes amniocentesis. An important element before amniocentesis is determining the position of each fetus, which is achieved by mapping the site of the placenta that is feeding the specific fetus with blood and nutritional substances, because the position of the placenta changes very little over time while the position of the fetus never remains stable. Consequently, in the case where after amniocentesis the problem of selective feticide arises due to a harmful result, we must know which is the specific fetus in question and its reference point so that we can pinpoint it, and this is nothing more than determining the position of the placenta, as determined by the mapping that was carried out before amniocentesis.

Three different methods for performing amniocentesis in twin gestations have been described.[44-46] In the first and most common technique method, amniocentesis is performed on each gestation sac separately and sequentially (Figures 13.2 and 13.3). Misdiagnosis is the main disadvantage of this method which is reported up to 3.5% of samples and in order to reduce the possibility of sapling one of the sacs twice some have suggested the use of methylene blue or other dye as a marker.[46-49] However the high-resolution ultrasound equipment available today, as well as the experience gained throughout the years, makes instillation of dye unnecessary. This method could be used in case that is difficult to define the septum and for higher-order pregnancies. Another is the single needle technique. During this technique the septum is identified, and the needle is inserted into the first sac close to the septum. After the aspiration of amniotic fluid, the needle is inserted through the septum into the second sac. In the third method is the insertion of two different needles with simultaneous ultrasound visualization of both sides of the dividing membranes.

The percentage of total fetal loss, as expressed by spontaneous abortions, stillbirths and neonatal deaths, is approximately 10.8%, a percentage that is almost the same as the statistical miscarriage percentage that is observed in every twin gestation after the 17th week of gestation.[42,50] According to other studies, the percentage of fetal losses up to the 28th week of gestation in twin gestations after amniocentesis ranges from 3.57% to 3.78% versus 0.6% for single gestations.[21,22] In other words, this means that the comparatively increased fetal losses observed in twin gestations versus single gestations after amniocentesis is not due to amniocentesis, but rather to the normally increased statistical percentage for abortions seen in twin gestations. In a recent review by Weisz and Rodeck[51] the pooled data regarding the pregnancy loss rate after amniocentesis are comparable to these background loss rates for twin pregnancies (Table 13.3).

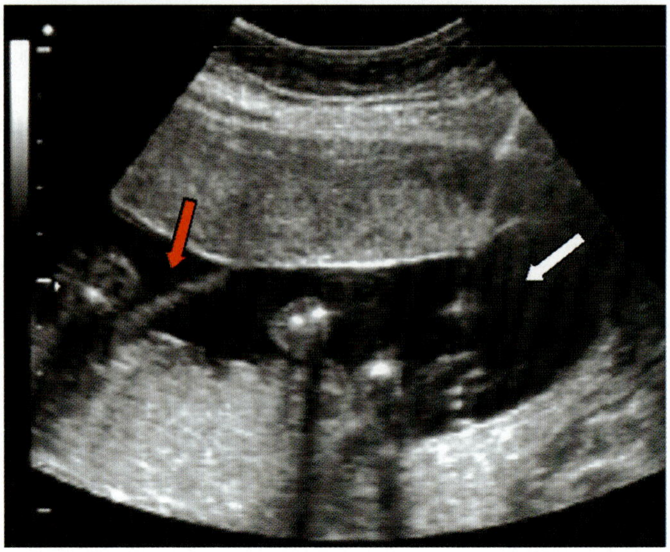

Figure 13.2: Amniocentesis in twin gestation which is performed on each gestation sac separately and sequentially (white arrow tip of the needle in the one sac, red arrow septum)

Finally, amniocentesis post multifetal pregnancy reduction MFPR does not seem to significantly increase the rate of fetal loss. But, one group has shown that amniocentesis post-MFPR was significantly associated with increased risk of preterm delivery at 25 to 28 weeks.[52]

Early Amniocentesis

Early amniocentesis was thought as an alternative proposal for early prenatal diagnosis in centres in which CVS was not offered. It was suggested to be performed between the 12th and 15th gestation weeks. The technique used for performing early amniocentesis is similar to that used in classical amniocentesis and the amount of amniotic fluid that is removed is equal in ml to the gestation weeks.[53] Failure or difficulty in taking out the amniotic fluid was due to the tenting of the membrane caused by

Table 13.3: FLR in twin pregnancies following amniocentesis

References	*No. of twin pregnancies*	*Fetal loss (%) <20 w gestat*	*Total fetal loss (%)*	*Control group (%)*	*Comments*
Anderson et al 1991	339	——	3.57	—	Compared to 0.6% miscarriage
Beekhuis et al 1992	63	——	4.0	——	A study evaluating maternal Hb as marking dye
Pruggmayer et al 1991	529	3.7	8.7	——	
Ghidini et al 1993	101	——	3.5	3.2	Control group of twins without amniocentesis
Wapner et al 1993	81	——	9.3	——	Compared to 3.9% fetal loss rate after CVS
Tabsh and Theroux, 1995	53	——	9.4	——	All amniocentesis post-MFPR
Sebire et al 1996	176	2.55	4.0	——	Single needle technique. Total loss attributed to procedure: 2.8%
McLean et al 1998 —	79	5.6	——	——	All amniocentesis post-MFPR
Zoppini et al 1993	50	2	——	——	
Horger et al 2001	71	——	7.6	——	
Yukobowich et al 2001	476	2.73	7.73	0.63	Two control groups. Twins, without amniocentesis and singletons
Antsaklis et al 2002	347	347	——	8.77	——

From B Weisz, CH Rodeck. Invasive diagnostic procedures in twin pregnancies (review). Prenat Diagn 2005; 25: 751-8.

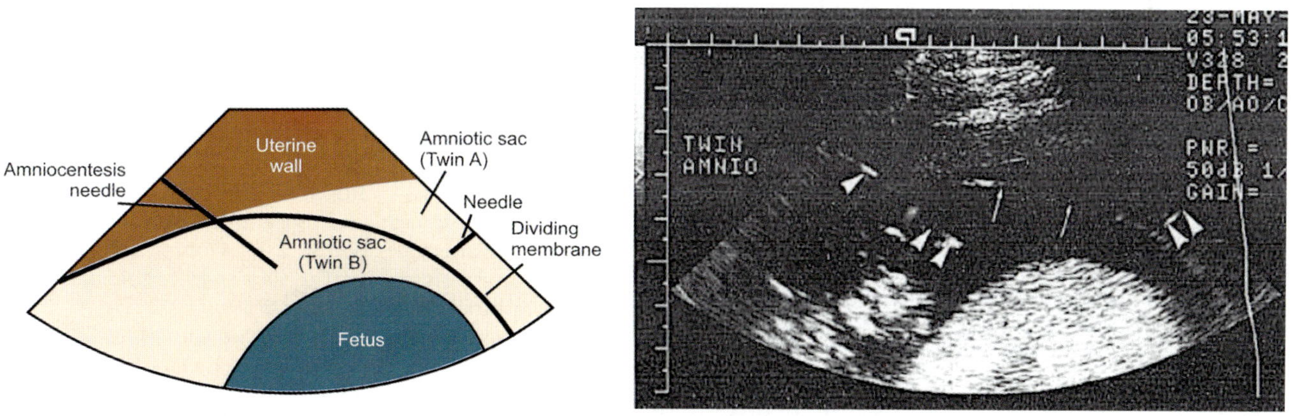

Figure 13.3: Double needle technique (from Bahado-Singh R, Schmitt R, Hobbins JC New technique for genetic amniocentesis in twins. Obstet Gynecol 1992;79:304)

the needle.[54] Since it was performed quite early, it was though that could give the opportunity to examine the karyotype of the fetus, determine the α-fetoprotein (AFP) and acetylcholinesterase for the early detection of those cases that show increased risk for nervous system abnormalities[55-57] with the same safety as mid-trimester amniocentesis. These expectations were confirmed by observational studies although definite conclusions could not be drown because of the small numbers.[58]

The safety of early amniocentesis was not completely clear until the Canadian trial. In two randomized studies[59,60] fetal loss rate was significantly higher for early amniocentesis when compared with TA-CVS. In another randomized trial[61] which compared first-trimester and mid-trimester amniocentesis fetal losses were more frequently observed after first-trimester than after mid-trimester amniocentesis. Additionally early amniocentesis had a significantly higher rate of amniotic fluid leakage than TA-CVS and mid-trimester amniocentesis.

Excessive risk for talipes equinovarus has been uniformly observed in all early amniocentesis studies, with an even greater likelihood with physician confirmation of amniotic fluid leakage (17.7% versus 0.5%).[59] Talipes can occur without apparent leakage of amniotic fluid, which likely results from a reduced amniotic fluid volume via transfer of amniotic fluid to the extraembryonic celomic space. TA-CVS did not have any affect on malformation rate. The Canadian study therefore indicated that early amniocentesis should be performed only if there is no alternative.

In 2005 Z Alfirevic et al conducted a systematic review[62] for the Cochrane collaboration and the pooled total pregnancy loss after early amniocentesis was 7.6% compared to 5.9% after mid-trimester amniocentesis. Similarly, the number of talipes equinovarus was higher in cases of early amniocentesis (1.3% versus 0.09%). In the same review combined total loss of pregnancy after early amniocentesis was 6.3% compared to 5% after CVS.

It is therefore justified to say that early amniocentesis should be performed only in extenuating circumstances, especially since transabdominal CVS has undoubtedly been proved as a safe and more effective alternative.

REFERENCES

1. Von Schatz F. Gine besondere art von einseitiger polyhydramnie mit anderseitiger oligohydramnie bie eineiigen zwillingen. Arch Gynaecol 1882;19:329.
2. Beris DCA. Composition of liquor amnii in haemolytic disease of newborn. 1950;Lancet 2:443.
3. Fuchs F, Riis P. Antenatal sex determination. Nature 1956;177:330.
4. Steele MW, Breg WR. Chromosome analysis of human amniotic fluid cells. Lancet 1966; 1:383.
5. Dodson MG, Forrtunat SJ. Microorganisms and premature labor. J Reprod Medicine 1988; 33: 87-96.
6. Emery AEH. Antenatal diagnosis of genetic disease. Modern Trends Hum Genet 1970; 1:267.
7. Jeanty P, Rodesch F, Romero R, et al. How to improve your amniocentesis technique. Am J Obstet Gynecol 1983; 146:593.
8. Romero R, Jeanty P, Reece EA, et al. Sonographically monitored amniocentesis to decrease intraperative complication. Obstet Gynecol 1985; 65:426.
9. NICHD National Registry for amniocentesis study group: Mid trimester amniocentesis for prenatal diagnosis: safety and accuracy. J Am Med Assoc 1976;236:1471.
10. Cassell GH, Davis RO, Waiter KB, et al. Isolation of *Mycoplasma hominis* and *Ureaplasma urealyticum* from amniotic fluid at 16-20 weeks of gestation: potential effect on outcome of pregnancy. Sex Transm Dis 1983;10:294.
11. Gray DJ, Robinson H, Malone J, et al. Adverse outcome in pregnancy following amniotic fluid isolation of ureaplasma urealyticum. Prenat Diagn 1992;12:111-7.
12. Simpson NE, Dallaire L, Miller JR, et al Prenatal diagnosis of genetic disease in Canada: report of a collaborative study. Canadian Medical Association Journal 1976:115; 739-48.
13. Medical Research Council. An assessment of the hazards of amniocentesis. Br J Obstetr Gynecol 1978; 85:1-41(sup 2).
14. Tabor A, Philip J, Madsen M, Bang J, Obel EB, Norgaard-Pedersen B. Randomised controlled trial of genetic amniocentesis in 4606 low-risk women. Lancet 1986;1:1287-93.
15. John W Seeds. Diagnostic mid trimester amniocentesis: How safe? Am J Obstet& Gynec 2004;191: 608-16.
16. FASTER Trial Research Consortium. Pregnancy loss rates after midtrimester amniocentesis. Obstet and Gynec 2006;108(5):1067-72.
17. F Mujezinovic, Z Alfirevic. Procedure-related complications of amniocentesis and chorionic villous sampling: a systematic review. Obstet Gynecol 2007;110:687-94.
18. E Salvador, J Bienstock, KJ Blakemore, E Pressman. Leiomyomata uteri, genetic amniocentesis, and the risk of second-trimester spontaneous abortion. Am J Obstet Gynecol 2002;186:913-5.
19. E Medda, S Donati, A Spinelli, GC Di Renzo EUROPOP Group. Genetic amniocentesis: a risk factor for preterm delivery? Eu J Obstetr and Gynecol Reprod Biol 2003;110: 153-8.
20. Williamson RA, Varner MW, Grant SS. Reduction in amniocentesis risks using a real-time needle guide procedure. Obstet Gynecol 1985;65:751-5.
21. Therkelsen AJ, Rehder H. Intestinal atresia caused by second trimester amniocentesis. BJOG 1981;88:559-62.
22. Admoni MM, BenEzra D. Ocular trauma following amniocentesis as the cause of leukocoria. J Pediatr Ophthalmol Strab 1988;25:196-7.
23. Youroukos S, Papadelis F, Matsaniotis N. Porencephalic cysts after amniocentesis. Arch Dis Child 1980;55:814-5.
24. Stock RJ. Fetal death secondary to needle laceration during 2nd trimester amniocentesis : a case report. Prenat Diagn 1982;2:133-7.
25. Bruce S, Duffy JO, Wolf JE. Skin dimpling associated with midtrimester amniocentesis. Pediatr Dermatol 1984;2:140-2.
26. Raimer SS, Raimer BG. Needle puncture scars from midtrimester amniocentesis. Arch Dermatol 1984;120:1360-2.
27. Finegan JK, Quarrington BJ, Hughes HE, Rudd NL, Stevens LJ, Weksberg R, Doran TA. Infant outcome following midtrimester amniocentesis: development and physical status at age six months. BJOG 1985;92:1015-23.
28. BenEzra D, Sela M, Peer J. Bilateral anophthalmia and unilateral microphthalmia in two siblings. Ophthalmologica 1989;198: 140-4.
29. Chong SKF, Levitt GA, Lawson J, Lloyd U, Newman CGH. Subarachnoid cyst with hydrocephalus—a complication of midtrimester amniocentesis. Prenatal Diagn 989;9:677-9.
30. Eller KM, Kuller JA. Porencephaly secondary to fetal trauma during amniocentesis. Obstet Gynecol 1995;85:865-7.
31. Raymond GV. Rare neurologic injury from amniocentesis.

Birth Defects Res Clin Mol Teratol 2003;67:205-6.
32. EM Clayton, WD Feldhaus, FE Whitacre. Fetal erythrocytes in maternal circulation of pregnant women. Obstet Gynecol 1964; 23:915-9.
33. A Tabor, J Bang, B Norgaard-Pedersem. Feto-maternal Haemorrhage associated with genetic amniocentesis: results of a randomized trial. Br J Obstet Gynecol 1987;94:528-35.
34. Murray JC, Karp LE, Williamson RA, Cheng EY, Luth DA. Rh isoimmunization related to amniocentesis. Am Journal of Medical Genetics 1983:16:527-34.
35. American College of Obstetricians and Gynecologists: Prevention of D Isoimmunization. ACOG Tech Bull No 147, 1990.
36. WHO .Prevention of rhesus sensitization. Who Technical Report Series1971; No 468.
37. Hunter AG. Neonatal lung function following mid-trimester amniocentesis. Prenatal Diagnosis 1987;7;433-41.
38. V Maiques, A Garci´a-Tejedor, A Perales, J Co´rdoba, RJ Esteban. HIV detection in amniotic fluid samples. Amniocentesis can be performed in HIV pregnant women? Eur J Obstetr Gynec Reprod Biology 108:137-41.
39. Borgida AF, Mills AA, Feldman Dm, Rodis JF, Ergan JF. Outcome of pregnancies complicated with rupture of membranes after genetic amniocentesis. Am J Obstet Gynecol 2000; 183:937-9.
40. Milunsky A. The of neural tube and other congenital defects. In Milunsky A (Ed): Genetic Disorders and the Fetus. New York, Plenum Press, 1986; p 453.
41. Karpa E, Schiller HS. Meconium staining of amniotic fluid of mid trimester amniocentesis. Obstet Gynecol 1977;50:475.
42. Imaizumi Y, Asaka A, Inouye E. Analysis of multiple birth rates in Japan. Rates of spontaneous and induced termination of pregnancy in twins. Jpn J Hum Genet, 1982;27:235.
43. A Antsaklis, N Papantoniou, A Xygakis, S Mesogitis, E Tzortzis, S Michalas. Genetic amniocentesis in women 20±34 years old: associated risks. Prenat Diagn 2000; 20: 247-50.
44. Elias S, Gerbie AB, Simpson JL, et al. Genetic amniocentesis in twin gestations. Am J Obstet Gynecol 138:169, 198.
45. Bahado-Singh R, Schmitt R, Hobbins JC. New technique for genetic amniocentesis in twins. Obstet Gynecol 1992;79:304.
46. Fribourg S. Safety of intra-amniotic injection of indigo carmine. Am J Obstet Gynecol 1981;140:350.
47. Tabsh KMA, Cramdall B, Lebherz TB, et al. Genetic amniocentesis in twin pregnancy. Obstet Gynecol 1985;65:843.
48. Bovicelli L, Michelacci L, Rizzo N, et al. Genetic amniocentesis in twin pregnancy. Prenat Diagn 1983;3:101.
49. Wolf DA, Scheible FW, Young PE, et al. Genetic amniocentesis in multiple pregnancies. J Clin Ultrasound 1979; 7:208.
50. Ager RP, Oliver RWA. The risk of mid trimester amniocentesis. Lancashire, UK: University of Salford. Monograph, 1986.
51. B Weisz, CH Rodeck. Invasive diagnostic procedures in twin pregnancies (review) Prenat Diagn 2005; 25: 751-8.
52. Antsaklis A, Daskalakis G, Papantoniou N, Mesogitis S, Michalas S. Genetic amniocentesis in multifetal pregnancies reduced to twins compared with nonreduced twin gestations. Fertil Steril 74: 1051-2.
53. Simpson JL, Elias S: Essentials of Prenatal Diagnosis Churchill Livingstone 1993;39.
54. Henry GP, Miller WA. Early amniocentesis. J Reprod Med 1992;37:396.
55. Elejalde BR, de Elejlde MM, Acuna JM, et al. Prospective study of amniocentesis performed between weeks 9 and 16 of gestation: 1st feasibility, risk, complications and use in early genetic prenatal diagnosis. Am J Med Genet, 1990;35:188-96.
56. Penso CA, Sandstrom MM, Garber MF, et al. Early amniocentesis: report of 407 cases with neonatal follow-up. Obstet-Gynecol 1990;76:1032.
57. Jorgensen FS, Bang I, Lind A, et al. Genetic amniocentesis at 7-14 weeks of gestation. Prenat Diagn 1992;12:277.
58. Elias S, Simpson JL. Amniocentesis and fetal blood sampling. In Milunsky A (ed): Genetic Disorders and the Fetus (5th ed). Baltimore and London: The Johns Hopkins University Press; 2004; 66-99.
59. Philip J, Silver RK, Wilson RD, et al. Late first-trimester invasive prenatal diagnosis: results of an international randomized trial. Obstet Gynecol 2004; 103:1164-73.
60. Nicolaides K, Brizot M de L, Patel F, Snijders R. Comparison of chorionic villus sampling and amniocentesis for fetal karyotyping at 10-13 weeks' gestation. Lancet 1994;344:435-9.
61. The Canadian Early and Mid-trimester Amniocentesis Trial (CEMAT) Group. Randomized trial to assess safety and fetal outcome of early and midtrimester amniocentesis. Lancet 1998; 351:242-7.
62. Z Alfirevic, K Sundberg, S Brigham. Amniocetesis and chorionic villus sampling for prenatal diagnosis (Review) the Cochrane Collaboration 2005 (issue 1).
63. B Brambati, L Tului. Chorionic villus sampling and amniocentesis. Curr Opin Obstet Gynecol 17:197-201.

CHAPTER 14

Chorionic Villus Sampling

T Grigoriadis , S Mesogitis, AJ Antsaklis

INTRODUCTION

Chorionic villus sampling is an invasive prenatal diagnostic procedure which was firstly introduced in the early 1980s and subsequently developed over the last 25 years. The distinct characteristic of CVS is the provision of genetic diagnosis in the first trimester of pregnancy. Early diagnosis has multiple individual and clinical advantages over the methods for prenatal diagnosis in later stages of pregnancy. The extensive research on this field has showed a comparable safety profile and reliability with the other methods, making CVS the only established method for prenatal diagnosis in the first trimester.

History of Chorionic Villus Sampling (CVS)

In 1968 Mohr[1] in Scandinavia introduced for the first time the concept of antenatal genetic diagnosis using chorionic villi sampled through the transvaginal-transcervical route. One year later, Hahnemann and Mohr[2,3] attempted to retrieve transcervically trophoblastic tissue under direct monitoring with a 4 mm diameter hysteroscope, but without achieving good results.

In 1973 Kullander and Sandahl[4] used the same technique that was used by previous researchers to take samples of trophoblastic tissue, achieving a 50% success rate. In 1974 Hahnemann[5] described his experience with respect to the taking of samples of trophoblastic tissue through a 2.5 mm diameter hysteroscope, but the results were still disappointing due to significant post-invasive complications.

The first successful prenatal diagnostic use of chorionic villi biopsy was reported in 1975 from the Department of Obstetrics and Gynaecology at the Tietung Hospital in Anshan, China. This team performed blind aspirations using a 3 mm metal cannula on a group of 100 patients, successfully diagnosing the sex of 93 out of 99 embryos.[2] However, other investigators in the United States failed to reproduce these promising results and the idea of first trimester diagnosis was therefore abandoned. At that time, in the late 1970s, amniocentesis was proving to be a safe and reliable procedure gaining popularity among health care practitioners. At the beginning of the 1980s with the advent of improved ultrasound equipment offering realtime sonography and allowing the possibility of the ultrasound guidance of tropoblast sampling, diagnosis during the first trimester become feasible. Kazy et al[3] in 1982, in the USSR reported fetal sexing and enzyme assay on chorion biopsies taken at 6 to 12 weeks' gestation, using either an endoscopic or ultrasound-guided approach. Biopsy forceps were used instead of cannulas. During the same year, Old[8] reported the feasibility of diagnosing β-thalassemia with trophoblastic cells obtained by ultrasound guided transcervical aspiration with a 1.5 mm diameter polyethylene catheter.

In 1983, Brambati et al in Milan demonstrated that with ultrasound guidance, success rate of obtaining chorionic material rose from 75 to 96%.[4,5] Brambati used a 1.5 mm polyethylene tube with a soft stainless steel malleable obturator inserted into the 1 mm internal barrel. This technique has been the basis for the transcervical sampling till our days. In 1984, Smidt-Jensen and Hahnemann[6] in Copenhagen introduced the transabdominal technique with a fine-needle villus aspiration under ultrasound guidance. With less rates of infective complications and re-insertions this procedure has become more popular than the transcervical counterpart in many prenatal diagnostic centers today.

Indications

As the trophoblast is a fetal organ, any examination of this tissue is considered to be also an examination of the fetus. Indications for trophoblastic tissue sampling and subsequent examination for fetal abnormalities are numerous and seen on Table 14.1.

Table 14.1: Indications for chorionic villus sampling

• Chromosomal abnormalities
• Advanced maternal age • High risk after prenatal screening of 1st or 2nd trimester • Previous pregnancy with chromosomal abnormality • Family history of chromosomal rearrangement • Ultrasound marker for chromosomal abnormalities
• Monogenic disorders
• Thalassemia • Duchenne/Becker muscular dystrophy • Hemophilia A/B • Cystic fibrosis • Congenital adrenal hyperplasia • Other monogenic diseases • Paternity testing
• Metabolic disorders
• Mucopolysaccharidoses • Lipidoses • Amino acid disorders • Carbohydrate metabolism disorders

Contraindications

There are only a few contraindications for CVS. Women with hepatitis B or C, should avoid invasive procedures, although the few studies that have been published so far did not show a significantly increased risk of transmission. A review article[7] showed that the overall risk is low, suggesting also that the levels of antigen 'e' might be an important factor for the risk of transmission. There are no specific published articles regarding CVS, and the majority of them assess the risk following genetic amniocentesis.

Regarding HIV, studies performed before the use of antiretroviral treatment reported an increased risk of vertical transmission of the human immuno-deficiency virus following antenatal invasive procedures with a relative risk RR=4.[8,9] However, studies published after the introduction of anti-retroviral treatment schemes in pregnancy, showed that invasive prenatal diagnosis might be safer, particularly during the first trimester of pregnancy and when the viral load is low. A recent Italian multicenter study,[10] found a small increase of the risk of vertical transmission in a group (n=63) of seropositive women who underwent amniocentesis or CVS compared to a larger group of seropositive women who did not have any of these procedures (n=712). The risk of transmission was respectively 3.3% and 1.7% which did not reach statistic significance. All women had a protocol based antiretroviral treatment. Despite these promising results, the lack of conclusive information regarding the risk of vertical viral transmission should be discussed with the woman on an individual basis and if possible these procedures should be avoided.

Specific contraindications for the transcervical CVS, are generally considered cases of active transvaginal bleeding or active cervicovaginal infections. For the transabdominal approach care should be taken in cases where there is a high suspicion of bowel adhesions between the abdominal wall and the uterus and cases where the placenta is posterior, making the sampling hazardous as it could cause trauma to the membranes and/or the fetus.

The potential for a CVS-induced maternal-fetal transfusion to worsen an already existing Rh immunization has been described, suggesting that sampling sensitized patients represents a contraindication to the procedure.[11] For such patients, amniocentesis or cordocentesis in the 2nd trimester should be considered as a safer alternative. It has been calculated that in 6 to 18% of the procedures the transfused fetal blood exceeds 0.1 ml, amount which could initiate an immune response in RhD-negative women bearing a rhesus positive fetus. A recent study found that none of the 61 cases undergoing CVS had more than 3.5 ml fetomaternal hemorrhage,[12] concurring with the American College of Obstetricians and Gynecologists (ACOG) recommendation, that 50 µg of anti-D are sufficient to prevent a rhesus immunization following CVS.

Techniques of Chorionic Villus Sampling

Chorionic villi cover the whole surface of the foetal sac up until the 9th week. As the gestation proceeds, the villi begin to regress with the exception of the implantation site. This site is characterised by a rapid growth of trophoblastic tissue (the chorion frondosum), easily recognizable with ultrasound after the 9th week of gestation.

There are two routes for CVS sampling, the transcervical (TC-CVS) and the transabdominal (TA-CVS) (Figure 14.1). Both of these procedures can be performed in an outpatient clinic setting. Continuous realtime ultrasound monitoring is mandatory for all the procedures. A careful medical history is taken before starting, and particular attention should be given to issues related with the current pregnancy such as, PV bleeding, symptoms of vaginal infections, or the presence of fibroids. The rhesus status should be confirmed and the indication for the procedure should be reviewed. The mother should be fully informed about the technical aspects of the procedure and of the relative risks such as fetal loss rates, bleeding, premature rupture of membranes, etc. It is important to discuss the fact that not always it is possible to have a definite diagnosis and a second procedure might be considered later in pregnancy. A detailed consent form should be signed prior to the procedure.

Transcervical CVS

For this technique the mother is placed in lithotomy position and the external genitalia are cleaned with an antiseptic solution. The cervix is then visualized with a Cusco's speculum and cleaned with a broad-spectrum antiseptic preparation. The cervix maybe gently grasped with a tenaculum to straighten the cervical canal, although this usually produces discomfort and maybe sometimes painful.[20] A 26 cm long polyethylene catheter with a 5 mm in outer diameter and a soft stainless still blunt obturator, is the instrument of choice for most operators performing TC-CVS. In 2003, a Cochrane systematic review[13] found no significant differences between the various instruments used for this approach.

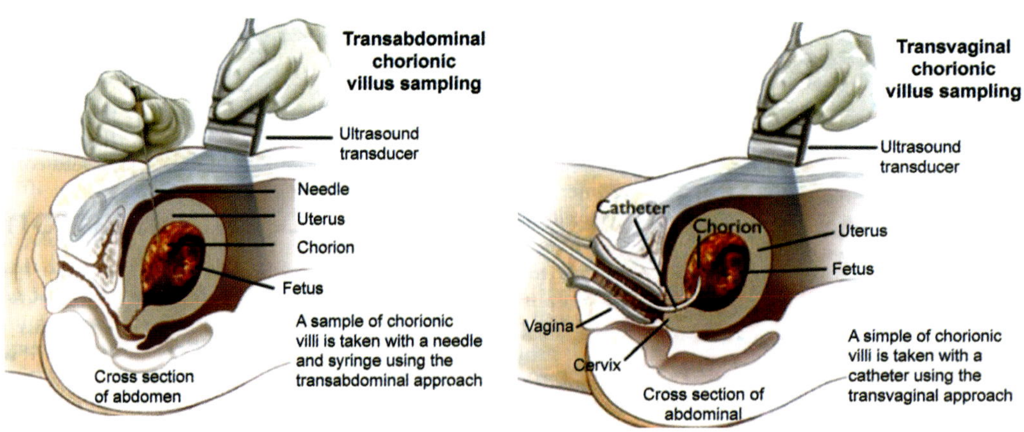

Figure 14.1: TA-CVS and TC-CVS

Transabdominal CVS

The technique for transabdominal CVS is very similar to amniocentesis. Two techniques have been described, the 'two-needle technique' and the 'free-hand' (or single needle) technique as described by Brambati.[20] With the first one, a double coaxial needle system can be inserted percutaneously through a needle guide attached to the ultrasound probe. An 18-gauge, 15 cm guide needle is first introduced and then stopped at the edge of the placenta. Thereafter, a thinner 22- or 20-gauge 20 cm needle is passed through the outer needle and repeatedly inserted in the chorion frondosum until an adequate sample is obtained.

As an alternative, a single 20 g, 9 or 12 cm spinal needle can be used and inserted by a free hand ultrasound guided approach. The needle tip is first inserted into the myometrium and then redirected parallel to the membrane. As with cervical sampling, the needle should be passed through as much villus tissue as possible and remain parallel to the chorionic membrane to avoid inadvertent puncture. Once within the placenta, the stylet is removed and a syringe containing 5 ml of media attached. Under continuous suction, four or five to and fro passes within the frondosum are made. The needle is then removed from the abdomen while suction is continued.

Rapid karyotyping may be performed by direct analysis of syncytiotrophoblastic cells arrested in metaphase, either immediately (a few hours) after sampling or after short-term (24-48 hr) culture. During the last years it has been possible to have a rapid reply for the most common trisomies (chromosome 21, 18 and 13) within 24 hours with the FISH method (Fluorescent *in situ* hybridization), whereas the PCR (Polymerase chain reaction) technique provides diagnosis for monogenic disorders. However, for a definite diagnosis, culture of the mesenchymal cells is required, taking 7 to 10 days.

Transcervical vs Transabdominal CVS

Five randomized trials have so far compared the TC-CVS with the TA-CVS.[14-18] Both techniques appear to be equally effective with more than 99% success of sampling rate. As far as safety is concerned transabdominal CVS appears to be safer than the transcervical route. A meta-analysis review by Cochrane collaboration[19] showed that the total pregnancy loss and spontaneous miscarriages rates were higher after TC-CVS compared to TA-CVS (9% versus 7.4% and 7.9% versus 4.5%, respectively). However, this observation was heavily influenced by the Danish Trial[15] which probably reflected the fact that this center was far more experienced with the TA-CVS technique compared with the TC-CVS technique. The fetal loss rates of the other 4 trials were similar. This meta-analysis concluded that after taking into account various statistical corrections for the observed heterogeneity of the results, the differences in pregnancy loss and miscarriage between these two methods were not statistically significant.

Nowadays, the TA-CVS appears to be the method of choice for sampling, not only because of the safety profile but also because it is better accepted by women. Transcervical CVS appears to be more technically demanding requiring more multiple insertions (11.2% versus 4.1%) and causing more vaginal bleeding (10%versus 1.6%). TC-CVS is reserved for cases where TA-CVS can be hazardous to the pregnancy, i.e. where the placenta is low posterior or if there are bowel adhesions on the anterior aspect of the uterus. As far as cytogenetic analysis is concerned both procedures are comparable. Every prenatal diagnostic center should have the resources to cope with all clinical scenarios and every operator should be appropriately trained for both procedures.

TECHNIQUES OF CVS

Timing

It is generally accepted that CVS should be undertaken between 10 and 13 completed weeks of pregnancy, the optimal being the 11th week. During this period fetal viability can be easily detected, embryogenesis has been completed, and the placenta has a sufficient thickness for safe sampling. After the end of the first trimester, the gestational sac becomes attached to the decidual wall which means that any attempt to insert either a catheter or a biopsy forceps carries a slightly higher risk of indenting and damaging the membranes. These difficulties become more evident when performing a transcervical sampling in cases where the proximal placental edge has moved away from the internal os.[20] The feasibility of CVS beyond the first trimester through the second trimester can be a valid alternative to amniocentesis for a prompt answer in cases of late booking, suspicious ultrasound findings, or increased risk of chromosomal abnormalities as a result of 1st trimester screening. A study done by Brambati,[21] showed comparable fetal loss rates after CVS at 11 to 12 weeks, 13 to 15 weeks and 15 to 20 weeks (fetal loss rates 1.02%, 0.86%, and 0.46% respectively) with no statistical significance. However, in the 15 to 20 weeks group, it was not possible to perform CVS in 4.2% of the cases, mainly due to a posterior unreachable placenta. In these cases a midtrimester amniocentesis was performed.

Efficiency of CVS

Successful sampling can be obtained from more than 99% of the cases. Various studies showed that the rate of sampling failure during the first trimester varies between 0.04% and 0.8% of the cases.[22,23] For most of these cases adequate samples can be obtained after a single device insertion. A recent review found that the average multiple insertion rate was 5.5%.[24] The fetal loss rate increases significantly after 3 consecutive insertions and according to some papers the rate can be as high as 10%.[25, 26] After a failed 2nd attempt the need for invasive prenatal diagnosis must be reviewed again and factors (such as placental location, contractions of the uterus, and presence of fibroids) which can make sampling difficult must be excluded. If there is no immediate need for fetal diagnosis, alternative methods of sampling should be considered.

Reliability of CVS

Despite a successful trophoblastic tissue sampling, a definite diagnosis is not always possible and there are cases that require further investigation. It has been calculated that the need for a second invasive procedure later in pregnancy is at the order of 1.1 to 3%.[23,27] The reason for a failed cytogenetic interpretation includes cases of maternal contamination, placental confined mosaicism and culture failures.

Maternal Contamination

After the retrieval of chorionic tissue, the quantity and quality of the sample should be checked in the clinic before the mother leaves the hospital. This can be done under direct vision, in order to confirm the presence of adequate amount of the characteristic branched villi. In case of doubt, an optic microscope can be very helpful. Contamination of samples with significant amounts of maternal decidual tissue occurs more frequently with a small sample size. This could lead to diagnostic errors and potentially to false-negative results, although there are no published reports of the latter. In a large retrospective article,[28] maternal contamination was found in 0.9% of the cases.[23] Biopsies with more than 10 mg are considered enough for accurate analysis.

Placental mosaicism

The second cause of potential diagnostic errors is mosaicism confined to the placenta. Placental mosaicism is defined by Hahnemann as:[29](i) the presence of at least two cells with identical chromosomal aberration, concomitant with a cell line with a normal diploid karyotype or with another chromosomal aberration in either direct CVS preparation/short-term incubation, CVS culture or both; (ii) the presence of a non-mosaic aberration in all mitoses analyses after direct CVS preparations/ short-term incubation, concomitant with a cell line with a normal, diploid karyotype or with another chromosomal aberration on CVS culture or vice versa.

Soon after the introduction of CVS in routine practice, it turned out that the cytogenetic diagnosis from direct preparations did not always reflect the chromosomal constitution of the fetus. A model of Crane and Cheung[30] can explain the discrepancy between the chromosomal constitutions of fetus and placenta. According to their model (Figure 14.2), from the first five cell divisions following fertilization only 2 of the 32 resulting cells will give rise to the formation of the embryo. All other cells are responsible for the formation of the trophoblast and the extraembryonic tissues.

Mosaicism can develop through two possible mechanisms.[31] The first mechanism involves a meiotic error in one of the two gametes leading to a formation of a trisomic conceptus. In subsequent early mitotic divisions one of the cells may lose the extra-chromosome, 'rescuing' the trisomic zygote, forming a normal disomic cell line (meiotic origin and trisomy rescue). A mosaic morula is the result of this process with the percentage of normal cells dependent on the cell division at which the rescue occurred. At approximately the 32- to 64-cell stage, only 3 or 4 cells become part of the inner cell mass and later form the embryo, whereas the remainders become precursors of the extraembryonic tissues. It is therefore more probable that the extraembryonic tissues will contain the trisomic cells and not the embryo. The condition where the abnormal cell lines are found to the placenta only is called confined placental mosaicism (CPM). The problem with CPM from mitotic rescue is that it could lead to uniparental disomy, when the trisomic embryo is left with a pair of chromosomes originating from the same parent. The theoretical probability of uniparental disomy in the 'rescued' diploid fetus is 33.3% because of the presence of one chromosome pair derived from only one parent. This may have clinical consequences if the chromosomes involved carry imprinted genes (that is, genes whose expression depends on whether they are inherited from the mother or father) or if the chromosomes carry a recessive gene that is now homozygous. For example, 15% of Prader-Willi syndrome cases result from uniparental, maternal disomy for chromosome 15.[32] In addition, chromosomes 7, 11,14 and 22 are believed to be imprinted. In all these cases evaluation of UDP by amniotic fluid analysis is required.[28]

In the second mechanism,[28] mitotic post-zygotic errors produce a mosaic morula or blastocyst with the distribution and percent of aneuploid cells dependent on the timing of non-disjunction. If mitotic errors occur early in the development of the morula, they may segregate to the inner cell mass and have the same potential to produce an affected fetus as do meiotic errors. Mitotic errors occurring after primary cell differentiation and compartmentalization has been completed lead to cytogenetic abnormalities in only one lineage.

Based on the position of the different cell lines and on the chromosomal constitution of the fetus three categories of placental mosaics can be distinguished. In type I, the abnormal cell line is confined to the cytotrophoblast; in type II, it only affects the stromal villous core (mesenchyme); and in type III, it involves both tissues. The karyotype of the two placental cell lineages can be obtained by means of direct preparations or short-term cultures (cytotrophoblast), or long-term incubations (mesenchyme) of the chorionic villi.

A large series of 15000 CVS which were evaluated by one single laboratory, mosaicism was found in 1.8% of the cases.[33] Mosaicism confined only to the placenta was found in 88.2%, meaning that the fetus was affected in only 12.8%. When a mosaic trisomy is detected the likelihood of this being confined to the placenta depends on the type of mosaicism and the chromosome involved. Definite diagnosis can be provided with the analysis of fetal cells by amniocentesis or cordocentesis.

During the first years of CVS, mosaicism created concerns about the validity and reliability of the trophoblastic cytogenetic results. The better understanding of the biology of the early placenta allowed not only the elimination of such concerns but also the addition of clinically important information. It has been shown that pregnancies with a CPM are at a higher risk for IUGR and perinatal death.[31] A more sticking finding is that pregnancies with CPM for chromosome 16 have a less than 35% chances of having a normal, appropriate-for-gestational-age, full-term infants.[34-36]

SAFETY OF CVS

Fetal Loss

The risk of fetal loss following an invasive procedure is the result of two parameters: (i) the background risk for fetal loss, and (ii) the risk related to the procedure itself. The background risk for fetal loss is the result of the following factors: (a) maternal age, (b) gestational age, (c) past medical history, and (d) the presence of congenital and/or chromosomic abnormalities of the fetus. In all cases, the risk for fetal loss should be balanced against the likelihood for having a fetal abnormality detected by the invasive procedure.

The best way to evaluate the added risk for fetal loss following a CVS would be with a randomized controlled trial in which women would be allocated to a CVS-group and a control group with no invasive procedures. A similar study for the assessment of fetal loss following 2nd trimester amniocentesis was published in 1986 by Tabor et al.[37] This randomized trial found that amniocentesis carried an added risk for fetal loss of 1% (1.7 % for the amniocentesis group compared to 0.7% for the control group, with a relative risk of 2.3). So far there are no such studies assessing CVS related fetal loss rates, and it is highly unlikely that they will ever be carried out, due to serious moral and ethical issues.

In view of these facts, the safety of CVS can be estimated indirectly by comparing post-CVS fetal losses with fetal losses observed after other prenatal invasive procedures such as midtrimester amniocentesis. However, in order to determine the incidence of procedure-induced pregnancy loss, adjustments for the relatively high background loss at the 1st trimester compared with the 2nd trimester must be made. All patients should be enrolled prior to the gestational age at which CVS is performed, and then the total loss rates compared, including spontaneous miscarriages and induced terminations of pregnancies. Only 6 RCTs comparing CVS to amniocentesis have been published to date, and the three largest of these studies were performed in late 1980s, soon after the introduction of this procedure (Table 14.2). In 1989, The Canadian Collaborative CVS/Amniocentesis Clinical Trial group[38] reported a 7.6% loss rate in the CVS group, compared to 7.0% loss rate in the amniocentesis group, with no statistical significance. The Danish randomized trial in 1992[15] found no difference between TA-CVS and midtrimester amniocentesis and similar results with no significant differences were observed from the other 3 studies. In the US, a nonrandomized study found a 0.8% increase in fetal loss after CVS as compared with midtrimester amniocentesis which was not statistically significant. On the contrary, a prospective randomized collaborative trial sponsored by the European Medical Research Council,[39] reported that CVS had a 4.6% greater pregnancy loss rate than amniocentesis, which was statistically significant. However, the general consensus is that low operator experience with CVS accounts for this increased risk. On average there were 52 cases per center, compared to 400 cases per center in the Finnish study, 325 cases per center in the US study and 106 in the Canadian study.

Table 14.2: RCTs comparing first trimester CVS vs midtrimester amniocentesis

Randomised trials CVS vs 2nd trimester amniocentesis				*Fetal loss rates (%)*	
Study	*No. of centers*	*CVS*	*Amnio*	*Difference (%)*	*Relative risks*
Canada 1990 *Lancet*	11	7.6	7.0	+0.6	1.1
USA 1989[26] *NEJM*	7	7.2	5.7	+1.5	
Denmark 1992[15] *Lancet*	2	6.4		+0.1	1.3
• TC-CVS		6.2		-0.1	0.9
• TA-CVS		10.1		+3.8*	1.7
• AMNIO			6.3		
Europe MRC1992[39] *Lancet*	31	13.6	9.0	+4.6*	1.51
Finland 1993[40] *Prenat Diagn*	1	78	8.3	–0.5	
Spain 1999[41]	1	2,2	2.8	–0.6	

The impact of operator experience has been demonstrated by various studies. It has been suggested that post-CVS fetal loss rates from operators with experience of less than 100 cases, can be 2 or 3 times higher compared to more experienced operators.[42-44] A recent retrospective cohort study[45] of women who underwent CVS or amniocentesis from 1983 to 2003 found that the difference in pregnancy loss rates before 24 weeks, between these two procedures decreased over time. From 1998 to 2003, the authors found no statistical significant difference between CVS and amniocentesis, underlying the importance of the experience factor and the relatively longer learning curve for CVS.

Similar findings were also found at our institution (Figure 14.2) where the overall pregnancy loss rate following CVS including miscarriages and endometrial deaths between 1991 and 2005 decreased significantly from 5 to 1.4% (p=0.023), a rate which was comparable to the overall amniocentesis loss rate 1.6% (p=0.752) (see Figure 14.1).

A recently published systematic review by Mujezinovic and Alfirevic[46] analyzed fetal loss rates and complications following amniocentesis after 14 weeks of pregnancy and CVS carried out transabdominally between 10 and 14 weeks. The authors included 29 and 16 papers assessing complications following amniocentesis and CVS respectively. There was a marginally higher total pregnancy loss following CVS compared to amniocentesis (2.0% vs. 1.9% respectively) which is to be expected given the difference in gestational age when the procedures are performed.

Procedure related reviews from centers performing CVS can also be a source of interesting information as seen in Table 14.3. Brambati et al[22] published the results from a large series of 9,471 cases sampled by the same operator, and found that the fetal loss rate including spontaneous miscarriages and endometrial deaths was 3.01%, with a 2.69% of these losses occurring before 28 weeks. Papp et al[50] found a fetal loss rate within the first 10 weeks after TA-CVs of 2.5%, whereas Brun et al[23] reported a total fetal loss rate of 1.9%. It is mandatory to look critically to every report mentioning fetal loss rate as there are significant differences that can affect the interpretation of the results, such as differences of the indications for sampling, the gestational age and maternal age.

Limb Reduction Defects

In 1986 Planteydt[51] published the first case report describing finger malformations of the hand of a child born after CVS on the 68th day of pregnancy. Three years later, Christiaens[52] published the second case report describing a fetus which was born at 18 3/7 weeks with an annular constriction of one of the arms as seen in the amniotic band sequence, suggesting that congenital defects might be one of the complications of chorionic villus sampling. In March 1991 Firth et al[53] published a paper describing 5 children showing severe limb deficiencies among 289 pregnancies sampled between 8.0 and 9.3 weeks of pregnancy. A few other reports followed, describing fetal abnormalities following CVS and in 1994 Firth et al[54] reviewed 75 cases with similar fetal limb deficiencies, suggesting a strong correlation between the severity of the defects and the gestational age of the CVS.

After these initial alarming reports in 1994, WHO performed a detailed analysis of infants or fetuses with limb defects, by standardized methods, of 138.996 CVS procedures, comparing them with the British Columbia Registry for malformations. This study did not indicate an increased risk of LRDs after CVS[55] (5.2 to 5.7 per 10,000 cases in the CVS group vs. 4.8 to 5.97 per 10,000 of the general population) and this was later confirmed by an update analysis

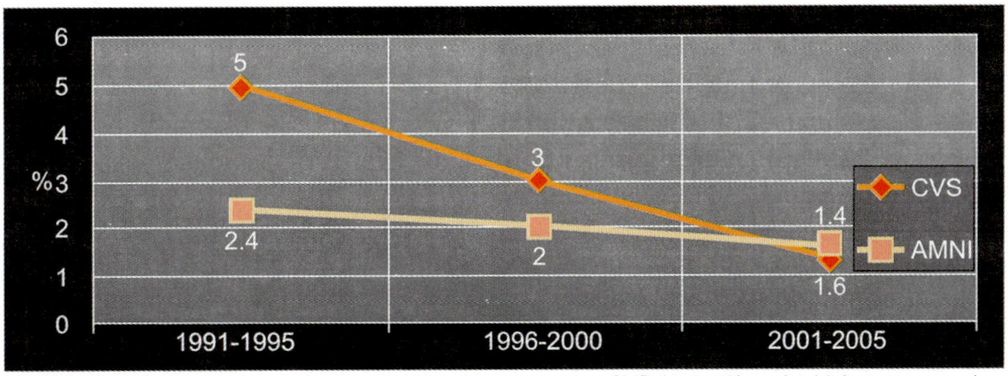

Figure 14.2: Total fetal loss rates (%) following first trimester CVS (n=3132) and midtrimester genetic amniocentesis (n=6448). For CVS p=0.023 'Alexandra' University Hospital, Athens

Table 14.3: Total fetal loss=spontaneous miscarriages and endometrial deaths, FLR= Fetal loss rates

Study	*(n)*	*Maternal age*	*Gestational age*	*FLR % Total*	*FLR % (weeks)*	*Comments*
Hogge 1986[47]	1000			3.8		Mosaicism 1.7%
Papp 2002[50] *Fetal Diagn Ther*	1044	ΔA	15		5.7	10 weeks Post-CVS TA-CVS=2.5%
Brun 2003[23] *Prenat Diagn*	4552	36	15	1.9		↑↑gest. age
Caughey 2006[45] *Obstet Gyn*	9886	37.1	9-15		3.12 (<24/40)	
Philip 2004[48] *Am J Obst Gyn*	1878	37	11-14		1.4 (<28/40)	
Akhlaghpoor 2006[49] *Prenat Diagn*	1381	26.2	11+4		1.45	2 weeks post-CVS
Brambati 1998[22] *Prenat Diagn*	9365	36	10	3.01	2.69 (<28/40)	
Mujezinovic 2007[46] *Obstet Gynecol*	NA	NA	NA	2	1.3	Systematic review
Our experience 'Alexandra Hospital' 1991-2005	3132	30	11+1	3.34 (1.7% for 2001-2005)	2.88 (<24/40)	1.4% for 2005

in 1999 of 2,02,682[56] cases, as well as by the results of many other studies. The theory behind structural abnormalities after CVS is based on the fact that the placental trauma can lead to local bleeding, hemodynamic changes, vasoconstriction, peripheral hypoxia and eventually cellular and tissue loss. However, parents can be reassured that there is good evidence showing that when CVS is performed after 10 weeks of pregnancy the risk of limb deficiencies is similar with the background risk of 1:3000.

Other Complications

Bleeding

Vaginal bleeding is more common after the TC-CVS compared to TA-CVS. In most cases, the bleeding is self-limited and the pregnancy outcome is excellent with no maternal adverse effects. Other complications such as PROM and post CVS infections occur rarely in less than 1% of the cases.

Pain

Various studies that have assessed the issue of pain during CVS found that in most cases the pain felt by the mothers is mid and comparable to the pain caused by amniocentesis. Young primiparous and women with high levels of stress before the procedure should be adequately counseled and reassured that this procedure is well tolerated by the majority of women.

Pre-eclampsia

In 2005 Silver et al[57] suggested a possible relation between the histological disturbance caused by late CVS (weeks 13 to 14) and the increased risk for pre-eclampsia later in pregnancy. This study used subjects recruited during a randomized trial funded by the NICHD, which compared early amniocentesis and late transabdominal chorionic villus sampling (CVS) in weeks 13 and 14, rates of gestational hypertension and preeclampsia were compared between cases with varying degrees of placental disruption. A significantly higher rate of hypertension/pre-eclampsia was observed in the late CVS group (5.4%, n = 1,878) compared with the early amniocentesis cohort (3.5%, n = 1,820; P = 0.005). Unfortunately, the criticism for this study is the lack of a standardized classification for the definition of pregnancy-induced hypertension and pre-eclampsia. In a more recent article, Adusumalli et al[58] compared women undergoing first trimester CVS with women having a nuchal translucency and biochemical screening test. Although the overall rates of pregnancy-induced hypertensive disorders were similar. There appears to be an association between chorionic villus sampling and severe hypertensive disorders including severe pre-eclampsia, eclampsia, and hemolysis, elevated liver enzymes, and low platelet count syndrome (2.7% vs 1.1% respectively, RR=2.48).

Perinatal Complications

There is no evidence from the available randomized and clinical control studies of an increased risk for perinatal maternal or fetal complications following CVS such as preterm labor, premature rupture of the membranes, IUGR, antepartum hemorrhage, maternal morbidity or other obstetric complications.[15, 26, 38-40]

Two population-based cohort studies from Sweden found no increased maternal complications and infant morbidity following CVS.[59, 60]

CVS in Multiple Pregnancies

Improvement in assisted reproductive techniques and an increasing mean maternal age are the main factors which led to the dramatic increase in the incidence of multiple pregnancies during the last 20 years. Nowadays, CVS is considered to be a valid and safe alternative to midtrimester amniocentesis for prenatal genetic diagnosis in multiple pregnancies. As for singleton pregnancies, the advantage of having an early diagnosis in late first trimester is also supplemented by the fact that fetal reduction can be performed for the affected twin during the first trimester. There is evidence that fetal reduction in the early stages of pregnancy compared to a fetal reduction later in pregnancy carries less clinical risks[61] not only for the mother but also for the unaffected twin.[62]

CVS for multiple pregnancies is performed after 10 weeks of pregnancy in order to avoid the already mentioned risks of fetal limb defects. It is imperative to determine the chorionicity of the pregnancy before the procedure (based on first trimester ultrasound using the 'Lambda' sign) and the preliminary scanning will be completed with a detailed mapping of the relative fetal and placental locations. Either TA-CVS or TC-CVS can be used based on the principles for singletons. Two sampling needles are used for the dichorionic pregnancies whereas for monochorionic twins only one needle is required. In order to minimize the risk of sampling errors the needles should be directed close to the insertion of each umbilical cord to the placenta or alternatively to the most distant placental sites from the point where the 2 placentas are fused. In cases where sampling from each placenta is difficult, both TC and TA technique can be used particularly in cases with both high and low placentas.[63]

It is recommended that these procedures be done by experienced operators to ensure correct ultra sound-guided placement of the instrument into each placenta.

Reliability of CVS in Multiple Pregnancies

In the hands of experienced operators and by appropriate methological approach, CVS has been reported to be highly effective in multiple gestations: In a study done by Brambati et al[64] genetic diagnosis was correct on all 338 fetuses sampled from 169 twin pregnancies, while sampling was incorrect in only three out of 771 fetuses (0.4%) sampled in 424 multiple pregnancies undergoing fetal reduction to a single fetus or twins from the same center.[65] Moreover, in both studies sampling was successfully performed in all cases by single needle insertion. It must be mentioned that these results come from one of the most experienced centers for CVS. Another study by van den Berg et al,[66] compared the diagnostic accuracy of 2nd trimester amniocentesis (n=297) and CVS (n=163) in twins and triplets. Successful sampling using a two pass approach was achieved in 99.3% vs. 99.7% respectively. Uncertain results were present in 7 CVS cases (5 with placental mosaicism). No uncertain results were found in the amniocentesis group. Four of the 15 triplet sets were sampled by CVS and 11 underwent amniocentesis. However, one from each group required further amniocentesis because of abnormal results. The authors concluded that fetal cell contamination and confined mosaicism could be kept to a minimum with CVS and did not lead to critical mistakes.

In fetuses of the same sex, it is impossible to spot these errors by routine analysis of the sampled

Table 14.4: Chorionic villus sampling in twin pregnancies

	n	*Study period*	*Gestation (weeks)*	*Miscarriage (%)*	*Total fetal loss (%)*	*Amniocentesis (Miscarriage/TFL)*
Pergament et al 1992[74]	126	1983-89	9-12	2.38	4.10	
Wapner et al 1993[72]	161	1984-90	<12	3.20	4.90	2.9 / 9.3
Appelman et al 1999[75]	28	1989-97	9-23	0	0	
De Catte et al 2000[77]	262	1988-98	9-13	3.10	5.50	
Brambati et al 2001[71]	198	1991-98	7-12	0.50	3.19	
Antsaklis et al 2002[73]	44	1986-2000	9-15	4.54	10.22	4.17/8.77
Casals et al 2002[76]	23	Period A			8.7	
Casals et al 2002	30	Period B			6.6	

material. Brambati et al[67] suggests that in case of same-sex dichorionic twins, DNA polymorphism markers can be easily checked to assure retrieval of villi from the individual placentas.

The impact of placental mosaicism can largely be reduced by the use of both short-term and long-term villi preparations. Since in long-term preparations mesenchyme cells of the villous core are cultured, the results are not influenced by the higher incidence of numerical chromosomal aberrations in trophoblastic tissue. In the minority of cases in which inconclusive results after long-term culture persist, amniocentesis must be performed. Whenever maternal cell contamination is responsible for the mosaic results, long-term cultures are not very helpful. It is generally advised to include in the pre-procedure counseling that about 2 to 3% of patients having CVS with twin pregnancies will need resampling because of uncertainty of results.[68]

Fetal Loss after CVS in Twins

There are a few published articles showing that CVS in multiple pregnancies is a safe method for genetic prenatal diagnosis. The reported post-CVS fetal loss rates range between 0.6 and 4%. Those studies that have compared fetal loss rates in singletons and twins within the same prenatal diagnostic institution found that CVS was not associated with an increased risk of either total pregnancy losses or single fetal losses (De Catte et al,[69] Aytoz et al,[70] Brambati et al[71]). Other studies show that CVS is as safe as amniocentesis when performed by experienced operators. Wapner et al[72] compared the fetal loss rates between a CVS group at 10 to 12 weeks (n=161) with a midtrimester amniocentesis group (n=72). No differences were observed between procedures in the rate of spontaneous abortion and perinatal mortality. The fetal loss rate following the procedure until 28/40 was 2.9% following amnio and 3.2% following CVS. However, if only cases with chromosomally normal fetuses and placentae were considered, the total fetal loss rate was significantly lower in the CVS series (3.9 in the CVS group vs 9.3% in the amniocentesis group). It was therefore concluded that CVS was at least as safe and as reliable as amniocentesis for prenatal diagnosis of twin pregnancies. Another article by Antsaklis et al[73] (Table 14.4), compared first trimester CVS to midtrimester amniocentesis. This study found comparable fetal loss rates and the authors emphasized the fact that CVS requires a more advanced level of expertise.

In a review paper by Furman et al, which included four articles found that in 614 twin pregnancies, the mean rate of pregnancy loss before 22 weeks was 3.1%, and the mean total pregnancy loss was 4.6%.[77] De Catt et al[69] found no differences between the two procedures of fetal losses up to the 28th week and in the perinatal obstetric outcomes such as preterm delivery, low birth weight and perinatal mortality were also comparable between the CVS and control groups.

REFERENCES

1. Mohr J. Foetal genetic diagnosis: development of techniques for early sampling of foetal cells. Acta Pathologica Microbiolabic Scandinavia 1968;73:7377.
2. Tietung Hospital on Ansham Iron and Steel Co. Fetal sex prediction by sex chromatin of chorionic villi cells during early pregnancy. Chin Med J 1975;1117-26.
3. Kazy Z, Rozovsky, Bakharev VA. Chorion biopsy in early pregnancy: a method of early prenatal diagnosis for inherited disorders. Prenat Diagn 1982;2:39-45.
4. Brambati B, Oldrini A, Aladerun SA. Transcervical specimen of chorionic villi in the 1st trimester of pregnancy. Pathologica. 1983;75 (Suppl):179-83.
5. Simoni G, Brambati B, Danesino C, Rossella F, Terzoli GL, Ferrari M, Fraccaro M. Efficient direct chromosome analysis and enzyme determinations from chorionic villi samples in the first trimester of pregnancy. Hum Genet 1983;63:349-57.
6. Smidt-Jehnsen S, Hahnemann N. Transabdominal fine-needle biopsy from chorionic villi in the first trimester. Prenat Diagn 1984;4:163-9.
7. Davies G, Wilson RD, Desilets V, Reid GJ, Shaw D,Summers A, et al. Society of Obstetricians and Gynaecologists of Canada. Amniocentesis and women with hepatitis B, hepatitis C,or human immunodeficiency virus. J Obstet Gynaecol Can 2003;25:145-52.
8. Mandelbrot L, Mayaux MJ, Bongain A, et al. Obstetric factors and mother-to-child transmission of human immunodeficiency virus type 1: the French perinatal cohorts. SEROGEST French Pediatric HIN Infection Study Group. Am J Obstet Gynecol 1996;175:661-7.
9. Tess BH, Ridrigues LC, Newell ML, Dunn DT, Lago TD. Breastfeeding, genetic, obstetric and other risk factors associated with mother-to-child transmission of HIV-1 in Sao Paulo State, Brazil. Sao Paulo Collaborative Study for Vertical Transmission of HIV-1. AIDS 1998;12:513-20.
10. Somigliana E, Bucceri AM, Tibaldi C, Alberico S, Ravizza M, Savasi V, Marini S, Matrone R, Pardi G; Italian Collaborative Study on HIV Infection in Pregnancy. Early invasive diagnostic techniques in pregnant women who are infected with the HIV: a multicenter case series. Am J Obstet Gynecol 2005;193(2):437-42.
11. Moise KJ, Carpenter RJ. Increased severity of fetal hemolytic disease with known rhesus alloimunisation after first trimester transcervical chorionic villus biopsy. Fetal Diagn Ther 1990;5:76.
12. Katiyar R, Kriplani A, Agarwal N, Bhatla N, Kabra M. Detection of fetomaternal hemorrhage following chorionic villus sampling by Kleihauer Betke test and rise in maternal serum alpha feto protein. Prenat Diagn 2007;27(2):139-42.
13. Alfirevic Z, von Dadelszen P. Instruments for chorionic villus sampling for prenatal diagnosis. Cochrane Database Syst Rev 2003;(1):
14. Brambati B, Terzian E, Tognoni G. Randomised clinical trial of transabdominal versus transcervical chorionic villus sampling methods. Prenat diagn 1991;11:285-93.
15. Smidt-Jensen S, Permin M, Philip J, et al. Randomised comparison of amniocentesis and transabdominal and transcervical chorionic villus sampling. Lancet 1992;340:1237-44.
16. Jackson GL, Zachary JM, Fowler SE, et al. A randomized comparison of transcervical and transabdominal chorionic villus sampling. N Engl J Med 1992;327:594-8.
17. Bovicelli L, Rizzo N, Montacuti V, Morandi R. Transabdominal vs transcervical routes for chorionic villus sampling. Lancet 1986;2:290.
18. Tomassini A, Campagna G, Paolucci M, Ferrario D, Zarini E, Tibiletti MG, et al. Transvaginal CVS vs transabdominal CVS (our randomized cases). XI European Congress of Perinatal Medicine; 1988 April 10-13; Rome, Italy, 1988:1101-4.
19. Alfirevic Z, Sundberg K, Brigham S. Amniocentesis and chorionic villus sampling for prenatal diagnosis. Cochrane Database Syst Rev 2003;(3).
20. Brambati B, Tului L. Prenatal genetic diagnosis through chorionic villus sampling. In Milunsky A (Ed): Genetic Disorders and the Fetus (5th ed): Baltimore and London: The Johns Hopkins University Press; 2004; pp179-213.
21. Brambati B, Tului L, Camurri L, Guircilena S. Early second trimester (13 to 20 weeks) transabdominal chorionic villus sampling (TA-CVS): a safe and alternative method for both high and low risk populations. Prenat Diagn 2002;22:907-13.
22. Brambati B, Tului L, Cislaghi C, Alberti E. First 10,000 chorionic villus samplings performed on singleton pregnancies by a single operator. Prenat Diagn. 1998;18(3):255-66.
23. Brun JL, Mangione R, Gangbo F, Guyon F, Taine L, Roux D, Maugey-Laulom B, Horovitz J, Saura R. Feasibility, accuracy and safety of chorionic villus sampling: a report of 10741 cases. Prenat Diagn 2003;23(4):295-301.
24. Mujezinovic F, Alfirevic Z. Procedure-related complications of amniocentesis and chorionic villous sampling: a systematic review. Obstet Gynecol 2007;110(3):687-94.
25. Jackson LJ, Wapner RJ: Risks of chorionic villus sampling. Clin obstet Gynecol 1987;1(3):513.
26. Rhoads GG, Jackson LG, Schlesselman SE, et al: The safety and efficacy of chorionic villus sampling for early prenatal diagnosis of cytogenetic abnormalities. N Engl J Med 1989;320:609.
27. Ledbetter DH, Martin AO, Verlinsky Y, et al: Cytogenetic results of chorionic villus sampling: High success rate and diagnostic accuracy in the United States collaborative study. Am J Obstet Gynecol 1990;162:495-501.
28. Wapner RJ. Invasive prenatal diagnostic techniques. Semin Perinatol 2005;29(6):401-4.
29. Hahnemann JM, Vejerslev LO. Accuracy of cytogenetic findings on chorionic villus sampling (CVS) diagnostic consequences of CVS mosaicism and non-mosaic discrepancy in centers contributing to EUCROMIC 1986-1992. Prenat Diagn 1997;17:801-2.
30. Crane JP, Cheung SW. An embryogenic model to explain cytogenetic inconsistencies observed in chorionic villus versus fetal tissue. Prenat Diagn 1988;8(2):119-29.

31. Wolstenholme J. Confined placental mosaicism for trisomies 2, 3, 7, 8, 9, 16, and 22: their incidence, likely origins, and mechanisms for cell lineage compartmentalization. Prenat diagn 1996;16:511-24.
32. Cassidy SB, Lai LW, Erikson RP, et al. Trisomy 15 with loss of the paternal 15 as a cause of Prader-Willi syndrome due to maternal disomy. Am J Hum Genet 1992;51:701-8.
33. Grati FR, Grimi B, et al. Confirmation of mosaicism and uniparental disomy in amniocytes, after detection of mosaic chromosome abnormalities in chorionic villi. Eur J Hum Genet 2006;14:282-8.
34. Kalousek DK, Langlois S, Barrett I, et al. Uniparental disomy for chromosome 16 in humans. Am J Hum Genet 1993;52:8-16.
35. Phillips O, Tharapel A, Lerner J, et al. Risk of fetal mosaicism when placental mosaicism is diagnosed by chorionic villus sampling. Am J Obstet Gynecol 1996;174:850-5.
36. Benn P. Trisomy 16 and trisomy 16 mosaicism: a review. Am J Med Genet 1998;79:121-33.
37. Tabor A, Philip J, Madsen M, Bang J, Obel EB, Nørgaard-Pedersen B. Randomized controlled trial of genetic amniocentesis in 4606 low-risk women. Lancet 1986;1(8493):1287-93.
38. Multicentre randomised clinical trial of chorion villus sampling and amniocentesis. First report. Canadian Collaborative CVS-Amniocentesis Clinical Trial Group. Lancet 1989;7;1(8628):1-6.
39. Medical Research Council European trial of chorion villus sampling. MRC working party on the evaluation pf chorion villus sampling. Lancet 1991;337(8756):1491-9.
40. Ammälä P, Hiilesmaa VK, Liukkonen S, Saisto T, Teramo K, von Koskull H. Randomized trial comparing first-trimester transcervical chorionic villus sampling and second-trimester amniocentesis. Prenat Diagn 1993;13(10):919-27.
41. Borrell A, Fortuny A, Lazaro L, Costa D, Seres A, Pappa S, Soler A. First-trimester transcervical chorionic villus sampling by biopsy forceps versus mid-trimester amniocentesis: a randomized controlled trial project. Prenat Diagn 1999;19(12):1138-42.
42. Wapner RJ, Barr MA, Heeger S, et al. Chorionic villus sampling: a 10-year, over 13000 consecutive case experience. American college of Medical Genetics first Annual Meeting, Orlando, FL, 1994; March 15-17.
43. Nizard J, Duyme M, Ville Y. Teaching ultrasound-guided invasive procedures in fetal medicine: learning curves with and without an electronic guidance system. Ultrasound Obstet Gynecol 2002; 19:274-7.
44. Saura R, Taine L, Guyon F, et al. Safety and fetal outcome of early and midtrimester amniocentesis. Lancet 1998; 351:1434-35.
45. Caughey AB, Hopkins LM, Norton ME. Chorionic villus sampling compared with amniocentesis and the difference in the rate of pregnancy loss. Obstet Gynecol 2006;108(3Pt1):612-6.
46. Mujezinovic F, Alfirevic Z. Procedure-related complications of amniocentesis and chorionic villous sampling: a systematic review. Obstet Gynecol 2007;110(3):687-94.
47. Hogge WA, Schonberg SA, Golbus MS. Chorionic villus sampling: experience of the first 1000 cases. Am J Obstet Gynecol 1986;154(6):1249-52.
48. Philip J, et al. NICHD EATA Trial Group. Late first-trimester invasive prenatal diagnosis: results of an international randomized trial. Obstet Gynecol 2004;103(6):1164-73.
49. Akhlaghpoor S. Chorionic villus sampling for beta-thalassemia: the first report of experience in Iran. Prenat Diagn 2006;26(12):1131-6.
50. Papp C, Beke A, Mezei G, Tóth-Pál E, Papp Z. Chorionic villus sampling: a 15-year experience. Fetal Diagn Ther 2002;17(4):218-27.
51. Planteydt HT, van de Vooren MJ, Verweij. Amniotic bands and malformation in child born after pregnancy screened by chorionic villus biopsy. Lancet 1986;2:756-57.
52. Christiaens GC, Van Baarlen J, Huber J, Leschot NJ. Fetal limb constriction: a possible complication of CVS. Prenat Diagn 1989;9(1):67-71.
53. Firth HV, Boyd p, Chamberalin P, et al. Severe limb abnormalities after chorion villus sampling at 56 66 days gestastion. Lancet 1991;337:726-63.
54. Firth HV, Boyd PA, Chamberlain PF, et al. Analysis of limb reduction defects in babies exposed to chorionic villus sampling. Lancet 1994;343:1069-71.
55. Froster UG, Jackson L. Limb defects and chorionic villus sampling: results from an international registry, 1992–94. Lancet 1996; 347:489-94.
56. WHO/PAHO. Consultation on CVS. Evaluation of chorionic villus sampling safety. Prenat Diagn 1999;19:97-9.
57. Silver RK, Wilson RD, Philip J, Thom EA, Zachary JM, Mohide P, Mahoney MJ, Simpson JL, Platt LD, Pergament E, Hershey D, Filkins K, Johnson A, Wapner RJ, Jackson LG; NICHD EATA Trial Group. Late first-trimester placental disruption and subsequent gestational hypertension/pre-eclampsia. Obstet Gynecol 2005;105(3): 587-92.
58. Adusumalli J, Han CS, Beckham S, Bartholomew ML, Williams J 3rd. Chorionic villus sampling and risk for hypertensive disorders of pregnancy. Am J Obstet Gynecol 2007;196(6):591.e1-7.
59. Cederholm M, Haglund B, Axelsson O. Complications following amniocentesis and chorionic villus sampling for prenatal karyotyping. BJOG 2003;110:392-9.
60. Cederholm M, Haglund B, Axelsson O. Infant morbidity following amniocentesis and chorionic villus sampling for prenatal karyotyping. BJOG 2005;112:394-402.
61. Evans MI, Dommergues M, Wapner RK, et al. International collaborative experience of 1789 patients having multifetal pregnancy reduction: a plateauing of risks and outcomes. J Soc Gynecol Invest 1996;3:23-6.
62. Evans MI, Goldberg JD, Horenstein J, et al. Selective termination for structural, chromosomal, and mendelian anomalies: international experience. Am J Obstet Gynecol 1999;181:893-7.

63. Brambati B, Tului L, Lanzani A, et al. First-trimester diagnosis in multiple pregnancy: principles and potential pitfalls. Prenat Diagn 1991;11:676-4.
64. Brambati B, Tului L, Guercilena S, Alberti E. Outcome of first trimester chorionic villus sampling for genetic investigation in multiple pregnancy. Ultrasound Obstet Gynecol 2001;17:209-16.
65. Brambati B, Tului L, Camurri L, Guercilena S. First-trimester fetal reduction to a singleton infant or twins: outcome in relation to the final number and karyotyping before reduction by transabdominal chorionic villus sampling. Am J Obstet Gynecol 2004;191:2035-40.
66. van de Berg C, Braat APG, Van Ostal D, et al. Amniocentesis or chorionic villus sampling in multiple gestations: experience with 500 cases. Prenat Diagn 1999;19:234-44.
67. Brambati B, Tului L, Lanzani A, et al. First-trimester diagnosis in multiple pregnancy: principles and potential pitfalls. Prenat Diagn 1991;11:676-4.
68. Weisz B, Rodeck CH. Invasive diagnostic procedures in twin pregnancies. Prenat Diagn 2005;25(9):751-8.
69. De Catte L, Liebaers I, Foulon W, Bonduelle M, van Assche E. First trimester chorionic villus sampling in twin gestations. Am J Perinatol 1996; 13: 413-7.
70. Aytoz A, De Catte L, Camus M, et al. Obstetric outcome afterprenatal diagnosis in pregnancies obtained after intracytoplasmic sperm injection. Hum Reprod 1998;13:2958-61.
71. Brambati B, Tului L, Guercilena S, Alberti E. Outcome of first trimester chorionic villus sampling for genetic investigation in multiple pregnancy. Ultrasound Obstet Gynecol 2001;17: 209-16.
72. Wapner RJ, Johnson A, Davis G, et al. Prenatal diagnosis in twin gestations: a comparison between second trimester amniocentesis and first-trimester chorionic villus sampling. Obster Gynecol 1993;82:49-56.
73. Antsaklis A, Souka AP, Daskalakis G, Kavalakis Y, Michalas S. Second-trimester amniocentesis vs. chorionic villus samplingfor prenatal diagnosis in multiple gestations. Ultrasound Obstet Gynecol 2002;20:476-81.
74. Pergament E, Schulman JD, Copeland K, Fine B, Black SH, Ginsberg NA, Frederiksen MC, Carpenter RJ. The risk and efficacy of chorionic villus sampling in multiple gestations. Prenat Diagn 1992;12:377-84.
75. Appelman Z, Vinkler C, Caspi B. Chorionic villus sampling in multiple gestations. Eur J Obstet Gynecol Reprod Biol 1999; 85:97-9.
76. Casals G, Borrell A, Martinez JM, Soler A, Cararach V, Fortuny A.Transcervical chorionic villus sampling in multiple pregnancies using a biopsy forceps. Prenat Diagn 2002;22: 260-5.
77. De Catte L, Liebaers I, Foulon W. Outcome of twin gestations after first trimester chorionic villus sampling. Obstet Gynecol 2000; 96(5Pt 1):714-20.

CHAPTER

15

Invasive Diagnostic Procedures in Multiple Pregnancies

Aris J Antsaklis, George A Partsinevelos

INTRODUCTION

During the past four decades, since the widespread use of ultrasonography for diagnostic purposes, prenatal screening for chromosomal abnormalities has been recognized as an invaluable component of modern obstetrics. In singletons, nuchal translucency (NT) measurement together with maternal serum biochemistry determination have been uniformly accepted in first-trimester risk assessment for fetal aneuploidies. Additional sonographic markers, such as absent nasal bone, abnormal Doppler waveform in the ductus venosus and tricuspid regurgitation, have been recently validated, though others have been proven less reliable. In as much as early pregnancy risk assessment is rapidly gaining popularity, invasive testing procedures such as chorionic villus sampling and amniocentesis is gradually restricted in cases where rationale exists, rendering prenatal screening safer. It has been a common practice to extrapolate data derived from singletons to multiples. However, implementation of invasive prenatal diagnostic modalities in twins or higher-order pregnancies, seems to be more complex.

The rising rate of multiple pregnancies demonstrated over the past two decades is mainly attributed to the greater reliance on infertility treatment such as in vitro fertilization and ovulation induction with intrauterine insemination. Furthermore, delayed childbearing in progressively advanced maternal age currently adopted by many prospective mothers increases the chance of multiple gestations. There is no doubt that the incidence of chromosomal abnormalities is associated with maternal age. On the other hand, assisted conception has been claimed to result in an increase in the rate of monozygotic (MZ) twins to greater than 10-fold, the latter being at high risk of functional and structural abnormalities, affecting 10 to 15% of these twins.[1-3] Available data confirm that twin pregnancies per se are at increased risk for fetal chromosomal abnormalities than those with singletons.[4,5] Hence, the increasing incidence of multiple pregnancies highlights a concomitant increase in the need for invasive procedures in these pregnancies.

ZYGOCITY AND CHORIONICITY

The management and the prenatal diagnosis of a multiple pregnancy are challenging, not only related to the number of fetuses, but also strongly influenced by chorionicity. Chorionicity refers to the placentation whereas zygosity implies the genetic profile of the pregnancy and therefore determines the degree of risk and whether or not the fetuses may be concordant or discordant for chromosomal abnormalities. More than 30% of twin pregnancies are monozygotic and nearly 70% are dizygotic.

MZ twins originate from the division of a single fertilized ovum with an incidence rate of about 2.3 to 4/1000 pregnancies. The rate of spontaneous MZ twin pregnancies is constant contrary to the increased frequency reported among pregnancies derived from infertility treatment modalities. MZ twins may be dichorionic (DC) or monochorionic (MC), the chorionicity determined by the period of embryonic development zygotic splitting takes place. In about 20 to 30% of cases, splitting occurs within three days of fertilization resulting in separate fetuses with independent placental circulations, therefore being dichorionic-diamniotic (DC-DA), even if placentas may seem to be in continuity or fused. In the majority of cases (about 70%) splitting within the first week but later than the third day results in a single monochorionic plate and two distinct amniotic sacs, hence monochorionic-diamniotic (MC-DA) twins originate. Delayed zygotic splitting leads to monochorionic-monoamniotic (MC-MA) twins, accounting for 1% of MZ twins, though later than 13th day is extremely rare, resulting in the formation of the abnormal conjoined (Siamese) twins.

Dizygotic (DZ) twins arise from the fertilization of two distinct ova, thus may be of the same or different sex. The incidence rate varies significantly, influenced by race (higher in blacks, lower in Asians), heredity, maternal age (peak between 35 to 40 years of age), history of previous DZ twin pregnancy, nutrition habitus and anthropometric features (height and weight) of the woman.

Artificial reproductive technologies (ART) including in vitro fertilization and non-ART procedures such as ovulation induction and subsequent intrauterine insemination using human pituitary gonadotropic hormones increase the incidence of multiple pregnancy, while clomiphene citrate increases the occurrence rate of DZ pregnancies to about 5 to 10%.[1-3,6]

The categorical general rule by far having been recognized in obstetrics that MC twins are exclusively MZ[7] was irrevocably staggered when the first case of monochorionic-dizygotic twin pregnancy, possibly resulting from assisted reproductive technology (ART), was reported.[8] Thenceforth, ART-mediated monochorionic-dizygotic twin pregnancy was validated, though it is claimed to be very infrequent.

THE RISK OF STRUCTURAL ABNORMALITIES IN MULTIPLE GESTATIONS

The incidence of structural anomalies in twins is higher compared to singletons. However, the frequency of malformations in DZ twins is thought to be similar to that of singletons (2-3%) contrary to that observed to MZ, which has been reported to be 2 to 3 times higher.

Neural tube defects, anencephaly, holoprocencephaly, sirenomelia complex, cloacal exstrophy and abnormalities that fit into the expanded VATER/ VACTERAL associations are more common in MZ twins. However, the risk of fetal abnormalities in twins may be biased, because multiple pregnancies are intensively scanned, increasing the chances of detecting underlying anomalies. Moreover, twinning is much more common in women of advanced age, in whom prenatal screening is more likely to yield the diagnosis of fetal defects as far as aging is associated with increased risk for fetal abnormalities.

THE RISK OF ANEUPLOIDY IN MULTIPLE GESTATIONS

The general aspect that the incidence of multiple pregnancies is correlated with increasing maternal age stands for DZ twins. It is well established that the frequency of MZ twinning remains relatively constant, independent of the age of the woman.

As far as zygosity represents the genetic make-up of the developing entity, accurate determination of this parameter is considered a prerequisite in multiple pregnancy prenatal screening for aneuploidies. In the clinical setting, zygosity is usually inferred from the ultrasound diagnosis of chorionicity,[4] the latter best achieved in the first trimester. In DA pregnancies with fused placentas, measurements of the thickness of the dividing membrane using a cut-off value of 2 mm can differentiate MC from DC twinning, though a high inter and intraobserver variability has been reported. Sonographic detection of the "lambda" or "twin peak" sign is reported as a more reliable indicator of DC placentation with an accuracy of 100% in 10 to 14 weeks gestation.[9] Delayed in the second trimester sonographic evaluation is associated with a 10 to 12% chorionicity misinterpretation rate,[10,11] while after 20 weeks gestation the determination may turn out impossible. Therefore, in the absence of the "lambda" or "twin peak" sign in a DA twin pregnancy, single placentation and monozygosity is concluded, when the rare cases of MC-DZ gestations following ART reported are not taken into consideration. However, when a single amniotic sac is detected, monochorionicity is indisputable. Given that the great proportion (80-90%) of DC twins are DZ,[12,13] chorionicity may roughly correspond to zygocity.[14]

MZ twins are always of the same sex and genetically identical and therefore the risk for chromosomal abnormalities does not differ from that in singletons. Very infrequently, mutations can cause genetic discordance between MZ siblings, involving mosaicism, skewed-X-inactivation, differential gene imprinting and small scale mutation.[15] Heterokaryotypia, is used to define the rare karyotypic discordance, most commonly expressed by one fetus affected by Turner's syndrome whereas the other presents either a normal male or normal female karyotype.[16-18] MZ discordance for trisomy 21, Klinefelter's syndrome, Pateau syndrome, trisomy 1 and 22q11 delation syndrome has also been described.[18-22] However, these unusual discrepancies are not taken into consideration when calculating aneuploid risk, though should always be assumed when invasive prenatal diagnosis is performed dictating sampling from both sacs.

In DZ twins, each embryo has an independent risk for aneuploidy and therefore the risk that at least one fetus being affected will be almost twice the maternal age risk for a singleton. The probability of both fetuses being involved is minimal.[12] In cases with uncertain choronicity and thus zygocity, aneuploidy risk assessment requires an estimation of the most likely zygocity, which may vary according to maternal age and race. In general, given that one-third of all twin pairs are monozygotic, the risk for one twin being aneuploid in case of unknown zygosity is calculated to five-thirds that of the singleton risk.[10,14] Based on these estimations, a 33-year-old woman bearing twins has a risk for at least one aneuploid offspring, comparable to the risk of a 35-year-old woman bearing a singleton. On this assumption, such women should be offered prenatal testing.[23] However, despite these aspects, reported series show a lower risk for fetal chromosomal abnormalities in live-born twins.

PRENATAL SCREENING FOR FETAL ANOMALIES IN MULTIPLES

Methods validated for prenatal screening for chromosomal and structural fetal abnormalities in singletons has been also applied in multiple pregnancies. However, cautious interpretation of screening results has been considered mandatory in order to minimize possible erroneous high false-positive rate and subsequent high rate of undue invasive procedures.

In DC multiple pregnancies, fetal NT screening in the first trimester has yielded comparable results regarding detection rate as well as false-positive rate.[24] However, in MC twins, a cautious evaluation of increased NT thickness should be reserved in respect to the possible early twin-to-twin transfusion syndrome origin of this finding. A rational approach has been proposed to be the application of the average value of NT measurement of both fetuses in risk assessment in an effort to reduce misinterpretation.[25] The inability to determine the degree to which each fetus contributes to the overall maternal biochemistry level may reflect a significant shortcoming in first trimester biomarkers' sensitivity and specificity in multiple gestations. A reasonable model of "pseudo-risk" approach has been proposed based on the utilization of the quotient derived from the division of the biomarkers' levels as multiples of the median (MoM) by the corresponding medians for normal twins.[26-28] No adequate data has validated this approach so far. Maternal serum alpha-fetoprotein (MSAFP) level in the second trimester in twin pregnancy is twice as high as that of a singleton one and 40% of twins are associated with MSAFP levels of more than a 2.5 MoM at 16 weeks.[29] The presence of multiples may explain the elevation of this specific serum marker, though it cannot preclude the possibility of an open neural tube defect in one or more fetuses. Thereby, amniocentesis performed in twins where MSAFP exceeds 4.5 MoM seems to be reasonable.[30] Since the implementation of maternal biochemistry in risk assessment for aneuploidies in twin or higher-order multiple gestations remains arguable, ultrasound scan has been proven of great value for early determination of chorionicity and subsequent standardized NT measurement as well as genetic sonogram targeting to illuminate possible sonographic markers of fetal aneuploidy.

INVASIVE PROCEDURES FOR PRENATAL DIAGNOSIS

Amniocentesis

Second trimester amniocentesis performed later than 15 weeks of gestation has been proven a safe and accurate procedure for sampling all fetuses of a multiple gestation. Currently, there is little information regarding the risk of amniocentesis between 13 and 15 weeks though this invasive procedure has been associated with increased risk for fetal loss, amniotic fluid leakage and fetal talipes equinovarus and therefore is not recommended.[10,31,32]

Three methods of tapping multiple sacs have been described so far. The first one, initially described by Elias et al in 1980, involves two or more needle insertions, one for each sac, also called the technique of double amniocentesis.[33] In a twin or higher-order multiple pregnancy, two or more 22-gauge 3.5 inches spinal needles are separately and sequentially inserted transabdominally under ultrasound visualization into each sac and about 20 ml of amniotic fluid is readily aspirated and sent for cytogenetic evaluation or fetal karyotyping. A problem not infrequently faced with this technique is erroneously sampling twice the same amniotic sac. In order to eliminate this possibility, the sampled sac is marked with a blue dye ensuring that the sac is tapped only once. For this purpose indigo carmine has been successfully used without any adverse effects,[34] though a mild vasoconstrictive effect following intravenous injection has been described. However, the instillation of a foreign substance into the amniotic cavity is of concern. A technical disadvantage with the instillation of indigo carmine is that the dye tends to concentrate at the bottom of the sac taking some time before the stained fluid surrounds the fetus. Methylene blue used as a marker dye in the past has been linked to certain toxic manifestations such as fetal hemolysis, fetal small bowel atresias and fetal death.[35-40] Nevertheless, the high resolution ultrasound equipment currently available, in expertise hands, may ensure accurate sampling from each sac,[41,42] reserving the installation of dye for cases of amniotic volume discordance where detection of the septum is uncertain or high-order pregnancies where documentation and "labeling" of sacs turn out insecure.[43]

An alternative approach first described by Jeanty et al in 1990 is the single needle insertion technique.[44] The needle entry is made into the proximal sac near the insertion of the dividing membrane and 20 ml of amniotic fluid are retrieved. After the stylet is replaced, the needle is advanced through the second sac under direct ultrasound guidance. In order to avoid contamination the first few milliliters of amniotic fluid are discarded and aspiration of 20 ml from the second sac integrates the procedure. Many advantages linked to this technique have been reported: requiring only one needle insertion and being swifter and shorter reduces woman's discomfort as well as the risk of post-procedural complications. Moreover, advancing the needle through the septum between the two sacs under ultrasound guidance provides positive proof of tapping both of them, diminishing the need for dye insertion. However, potential disadvantages render this approach less popular. Possible contamination of the second sample with amniotic fluid and fetal cells from the first one, may lead to an incorrect diagnosis of mosaicism in the second fetus. This complication can be avoided by strictly adhering to the technique, by replacing the stylet prior to intertwin membrane penetration and by discarding the first few milliliters from the second sac. Besides, the possibility of converting DA to pseudo-MA twin preganancy with the correspondence risks for cord entanglement and the formation of the amniotic band syndrome cannot be precluded.[45] In addition, a technical difficulty in penetrating a "tenting" dividing membrane has been reported.

Another approach called double simultaneous amniocentesis, was introduced by Bahado-Singh et al in 1992.[46] This technique involves two needles inserted separately into the amniotic sacs under ultrasound visualization like in the technique of double amniocentesis. The difference is that after aspiration of the amniotic fluid from the first sac, the needle is left in place indicating the sampled cavity and the second insertion is made into the other sac. The main advantage seems to be the documentation of correct sampling from each sac. However, it is not widely used mainly because it is more time consuming and thereby the experience with this approach is limited.

Amniocentesis as well as all prenatal diagnostic invasive procedures must be preceded by a detailed ultrasound evaluation of the multiple pregnancy involving chorionicity and amnionicity determination and documentation of the location of the placenta(s). Moreover, relative position, size and anatomy of each fetus should be specified and "labeling" of the multiples using text and diagram should be performed to ensure correct sampling from each of them. Recently, the role of amniotic fluid alpha-fetoprotein (AFAFP) values was evaluated in confirmation of both sacs in a dichorionic pregnancy being sampled.[47]

Concern regarding potential post-amniocentesis increase in fetal loss rate in multiples has led to a plethora of studies evaluating this parameter. Early reports suggested a higher fetal loss rate in twin pregnancies than in those with singletons.[48-50] However, these studies did not take into account the possibility that the increased fetal wastage might be attributed to the twin pregnancy itself rather than the invasive procedure. Later on, it was reported that the maternal history of twins per se carries a pregnancy loss rate up to 24 weeks of about 6.3% and severe prematurity (24 to 28 weeks) rate of about 8%.[51] Most series of pregnancy outcome following second-trimester amniocentesis report loss rates before 20 weeks' gestation of between 1 and 2.5% and a much higher loss rate before 28 weeks. In a multicenter European study, the pregnancy loss rate was estimated to be 2.3% and 3.7% before 20 and 28 weeks' gestation respectively.[52] In a case control study, a similar fetal loss rate was reported between sampled twins and unsampled matched twin controls (3.5% vs 3.2%).[53]

In conclusion, amniocentesis in twin pregnancies is thought to be a relative safe and accurate diagnostic procedure providing that sampling involves both sacs regardless the zygocity and chorionicity.

Chorionic Villus Sampling

Chorionic villus sampling (CVS) is a safe alternative invasive procedure to amniocentesis for prenatal diagnosis in singletons. CVS has been shown to be safe and efficacious for sampling twin gestations as well.[54-56] The main advantage of CVS is early diagnosis, obtained in the first trimester of pregnancy. In particular, genetic results are feasible either within hours by direct preparations of the cytotrophoblast layer, or within 3 to 7 days by tissue culture of chorionic villus mesenchymal core. Early diagnosis provides earlier reassurance of fetal well being and thereby eliminates both maternal anxiety and uncertainty regarding the present gestation. On the other hand, the diagnosis of one or both abnormal fetuses allows subsequent selective reduction of the affected fetus or termination of pregnancy as early as in the first trimester where complication rates are lower. Moreover, fetal reduction performed earlier in pregnancy may be associated with a higher survival rate of the unaffected twin.[57] In terms of privacy and maternal psychology, the earlier an abnormal pregnancy is terminated the lesser the chance of being widely recognized.

CVS is best performed between 11 and 13 weeks' gestation. In general, first-trimester CVS in multiple gestations is technically more challenging than second-trimester amniocentesis. Transabdominal as well as transcervical aporoach have been widely used and certain advantages and disadvantages have been ascribed to each technique. Transcervical CVS is performed either by an aspiration catheter or by a biopsy forceps. Technically, it may be more difficult to perform and the "learning curve" appears to involve many patients. Transabdominal approach uses an aspiration needle and is technically more similar to mid-trimester amniocentesis. This maybe the reason for this technique being most widely adopted by obstetricians.

Since no marker is available to assure sampling from each chorion, continuous ultrasound localization of the tip of the needle or catheter is required. If in doubt, a follow-up procedure should be performed either by an immediate repeat CVS or by second trimester amniocentesis. A serious drawback of CVS is potential contamination of one sample by villi belonging to the other chorion leading to a confusing or even misleading diagnosis. Although early studies suggested a contamination rate as high as 4% more recent studies report a much lower rate, almost nullified.[58,59] Still, Weisz and Rodeck suggest that it would be prudent to counsel patients that about 2 to 3% of twin pregnancies having CVS will need re-sampling because of uncertainty of results.[43]

The combination of transcervical and transabdominal approach together with the increasing experience available today can eliminate such an unfortunate possibility. Furthermore, obtaining samples adjacent to the cord insertion site far away from the dividing membrane is reasonably recommended.

Since there is the possibility of a discordant abnormal result, detailed documentation and "labeling" of the fetuses and the chorions is equally as important with CVS as it is with amniocentesis. Although the position of sacs will remain unchanged during the 2 to 3 weeks-time following sampling, it is standard practice to re-confrim the original diagnosis in both fetal and chorionic tissues before selective reduction of the affected twin.

The estimated risk of CVS-associated fetal loss in singletons varies widely (1.3-4.3%). Two or more samplings during one procedure have been linked to increased risk of post-procedural miscarriage,[60,61] implying that the risk may be higher in twin sampling. Overall an estimated risk of 2 to 4% in twin pregnancies has been reported. However, available data demonstrate significant variations. In a study, the risk of CVS-associated fetal loss before 28 weeks' gestation did not seem to differ between twin and singleton pregnancies (4.9 vs 4%).[54] When only chromosomal normal pregnancies are considered, the overall loss rate found in a study of 202 twin pregnancies that underwent CVS became 3.7%, a figure that is considerably less than that of amniocentesis.[54] In another study, the pregnancy loss rate before 20 weeks following CVS was found 3.3% comparable to 2.8% in a control group of twin pregnancies undergone amniocentesis. Hence, It may be claimed that in experienced centers, CVS is as safe as amniocentesis for sampling twins.

Eventually, is there a clear benefit of performing CVS than amniocentesis or vice versa in invasive prenatal screening, that would render one procedure by far superior than the other? The answer is definitely no. Amniocentesis is technically easier and widely adopted, whereas CVS results are available about one month earlier thus therapeutic as well as selective terminations are safer. The ultimate choice depends on several factors, such as gestational age at referral date, placental location, operator's experience and the likelihood of selective feticide. It should be emphasized that if the center is not skilled and experienced in CVS, amniocentesis should be preferred. A rational approach may be as follows: the choice of invasive technique should be based on individual risk calculated from the combination of maternal age and fetal NT thickness measured in the first trimester. When the risk for a chromosomal defect, in at least one of the fetuses, is greater than 1 in 50, it may be preferable to perform CVS. For pregnancies with a lower risk, amniocentesis after 15 weeks may be more appropriate.

Fetal Blood Sampling

Prenatal diagnosis using fetal blood sample was previously mainly indicated when abnormal findings in amniocentesis or CVS necessitated confirmation. Another frequent indication was the need for a rapid chromosomal diagnosis (rapid karyotyping), inasmuch as results are offered in 2 to 3 days-time. Nowadays, novel molecular techniques allow rapid karyotype determination thereby limiting fetal blood sampling's indications.

From a technical point of view, fetal blood sampling in twins is not different from the procedure in singletons. Umbilical cord insertion must be identified before sampling under sonographic guidance. In a study conducted in 2003, involving 84 twin pregnancies, mainly screened for hemoglobinopathies, the overall procedure-related fetal loss (up to 2 weeks post-procedurally) was 8.2%, about fourfold higher than the correspondence risk in singletons. However, this technique can be used as an alternative to amniocentesis after 20 weeks' gestation to confirm an abnormal karyotype in a DC pregnancy, when selective feticide is considered a few weeks after the initial procedure.[62]

CONCLUSION

In conclusion, the increasing incidence of multiple pregnancies mainly due to the widely use of infertility treatment modalities has increased the need for invasive genetic studies in these pregnancies. Diagnosis of fetal aneuploidies and genetic defects can be achieved either by first-trimester CVS or by second-trimester amniocentesis, whereas it is claimed that they are equally safe in expertise hands. The choice of invasive procedure in twin pregnancies depends on several factors, but the experience of the center performing the modality should be emphasized in decision making. The indications of fetal blood sampling are currently limited and progressively surrogated by novel molecular techniques implemented in CVS or amniocentesis' specimen. High resolution ultrasound equipment available today, together with increasing operator experience gained throughout the years, results in more accurate and efficacious invasive prenatal diagnosis in twin or higher-order pregnancies, minimizing potential post-procedural fetal loss rate.

REFERENCES

1. Derom C, Vlietinck R, Derom R, van den Berghe H, Thiery M. Increased monozygotic twinning rate after ovulation induction. Lancet. 1987;1(8544):1236-8. Erratum in: Lancet 1987;2(8551):170.
2. Wenstrom KD, Syrop CH, Hammitt DG, van Voorhis BJ. Increased risk of monochorionic twinning associated with assisted reproduction. Fertil Steril 1993;60(3):510-4.
3. Blickstein I. Estimation of iatrogenic monozygotic twinning rate following assisted reproduction: pitfalls and caveats. Am J Obstet Gynecol 2005;192(2):365-8.
4. Kohl SG, Casey G. Twin gestation. Mt Sinai J Med 1975;42(6):523-33.
5. Nicolaides KH, Sebire NJ, Snjiders RJM (Eds): The 11-14 Week Scan. The Diagnosis of Fetal Abnormalities. New York, NY, Parthenon Publishing, 1999.
6. Benirschke K, Kim CK. Multiple pregnancy. N Engl J Med 1973;288(25):1329-36.
7. Quintero RA, Mueller OT, Martínez JM, Arroyo J, Gilbert-Barness E, Hilbelink D, Papenhausen P, Sutcliffe M. Twin-twin transfusion syndrome in a dizygotic monochorionic-diamniotic twin pregnancy. J Matern Fetal Neonatal Med 2003;14(4):279-81.
8. Souter VL, Kapur RP, Nyholt DR, Skogerboe K, Myerson D, Ton CC, Opheim KE, Easterling TR, Shields LE, Montgomery GW, Glass IA. A report of dizygous monochorionic twins. N Engl J Med 2003;349(2):154-8.
9. Sepulveda W, Sebire NJ, Hughes K, Kalogeropoulos A, Nicolaides KH. Evolution of the lambda or twin-chorionic peak sign in dichorionic twin pregnancies. Obstet Gynecol 1997;89(3):439-41.
10. Jenkins TM, Wapner RJ. The challenge of prenatal diagnosis in twin pregnancies. Curr Opin Obstet Gynecol 2000;12(2):87-92.
11. Wood SL, St Onge R, Connors G, Elliot PD. Evaluation of the twin peak or lambda sign in determining chorionicity in multiple pregnancy. Obstet Gynecol 1996;88(1):6-9.
12. Rodis JF, Egan JF, Craffey A, Ciarleglio L, Greenstein RM, Scorza WE. Calculated risk of chromosomal abnormalities in twin gestations. Obstet Gynecol 1990;76(6):1037-41.
13. Fisk NM, Bennett PR. Prenatal determination of chorionicity and zygosity. In Ward RH, Whittle W (Eds): Multiple Pregnancy. London, RCOG Press, 1995, pp 56-66.
14. Matias A, Montenegro N, Blickstein I. Down syndrome screening in multiple pregnancies. Obstet Gynecol Clin North Am 2005;32(1):81-96.
15. Machin GA. Some causes of genotypic and phenotypic discordance in monozygotic twin pairs. Am J Med Genet 1996;61(3):216-28.

16. Rogers JG, Voullaire L, Gold H. Monozygotic twins discordant for trisomy 21. Am J Med Genet 1982;11(2):143-6.
17. Dallapiccola B, Stomeo C, Ferranti G, Di Lecce A, Purpura M. Discordant sex in one of three monozygotic triplets. J Med Genet 1985;22(1):6-11.
18. Perlman EJ, Stetten G, Tuck-Müller CM, Farber RA, Neuman WL, Blakemore KJ, Hutchins GM. Sexual discordance in monozygotic twins. Am J Med Genet 1990;37(4):551-7.
19. Schmid O, Trautmann U, Ashour H, Ulmer R, Pfeiffer RA, Beinder E. Prenatal diagnosis of heterokaryotypic mosaic twins discordant for fetal sex. Prenat Diagn 2000;20(12):999-1003.
20. Wachtel SS, Somkuti SG, Schinfeld JS. Monozygotic twins of opposite sex. Cytogenet Cell Genet 2000;91(1-4):293-5.
21. Lespinasse J, Gicquel C, Robert M, Le Bouc Y. Phenotypic and genotypic variability in monozygotic triplets with Turner syndrome. Clin Genet 1998;54(1):56-9.
22. Nieuwint A, van Zalen-Sprock R, Hummel P, Pals G, Van Vugt J, van Der Harten H, Heins Y, Madan K. Identical' twins with discordant karyotypes. Prenat Diagn 1999;19(1):72-6.
23. Weinblatt V, Wapner RJ. Chorionic villus sampling and amniocentesis in multiple pregnancy. In Creasy RK, Resnik R (Eds): Maternal-Fetal Medicine Principles and Practice, (4th Ed). Philadelphia: WB Saunders, 1999; pp 201-11.
24. Sebire NJ, Snijders RJ, Hughes K, Sepulveda W, Nicolaides KH. Screening for trisomy 21 in twin pregnancies by maternal age and fetal nuchal translucency thickness at 10-14 weeks of gestation. Br J Obstet Gynaecol 1996;103(10):999-1003.
25. Vandecruys H, Faiola S, Auer M, Sebire N, Nicolaides KH. Screening for trisomy 21 in monochorionic twins by measurement of fetal nuchal translucency thickness. Ultrasound Obstet Gynecol 2005;25(6):551-3.
26. Spencer K, Salonen R, Muller F. Down's syndrome screening in multiple pregnancies using alpha-fetoprotein and free beta hCG. Prenat Diagn 1994;14(7):537-42.
27. Muller F, Dreux S, Dupoizat H, Uzan S, Dubin MF, Oury JF, Dingeon B, Dommergues M. Second-trimester Down syndrome maternal serum screening in twin pregnancies: impact of chorionicity. Prenat Diagn 2003;23(4):331-5.
28. Wald NJ, Rish S. Prenatal screening for Down syndrome and neural tube defects in twin pregnancies. Prenat Diagn 2005;25(9):740-5.
29. Gardner S, Burton BK, Johnson AM. Maternal serum alpha-fetoprotein screening: a report of the Forsyth County project. Am J Obstet Gynecol 1981;140(3):250-3.
30. Wapner RJ. Genetic diagnosis in multiple pregnancies. Semin Perinatol 1995;19(5):351-62.
31. Jenkins TM, Wapner RJ. First trimester prenatal diagnosis: chorionic villus sampling. Semin Perinatol 1999;23(5):403-13.
32. Cleary-Goldman J, D'Alton ME, Berkowitz RL. Prenatal diagnosis and multiple pregnancy. Semin Perinatol 2005;29(5):312-20.
33. Elias S, Gerbie AB, Simpson JL, Nadler HL, Sabbagha RE, Shkolnik A. Genetic amniocentesis in twin gestations. Am J Obstet Gynecol 1980;138(2):169-74.
34. Cragan JD, Martin ML, Khoury MJ, Fernhoff PM. Dye use during amniocentesis and birth defects. Lancet 1993;341(8856):1352.
35. Nicolini U, Monni G. Intestinal obstruction in babies exposed in utero to methylene blue. Lancet 1990;336(8725):1258-9.
36. Kidd SA, Lancaster PA, Anderson JC, Boogert A, Fisher CC, Robertson R, Wass DM. Fetal death after exposure to methylene blue dye during mid-trimester amniocentesis in twin pregnancy. Prenat Diagn 1996;16(1):39-47.
37. McEnerney JK, McEnerney LN. Unfavorable neonatal outcome after intraamniotic injection of methylene blue. Obstet Gynecol 1983; 61(3 Suppl):35S-37S.
38. McFadyen I. The dangers of intra-amniotic methylene blue. Br J Obstet Gynaecol 1992;99(2):89-90.
39. van der Pol JG, Wolf H, Boer K, Treffers PE, Leschot NJ, Hey HA, Vos A. Jejunal atresia related to the use of methylene blue in genetic amniocentesis in twins. Br J Obstet Gynaecol 1992;99(2):141-3.
40. Vincer MJ, Allen AC, Evans JR, Nwaesei C, Stinson DA. Methylene-blue-induced hemolytic anemia in a neonate. CMAJ 1987;136(5):503-4.
41. Antsaklis A, Souka AP, Daskalakis G, Kavalakis Y, Michalas S. Second-trimester amniocentesis vs. chorionic villus sampling for prenatal diagnosis in multiple gestations. Ultrasound Obstet Gynecol 2002;20(5):476-81.
42. Taylor MJ, Fisk NM. Prenatal diagnosis in multiple pregnancy. Baillieres Best Pract Res Clin Obstet Gynaecol 2000;14(4):663-75.
43. Weisz B, Rodeck CH. Invasive diagnostic procedures in twin pregnancies. Prenat Diagn 2005;25(9):751-8.
44. Jeanty P, Shah D, Roussis P. Single-needle insertion in twin amniocentesis. J Ultrasound Med 1990;9(9):511-7.
45. Megory E, Weiner E, Shalev E, Ohel G. Pseudomonoamniotic twins with cord entanglement following genetic funipuncture. Obstet Gynecol 1991;78 (5 Pt 2):915-7.
46. Bahado-Singh R, Schmitt R, Hobbins JC. New technique for genetic amniocentesis in twins. Obstet Gynecol 1992;79(2):304-7.
47. Delisle MF, Brosseuk L, Wilson RD. Amniocentesis for twin pregnancies: is alpha-fetoprotein useful in confirming that the two sacs were sampled? Fetal Diagn Ther 2007;22(3):221-5.
48. Palle C, Andersen JW, Tabor A, Lauritsen JG, Bang J, Philip J. Increased risk of abortion after genetic amniocentesis in twin pregnancies. Prenat Diagn 1983;3(2):83-9.
49. Pijpers L, Jahoda MG, Vosters RP, Niermeijer MF, Sachs ES. Genetic amniocentesis in twin pregnancies. Br J Obstet Gynaecol 1988;95(4):323-6.
50. Anderson RL, Goldberg JD, Golbus MS. Prenatal diagnosis in multiple gestation: 20 years' experience with amniocentesis. Prenat Diagn 1991;11(4):263-70.
51. Yaron Y, Bryant-Greenwood PK, Dave N, Moldenhauer JS, Kramer RL, Johnson MP, Evans MI. Multifetal pregnancy reductions of triplets to twins: comparison with nonreduced triplets and twins. Am J Obstet Gynecol 1999;180(5):1268-71.
52. Pruggmayer MR, Jahoda MG, van der Pol JG, Baumann P, Holzgreve W, Karkut G, Lettau R, Eiben B, Osmers R, Gola HW, Duda V, Polak P, Körner H, Schulte-Valentin

M, Schütte H. Genetic amniocentesis in twin pregnancies: results of a multicenter study of 529 cases. Ultrasound Obstet Gynecol 1992;2(1):6-10.

53. Ghidini A, Lynch L, Hicks C, Alvarez M, Lockwood CJ. The risk of second-trimester amniocentesis in twin gestations: a case-control study. Am J Obstet Gynecol 1993;169(4):1013-6.
54. Pergament E, Schulman JD, Copeland K, Fine B, Black SH, Ginsberg NA, Frederiksen MC, Carpenter RJ. The risk and efficacy of chorionic villus sampling in multiple gestations. Prenat Diagn 1992;12(5):377-84.
55. Brambati B, Tului L, Lanzani A, Simoni G, Travi M. First-trimester genetic diagnosis in multiple pregnancy: principles and potential pitfalls. Prenat Diagn 1991;11(10):767-74.
56. Wapner RJ, Barr MA, Heeger S, et al: Chorionic villus sampling: a 10-year over 13,000 consecutive case experience. American College of Medical Genetics, First Annual Meeting, Orlando, FL, 1994 (abstract).
57. Evans MI, Goldberg JD, Horenstein J, Wapner RJ, Ayoub MA, Stone J, Lipitz S, Achiron R, Holzgreve W, Brambati B, Johnson A, Johnson MP, Shalhoub A, Berkowitz RL. Selective termination for structural, chromosomal, and mendelian anomalies: international experience. Am J Obstet Gynecol 1999;181(4):893-7.
58. De Catte L, Liebaers I, Foulon W. Outcome of twin gestations after first trimester chorionic villus sampling. Obstet Gynecol 2000;96(5 Pt 1):714-20.
59. Brambati B, Tului L, Guercilena S, Alberti E. Outcome of first-trimester chorionic villus sampling for genetic investigation in multiple pregnancy. Ultrasound Obstet Gynecol 2001;17(3):209-16.
60. Rhoads GG, Jackson LG, Schlesselman SE, de la Cruz FF, Desnick RJ, Golbus MS, Ledbetter DH, Lubs HA, Mahoney MJ, Pergament E, et al. The safety and efficacy of chorionic villus sampling for early prenatal diagnosis of cytogenetic abnormalities. N Engl J Med 1989;320(10):609-17.
61. Kuliev A, Jackson L, Froster U, Brambati B, Simpson JL, Verlinsky Y, Ginsberg N, Smidt-Jensen S, Zakut H. Chorionic villus sampling safety. Report of World Health Organization/EURO meeting in association with the Seventh International Conference on Early Prenatal Diagnosis of Genetic Diseases, Tel-Aviv, Israel, May 21, 1994. Am J Obstet Gynecol 1996;174(3):807-11.
62. Antsaklis A, Gougoulakis A, Mesogitis S, Papantoniou N, Aravantinos D. Invasive techniques for fetal diagnosis in multiple pregnancy. Int J Gynaecol Obstet 1991;34(4):309-14.

Index

A

B

C